Clinics in Developmental Medicine No. 186
VISUAL IMPAIRMENT IN CHILDREN
DUE TO DAMAGE TO THE BRAIN

Clinics in Developmental Medicine No. 186

Visual Impairment in Children Due to Damage to the Brain

Edited by

GORDON N. DUTTON
Department of Vision Sciences, Glasgow Caledonian University;
Tennent Institute of Ophthalmology, Gartnavel General Hospital;
and Royal Hospital for Sick Children, Yorkhill, Glasgow, UK

and

MARTIN BAX
Department of Medicine and Therapeutics, Imperial College,
Chelsea and Westminster Hospital Campus, London, UK

2010
Mac Keith Press

Editor: Hilary Hart
Managing Editor: Caroline Black
Production Manager: Udoka Ohuonu
Project Manager: Catriona Vernal

The views and opinions expressed herein are those of the authors and do not necessarily represent those of the publisher

First published in this edition 2010
Reprinted 2011

British Library Cataloguing-in-Publication data
A catalogue record for this book is available from the British Library

Cover image used with permission from Sight-Sim™, courtesy of Drs Michael Bradnam, Aled Evans, and Ruth Hamilton, Department of Clinical Physics and Bioengineering, NHS Greater Glasgow and Clyde

ISBN: 978-1-898683-86-5

Typeset by Prepress Projects Ltd, Perth, UK
Printed by TJ International Ltd, Padstow, Cornwall, UK
Mac Keith Press is supported by Scope

CONTENTS

vii

AUTHORS' APPOINTMENTS

Stuart Aitken　　Sense Scotland, Glasgow; CALL Scotland, School of Education, University of Edinburgh, Edinburgh, UK

Susann Andersson　　Department of Ophthalmology, The Queen Sylvia Children's Hospital, Gothenburg, Sweden

Janette Atkinson　　Department of Developmental Science, University College London, London, UK

Martin Bax　　Imperial College (Chelsea and Westminister Hospital Campus), London, UK

Paolo E. Bianchi　　Department of Ophthalmology, IRCCS San Matteo Hospital, University of Pavia, Pavia, Italy

Oliver Braddick　　Department of Experimental Psychology, University of Oxford, Oxford, UK

Marianna Buultjens　　Monifieth, Dundee, UK

Julie Calvert　　Royal Hospital for Sick Children, Yorkhill, Glasgow, UK

Margot Campbell　　Armistead Child Development Centre, Dundee, UK

Giovanni Cioni　　Division of Child Neurology, University of Pisa, Stella Maris Scientific Institute, Pisa, Italy

Debbie Cockburn　　Southbank Child Centre, Glasgow, UK

August Colenbrander　　The Smith Kettlewell Eye Research Institute, San Francisco, CA, USA

Naomi Dale　　Department of Neurodisability, Great Ormond Street Hospital for Children, London, UK

Suzannah R. Drummond　　Tennent Institute of Ophthalmology, Gartnavel General Hospital, Glasgow, UK

Gordon N. Dutton

Tennent Institute of Ophthalmology, Gartnavel General Hospital; Department of Vision Sciences, Glasgow Caledonian University; The Royal Hospital for Sick Children, Yorkhill, Glasgow, UK

Heleen M. Evenhuis

Erasmus University Medical Center, Intellectual Disability Medicine, Department of General Practice, Rotterdam, the Netherlands

Elisa Fazzi

Mother and Child Department, Medical Faculty, University of Brescia, Brescia, Italy

Olof Flodmark

Department of Clinical Neuroscience, Karolinska Institute, Stockholm, Sweden

Roger D. Freeman

Department of Psychiatry and Department of Pediatrics, University of British Columbia; Neuropsychiatry Clinic, BC Children's Hospital, Vancouver, BC, Canada

Anne B. Fulton

Department of Ophthalmology, Children's Hospital Boston, Boston, MA, USA

William V. Good

Smith-Kettlewell Eye Research Institute, San Francisco, CA, USA

Melvyn A. Goodale

Centre for Brain and Mind, Department of Psychology, University of Western Ontario, London, ON, Canada

Andrea Guzzetta

Division of Child Neurology, University of Pisa, Stella Maris Scientific Institute, Pisa, Italy

Lea Hyvärinen

Faculty of Rehabilitation Sciences, Technical University of Dortmund, Dortmund, Germany; Faculty of Behavioural Sciences, University of Helsinki, Helsinki, Finland

Hussein Ibrahim

Royal Hospital for Sick Children, Yorkhill; Glasgow Caledonian University, Glasgow, UK

Lena Jacobson

Department of Clinical Neuroscience, Karolinska Institute, Stockholm, Sweden

Josée Lanners

Robert Hollman Foundation, Cannero Riviera (VB), Padova, Italy

Daphne L. McCulloch   Royal Hospital for Sick Children, Yorkhill; Glasgow Caledonian University, Glasgow, UK

Gillian McDaid   Royal Hospital for Sick Children, Yorkhill, Glasgow, UK

Elisabeth Macdonald   Tennent Institute of Ophthalmology, Gartnavel General Hospital; Royal Hospital for Sick Children, Yorkhill, Glasgow, UK

Catriona Macintyre-Beon   Royal Hospital for Sick Children, Yorkhill, Glasgow, UK

Carey Matsuba   British Columbia Children's Hospital, Vancouver, BC, Canada

Eugenio Mercuri   Paediatric Neurology Unit, Catholic University, Policlinico Gemelli, Rome, Italy

Katherine Mitchell   The Royal Hospital for Sick Children, Yorkhill, Glasgow, UK

Giorgio Porro   Department of Ophthalmology, Utrecht University Hospital, Utrecht, the Netherlands

Daniela Ricci   Paediatric Neurology Unit, Catholic University, Rome, Italy

Shohista Saidkasimova   Tennent Institute of Ophthalmology, Gartnavel General Hospital, Glasgow, UK

Alison Salt   Department of Neurodisability, Great Ormond Street Hospital for Children, London, UK

Jenefer Sargent   Department of Neurodisability, Great Ormond Street Hospital for Children, London, UK

Sabrina G. Signorini   Center of Child Neuro-ophthalmology, Child Neuropsychiatry Unit, IRCCS C. Mondino Institute, Pavia, Italy

Janet Soul   Harvard Medical School, Boston, MA, USA

Katherine M. Spowart   Royal Hospital for Sick Children, Yorkhill, Glasgow, UK

Peter Stiers   Faculty of Psychology and Neuroscience, Maastricht University, Maastricht, the Netherlands

Renate Walthes   Faculty of Rehabilitation Sciences, Technical
                            University of Dortmund, Dortmund, Germany

Dienke Wittebol-Post   Utrecht University Hospital, Utrecht, the
                            Netherlands

J. Margaret Woodhouse   School of Optometry and Vision Sciences,
                            Cardiff University, Cardiff, UK

FOREWORD

This book is a worthy sequel to the Castang Foundation meeting in November 2005 on visual impairment, bringing together experts in cognitive and perceptual dysfunction in children and how they can be helped. It is an 'eclection' of ideas and data on caring for children with visual brain damage, aimed at the medical and caring professions. The book starts with an authoritative statement by Mel Goodale on functional organization of the central visual pathways, and the important distinction between ventral and dorsal processing, which recurs throughout the book. Gordon Dutton discusses, with Elisabeth Macdonald, impairment of cognitive vision with issues of detection and measurement and, with others, cognitive dysfunction associated with brain damage in children.

Janette Atkinson and Oliver Braddick (Oxford, UK) discuss behaviour and electrophysiological measures for assessing visual brain function in infants and young children. The effects of impaired vision on development and visual impairment in the context of cerebral palsy are the themes of Elisa Fazzi's work. Recent experimental techniques have their place here, including correlations between imaging and early visual development by Eugenio Mercuri and colleagues in Italy. Central visual function and how it is assessed are examined by William Good and Anne Fulton.

Clinical features of cognitive and visual impairments are analysed by Gordon Dutton and his colleagues at the Tennent Institute of Ophthalmology in Gartnavel General Hospital in Glasgow, UK.

Aside from the clinical and philosophical issues, there are political implications, especially as financial and medical, as well as educational, resources are made available or are withheld according to complicated social factors. By increasing understanding and awareness of these issues, this book will be of direct help to children with visual impairments. Many of the issues that are raised are technical, but there is an underlying appreciation of the importance of understanding these problems at many levels, from clinical to social, with sensitivity to emotional issues.

There is a concern throughout of how to tap into normal or damaged systems in infants without the use of language. So, experiments with eye movements and accommodation changes are particularly significant. For normal adults, eye movements are controlled from all levels of brain activity, including subtle cognitive estimates of probabilities and dangers and rewards. Presumably, as knowledge grows, and as techniques become more powerful, it will be possible to gain richer insights into cognitive processing in infancy and childhood. Not only should this be of great clinical importance, but it should also tell us a great deal about human development and the effect of environment in home life and school. This clearly needs an interdisciplinary approach, which is just what emerges from the insights and future promises of this ambitious book.

Richard Gregory CBE, FRS[†]
Emeritus Professor and Senior Research Fellow
Department of Experimental Psychology
University of Bristol

[†]Sadly, Richard Gregory passed away on 17 May 2010.

PREFACE

Cerebral visual impairment (CVI) and optic neuropathy have become the most common causes of visual impairment in children in developed countries (Rogers 1996 [UK], Blohmé and Tornqvist 1997a [Sweden], Alagaratnam et al 2002 [Scotland], Flanagan et al 2003 [Ireland], Matsuba and Jan 2006 [Canada], Hatton et al 2007 [USA], Neilsen et al 2007 [Denmark], Bunce and Wormald 2008 [UK]), probably on account of a combination of successful treatment of cataract and glaucoma in children (McClelland 2007) combined with improving survival of both preterm-born children (Rudanko et al 2003) and those with life-threatening conditions with cerebral complications. The condition is also being increasingly recognized and acknowledged, and children with CVI are being registered as being visually impaired, when hitherto they were not (Bamashmus et al 2004).

Children with cerebral palsy have a high probability of additional visual dysfunction (Pennefather and Tin 2000, Matsuba and Jan 2006, Ghasia et al 2008). Moreover, CVI is a major cause of low vision in adults with intellectual disabilities (Warburg 2001, van Splunder et al 2004).

The complexity of visual processing is responsible for considerable heterogeneity of expression of visual impairment due to damage to the brain. Yet despite the high lifelong prevalence of CVI in at-risk children and those with intellectual disabilities and cerebral palsy, there is limited information available concerning this complex subject. This book is aimed at addressing this need.

Gordon Dutton and Martin Bax
January 2010

This book resulted from a meeting which was organised and funded by the Castang Foundation in November 2005.

INTRODUCTION

Gordon N. Dutton and Martin Bax

Increased awareness of cerebral visual impairment in children, combined with improved recognition of its wide-ranging manifestations, has led to it becoming the most common cause of visual impairment in children in the developed world. Yet the subject is in its infancy.

The development of a child's visual acuity from early childhood, and its measurement, are well described (Teller 1997), but despite longstanding evidence that the newborn infant has an inbuilt capability to identify a face compared with other patterns (Goren et al 1975) and an early ability to imitate facial movements (Meltzoff and Moore 1983), surprisingly little information about the functional use of vision by the infant has been collected. It is known that the fetus learns to discriminate sounds such as a female voice while in utero (Lecanuet 1989), and the newborn infant can use smell to discriminate between a mother's breast milk and that of a stranger (Macfarlane 1975). Given such very early facilitation of these senses to identify specific elements in the environment, it would be surprising if vision, with its larger allocation of dedicated brain function, does not play a major part in the child's social (and psychosocial) development at a very early stage.

Much theorizing about the early psychosocial development of the child remains fixated on the oral Freudian model, despite the fact that, from research, we know that the oral mechanism reaches its level of sophistication very early on, because it is essential to the infant's survival. The centres that control it are in the region of the midbrain and probably do not involve the cortex, in so far as the infant sucks and swallows satisfactorily from 34 weeks. The anencephalic child successfully swallows and survives for days, if not weeks. It appears much more likely that the early psychosocial developmental period for humans should be regarded as the visual rather than the oral period. Indeed, during breast feeding, once satiation is partially achieved, the child will break off from sucking and swallowing to gaze intently into the eyes of the mother (Blass et al 2001). The pacifier induces somnolence whereas the visual display excites interest. Visual identification of the face has been investigated in the classic studies of infants, and the importance of identification of the face leading to the development of the awareness of strangers (Piaget 1955) is self-evident. Here is not the place for a full review of the role of vision in early psychosocial development, but its importance cannot be over-emphasized. Vision certainly plays a role in disturbed social interactions, which are seen in many neurodevelopmental disorders, such as autism (Pellicano et al 2007), but its role has yet to be fully elucidated.

This book originates from a Castang Foundation workshop with the same title, held in London in late 2005. It links the work of a range of authors who have made significant contributions to the literature on the subject of cerebral visual impairment and provides a structured amalgam of the viewpoints of different specialists. The authors each have different perspectives, some of which, to the reader, may appear to be contradictory, or at least not complementary. This applies particularly to the last two chapters, which present different viewpoints concerning the classification of cerebral visual impairment. At this stage in the evolution of knowledge, we believe this is an appropriate approach, as it provides the substrate for the development of a consistent model, which will gradually be built up through exchanging ideas and concept frameworks about this complex and wide-ranging subject.

A large proportion of the brain serves vision, but, in contrast to movement of the body, vision is an internalized function. Early-onset damage to the brain can interfere with the development of movement and manifests as cerebral palsy, but when vision is affected the result is less evident in all but the most severely affected cases. Yet the adverse effects on development can be profound. The classic model of thinking about vision, in which a picture is somehow formed by the eyes and processed in the striate cortex, has long been recognized to be limited. Yet in medical practice this conceptual framework has continued to hold sway, with impairment of visual acuity considered a prerequisite for both diagnosis and the provision of assistance. Damage to the visual pathways and occipital cortex impairs visual fields and visual acuities, whereas damage to the higher centres serving vision interferes with visual processing. These visual manifestations may occur either in isolation or in combination. But a wider concept of how damage to the brain can give rise to multiple visual difficulties has yet to be fully recognized. Children with such visual problems may, in some cases, be seen as having one of the syndromic classifications such as autism, cerebral palsy, or simply intellectual disability, but the visual element in these children is rarely recognized and may even be judged irrelevant to the child's condition, despite potentially being pivotal.

When considering terminology, the term 'cortical visual impairment' has been defined as 'loss of or highly inefficient visual acuity, essentially due to occipital lobe disturbance' (J. Jan, British Columbia's Children's Hospital, BC, Canada; personal communication, 2009), whereas the term 'cerebral visual impairment' has been taken to encompass a wider range of disorders, including 'visual disturbance on account of oculomotor incoordination, and visual, cognitive, and perceptual impairment owing to pathology affecting the visual association cortices and their interconnecting pathways' (Fazzi et al 2004). Both terms are abbreviated in the literature to CVI, which can be a source of confusion. In this text, the term 'cerebral visual impairment' is predominantly used in view of its wider meaning. It also serves as a reminder that visual fields and visual acuities are rarely impaired in isolation and a search for evidence of visual–perceptual impairment in such children will usually be rewarded and will, in turn, lead to the implementation of a wider range of habilitative strategies. (The term 'habilitative' is chosen in preference to 'rehabilitative' because in most cases of cerebral visual impairment no function has been lost to rehabilitate. Similarly, the term 'loss of vision' can apply only to those who have lost vision. Thus, the term 'visual impairment' is preferable for those who have had low vision from birth.)

A wide spectrum of visual problems has now been described in children with cerebral visual impairment, which differs from that seen in adults, because the loss of a visual function is very different to impaired development of that same function. Moreover, early-onset damage to the brain is followed by brain growth and development, and the adult model – of damage to the visual system being immutable – does not apply. The fact that training is now known to lead to brain growth accompanied by greater cell size and greater numbers of synaptic connections in the occipital area indicates that strategies which optimize habilitation may affect ultimate visual outcome, and there is limited evidence that this is the case (Sonksen et al 1991). Simply the act of identifying, characterizing, and communicating the diagnosis of cerebral visual impairment to parents and carers can set the child on a new pathway of development. For example, lower visual field impairment is no longer attributed to clumsiness, but is managed appropriately; inability to copy from the 'blackboard' is understood to be a result of visual difficulties, and alternative measures are implemented; and impaired social interaction because of an inability to find someone in a group is recognized not as being caused by being socially aloof, but as a specific disability which can be managed appropriately. The resultant change in attitude of both parents and teachers can revolutionize a child's life. Unlike impairment of vision owing to eye pathology, cerebral visual impairment in children can vary from hour to hour and day to day, and recognition that this is a typical feature and is not a result of bad behaviour is essential. The adverse emotional consequences of failure of diagnosis, and the child having to tolerate unfounded criticism of fully explicable behaviour, can be profound.

Focal damage to the visual brain leads to specific visual difficulties, which can be specifically characterized. By contrast, diffuse damage which affects all aspects of brain function can adversely impact upon visual function in a manner which is much more difficult to characterize, yet still needs to be recognized if appropriate measures are to be taken. It may be impossible to fully characterize the visual dysfunction in those who are profoundly impaired, yet the knowledge gained from those with focal damage can be used to afford a greater philosophical understanding of the visual problems in such children, which underpins the practical basis for how best they can be managed.

It is remarkable that knowledge concerning the specific cortical areas serving visual function goes back to the studies of soldiers with brain injuries during the First World War. Not only was the anatomy of the afferent visual pathways determined with accuracy (Holmes 1918a), but the profound visual consequences of damage to the posterior parietal cortex were graphically described in a second, but less well-recognized, paper (Holmes 1918b). This second paper described six soldiers who sustained bilateral posterior parietal shrapnel injuries. These soldiers all had lower visual field loss, impaired visual guidance of movement (optic ataxia) of the limbs (despite intact stereopsis in four cases), and profound simultanagnosia (being unable to identify more than one or two objects at a time). (This symptom, complex in its severe form, came to be known as Balint syndrome, and in its milder form is beginning to be referred to as dorsal stream dysfunction.) It is no coincidence that the selfsame features of impaired lower visual fields – inability to handle complex visual scenes and impaired visual guidance of movement – are evident in children with posterior superior periventricular white matter pathology (Jacobson and Dutton 2000). Affected children have coordination difficulties and cannot see a friend in a group. They can appear antisocial and may be ascribed a range of alternative diagnoses if the visual origin of the behaviour is not recognized. While the ventral stream disorders are less clearcut, it is clear that they play a major role in visual function, and we can be sure that they have a large, as yet unrecognized, part to play in many of the syndromic neurodevelopmental disorders, such as cerebral palsy and autism.

Inevitably, the nature of service provision in different countries influences the thinking, with clinical experience constraining the patterns of visual disturbance seen by different practitioners. For example, those working in facilities for the visually disabled do not see how children with cerebal visual impairment manage in mainstream schooling or other special educational provision.

We were particularly aware that, while 'simple' problems affecting visual acuity, contrast sensitivity, and visual fields are identified, the role of perceptual and cognitive visual dysfunction in many disabilities may not be recognized or understood. We think particularly, for example, of the many children on the autistic spectrum who have problems with vision and visual interpretation, as these problems tend to be enveloped in the general description of the condition, such as autism, and not focused on diagnostic issues in their own right. The same applies to the field of cerebral palsy and is also probably of considerable importance in the field of intellectual disability. The possibility that such complex visual problems exist and may provide remediable explanations for some of the behavioural manifestations potentially renders this book important reading for those who look after such children, whether they be teachers, therapists, psychologists, doctors, or other health professionals. Simply thinking of children on the autistic spectrum as having fundamental visual problems, rather than purely behavioural issues, changes the cast of one's mind as one approaches such a child. We hope that this book will lead people to look at children with disabilities in a different way and constantly keep in mind the role of the visual system in their disorder (without neglecting all the other areas of function which will affect the child). This book is not aimed at the paediatric ophthalmologist; rather, it is aimed at a whole community of clinicians, from paediatric neurologists through to psychologists, therapists, and teachers. To this end, the chapters with a more technical content therefore include summaries written with less technical language. We hope that all these groups will actively consider vision (in its broadest sense) and its role in the wide range of disorders which may present to them.

1
THE FUNCTIONAL ORGANIZATION OF THE CENTRAL VISUAL PATHWAYS

Melvyn A. Goodale

Introduction: What is vision for? A brief discussion of the origins of vision

Visual systems first evolved not to enable animals to see, but to provide distal sensory control of their movements. Vision as 'sight' is a relative newcomer on the evolutionary landscape, but its emergence has enabled animals to carry out complex cognitive operations on perceptual representations of the world. Thus, vision in humans and other primates (and other animals as well) has two distinct but interacting functions: (1) the perception of objects and their relations, which provides a foundation for the organism's cognitive life and its conscious experience of the world and (2) the control of actions directed at (or with respect to) those objects, in which separate motor outputs are programmed and controlled online. These different demands on vision have shaped the organization of the visual pathways in the primate brain. Moreover, as we shall see, this distinction between 'vision for perception' and 'vision for action' provides a useful framework for understanding the functional organization of the human visual system, including the visual pathways within the cerebral cortex (for reviews see Goodale and Milner 2004, Milner and Goodale 2006). But before these different functions of vision are discussed in any detail, what is known about the organization of the projections from retina to different subcortical structures will be briefly reviewed.

From retina to brain

The retina not only transduces the electromagnetic radiation striking the photoreceptors into physiological signals that can be understood by the brain, but it also performs several computations on those signals, which involve combining information from a number of different photoreceptors (Masland 2001, Field and Chichilnisky 2007). Thus, by the time the sensory signals leave the eye on their way to the brain, a good deal of processing has already occurred. This processing, furthermore, is not uniform within the retinal system. The ganglion cells, whose axons leave the eye and constitute the optic nerve, are heterogeneous in the kinds of information they convey (Wässle 2004). Some ganglion cells, for example, carry information that is particularly useful for an analysis of the spatial distribution of light energy striking the retina; others carry information that is more related to the temporal dynamics of the retinal array, arising, for example, from the motion of a distal stimulus. Still others appear to be primarily concerned with the distribution of the different wavelengths of light entering the eye, leading ultimately to the perception of colour (Dacey and Packer 2003, Solomon and Lennie 2007). Moreover, across different species, the organization of the eye and the signal transformations that occur in the retina vary enormously, no doubt reflecting the range of ecological niches in which animals live (Lamb et al 2007).

It is often not appreciated that the neuronal projections from the retina travel to a number of distinct target areas in the vertebrate brain. In other words, they do not form a set of parallel lines of information projecting together from one complex processing station to another, but instead diverge to very different processing targets right from the outset (Fig. 1.1). These different projections reflect both the evolutionary origins of different visual pathways as well as the different behavioural functions to which vision contributes.

The earliest set of projections to leave the optic tract and terminate in the brain are those terminating in a structure in the hypothalamus called the suprachiasmatic nucleus (SCN), which, as the name implies, sits right above the optic chiasm. The SCN is a critical structure in the brain circuit that controls circadian rhythms, such as the sleep–wake cycle and the production and release of circulating hormones (Herzog 2007). The retinal projections to the SCN provide input about ambient light levels that locks the intrinsic circadian rhythm of SCN neurons to the local light–dark cycle. When the local light–dark cycle changes dramatically, as it does when one flies across the Atlantic, it takes some time for the SCN neurons to be retrained to the new light–dark cycle (hence, one experiences 'jet lag').

Another set of ancient retinal projections, the accessory optic tract, terminates in three separate nuclei in the brainstem, known collectively as the accessory optic system (AOS). Neurons in the AOS are driven by large moving patterns of optic flow on the retina. They project via premotor relay nuclei to the cerebellum and spinal cord, and play a critical role (together with the vestibular system and proprioception) in visual stabilization, the control of posture, and the regulation of locomotion and heading (Simpson 1984).

A prominent set of pathways from the retina also projects to the midbrain, to a laminated structure known in simpler vertebrates and birds as the optic tectum, and in mammals as the superior colliculus (Figs 1.1 and 1.2). The superior colliculus plays a central role in the initiation and control of orientating movements of the eyes, head, and body towards salient visual stimuli in the peripheral visual fields and the maintenance of fixation on those stimuli (Sparks 2002). Other collicular circuits mediate visually guided escape responses by generating rapid movements away from looming visual stimuli that could be potential predators (Dean et al 1989). The deeper layers of the superior colliculus project to premotor nuclei in the brainstem involved in the control of the eye muscles and to parts of the spinal cord involved in the control of the neck musculature and the trunk and forelimbs (Crawford et al 2003, May 2005). The superficial layers of the superior colliculus send projections to visual areas in the cerebral cortex, via thalamic nuclei such as the pulvinar and medial dorsal nucleus (May 2005). The exact role of these projections is not well understood, although it is thought that some of them might send an efferent copy signal (corollary discharge) about shifts in gaze that could modulate attention and the processing of visual motion in the cerebral cortex (Sommer and Wurtz 2006).

Other retinal projections include those to various pretectal nuclei, which, as the name suggests, are located just in front of the optic tectum (or superior colliculus). One of these

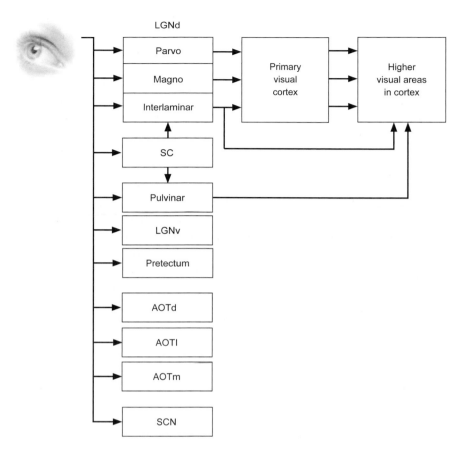

Fig. 1.1 Schematic drawing of the main retinal projection sites in the brain. LGNd, lateral geniculate nucleus, pars dorsalis; parvo, parvocellular layers of LGNd; magno, magnocellular layers of LGNd; interlaminar, interlaminar regions of LGNd; SC, superior colliculus; pulvinar, pulvinar nucleus of the thalamus; LGNv, lateral geniculate nucleus, pars ventralis; AOTd, dorsal terminal nucleus of the accessory optic tract; AOTl, lateral terminal nucleus of the accessory optic tract; AOTm, medial terminal nucleus of the accessory optic tract; SCN, suprachiasmatic nucleus. For more details see Milner and Goodale (2006).

pretectal nuclei, the nucleus of the optic tract, has strong links with the AOS; another, the olivary pretectal nucleus, is part of the circuit mediating the pupillary light reflex and other reflexive responses such as light-evoked blinking (Gamlin 2005). There is also evidence that retinal projections to (unspecified) pretectal nuclei might play a role in obstacle avoidance during locomotion in both amphibians and mammals (Ingle 1982, Milner and Goodale 2006). Nevertheless, much remains to be discovered about the functions of the different pretectal nuclei, as well as neighbouring thalamic nuclei such as the ventral part of the lateral geniculate

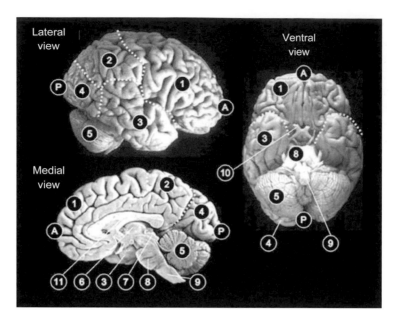

Fig. 1.2 The human brain, showing the lateral, medial, and ventral surfaces. A, anterior; P, posterior; 1, frontal lobe; 2, parietal lobe; 3, temporal lobe; 4, occipital lobe; 5, cerebellum; 6, thalamus; 7, superior colliculus; 8, pons; 9, medulla; 10, optic nerve; 11, corpus callosum.

nucleus (LGNv) and the retino-recipient region of the pulvinar (for a review see Kaas and Lyon 2007).

By far and away the most prominent visual pathway from the retina to the brain in humans and their primate cousins is the retinogeniculate projection, which terminates in the dorsal part of the lateral geniculate nucleus of the thalamus (LGNd). In other vertebrate classes, such as amphibians and reptiles, this pathway is barely evident. Even in birds, which are highly visual creatures, the homologue of the retinogeniculate projection is much smaller than the projection to their optic tectum. Only in mammals has this projection system become prominent. Neurons in the LGNd project in turn to the cerebral cortex, with almost all of the fibres, in primates at least, terminating in the primary visual area, or striate cortex (often nowadays called 'area V1') in the occipital lobe (Fig. 1.2). This geniculostriate projection and its cortical elabora-tions probably constitute the best studied neural 'system' in the whole of neuroscience. This fact is perhaps not unrelated to the general belief that subjective visual experience in humans depends on the integrity of this projection system.

Finally, it should be emphasized that almost all the subcortical structures discussed above receive not only direct input from the retina, but also inputs from other visual structures, including visual areas in the cerebral cortex. Thus, the superior colliculus, the pretectal nuclei, the pulvinar, and the lateral geniculate nucleus all receive inputs from area V1. In addition, many of the subcortical nuclei are highly interconnected. For example, the superior colliculus projects to pretectal nuclei, the pulvinar, and the lateral geniculate nucleus. Moreover, many of these structures receive input from other modalities, such as audition and somatosensation. Nevertheless, each of these different visual structures plays a critical role in the control of a particular set of visually guided and/or visually modulated patterns of behaviour.

Two cortical visual pathways

Beyond the primary visual cortex in the primate cerebral cortex, visual information is conveyed to a bewildering number of extrastriate areas (Van Essen 2001). Despite the complexity of the interconnections between these different areas, two broad 'streams' of projections from primary visual cortex have been identified in the macaque monkey brain: a ventral stream projecting eventually to the inferotemporal cortex and a dorsal stream projecting to the posterior parietal cortex (Ungerleider and Mishkin 1982; see Figs 1.2 and 1.3). Although some caution must be exercised in generalizing from monkey to human (Sereno and Tootell 2005), recent neuroimaging evidence suggests that the visual projections from early visual areas to the temporal and parietal lobes in the human brain also involve a separation into ventral and dorsal streams (Grill-Spector and Malach 2004, Culham and Valyear 2006).

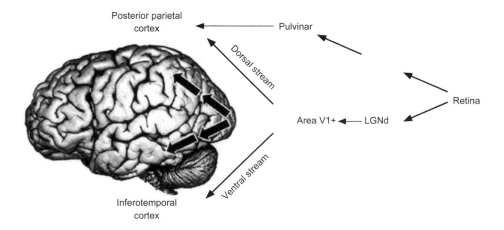

Fig. 1.3 Schematic representation of the two streams of visual processing in human cerebral cortex. The retina sends projections to the dorsal part of the lateral geniculate nucleus in the thalamus (LGNd), which projects in turn to primary visual cortex (V1). Within the cerebral cortex, the ventral stream arises from early visual areas (V1+) and projects to regions in the occipito-temporal cortex. The dorsal stream also arises from early visual areas but projects instead to the posterior parietal cortex. The posterior parietal cortex also receives visual input from the superior colliculus via the pulvinar. On the left, the approximate locations of the pathways are shown on an image of the brain. The routes indicated by the arrows involve a series of complex interconnections.

THE PERCEPTION–ACTION HYPOTHESIS

Traditional accounts of the division of labour between the two streams (e.g. Ungerleider and Mishkin 1982) focused on the distinction between object vision and spatial vision. This distinction between what and where resonated remarkably with not only psychological accounts of perception, but also nearly a century of neurological thought about the functions of the temporal and parietal lobes in vision (Ferrier and Yeo 1884, Brown and Schäfer 1888, Schäfer 1888, Holmes 1918a).

In the early 1990s, however, the 'what versus where' story began to unravel as new evidence emerged from work with both monkeys and patients with neurological disorders. It became apparent that a purely sensory/perceptual account of ventral–dorsal function could not explain these findings. The only way to make sense of them was to consider the nature of the outputs served by the two streams – and to work out how visual information is eventually transformed into motor acts. In 1992, Goodale and Milner proposed a re-interpretation of the Ungerleider and Mishkin account of the two visual streams. According to their proposal, the dorsal stream plays a critical role in the real-time control of action, transforming moment-to-moment information about the location and disposition of objects into the coordinate frames of the effectors being used to perform the action (Goodale and Milner 1992, Milner and Goodale 2006). The ventral stream (together with associated cognitive networks) helps to construct the rich and detailed representations of the world that allow us to identify objects and events, attach meaning and significance to them, and establish their causal relations. Such operations are essential for accumulating and accessing a visual knowledge-base about the world. Thus, it is the ventral stream that provides the perceptual foundation for the offline control of action, projecting action into the future and incorporating stored information from the past into the control of current actions. In contrast, processing in the dorsal stream does not generate visual percepts; it generates skilled actions (in part by modulating more ancient visuomotor modules described in the previous section). The division of labour proposed by Goodale and Milner not only accounts for the neurological dissociations observed in patients with damage to different regions of the cerebral cortex, but it is also supported by a wealth of anatomical, electrophysiological, and behavioural studies in the monkey.

NEUROPSYCHOLOGICAL EVIDENCE

It has been known for a long time that patients with lesions in the superior regions of the posterior parietal cortex, particularly lesions that invade the territory of the intraparietal sulcus (or IPS) and the parieto-occipital sulcus, can have problems using vision to direct a grasp or aiming movement towards the correct location of a visual target placed in different positions in the visual field, particularly the peripheral visual field. This particular deficit is often described as *optic ataxia* (following Bálint 1909). But the failure to locate an object with the hand should not be construed as a problem in spatial vision; many of these patients, for example, can describe the relative position of the object in space quite accurately, even though they cannot direct their hand towards it (Perenin and Vighetto 1988). Moreover, sometimes the deficit will be seen in one hand but not the other. (It should be pointed out, of course, that these patients typically have no difficulty using input from other sensory systems, such as proprioception or audition, to guide their movements.) Some of these patients are unable to use visual information to rotate their hand, scale their grip, or configure their fingers properly when reaching out to pick up an object, even though they have no difficulty describing the orientation, size, or shape of objects in that part of the visual field (see Fig. 1.4). Clearly, a 'disorder of spatial vision' (Holmes 1918a) fails to capture this range of visuomotor impairments. Instead, this pattern of deficits suggests that the posterior parietal cortex plays a critical role in the visual control of skilled actions (for more details see Milner and Goodale 2006).

The opposite pattern of deficits and spared abilities can be seen in patients with visual agnosia. Take the case of patient DF, who developed a profound visual-form agnosia following carbon monoxide poisoning (Goodale et al 1991). Although magnetic resonance imaging (MRI) showed evidence of diffuse damage consistent with hypoxia, most of the damage was evident in ventrolateral regions of the occipital cortex with V1 remaining largely spared. Even though DF's 'low-level' visual abilities are reasonably intact, she can no longer recognize everyday objects or the faces of her friends and relatives, nor can she identify even the simplest of geometric shapes. (If an object is placed in her hand, of course, she has no trouble identifying it by touch.) Remarkably, however, DF shows strikingly accurate guidance of her hand movements when she attempts to pick up the very objects she cannot identify. Thus, when she reaches out to grasp objects of different sizes, her hand opens wider midflight for larger objects than it does for smaller ones, just like it does in people with normal vision (see Fig. 1.4). Similarly, she rotates her hand and wrist quite normally when she reaches out to

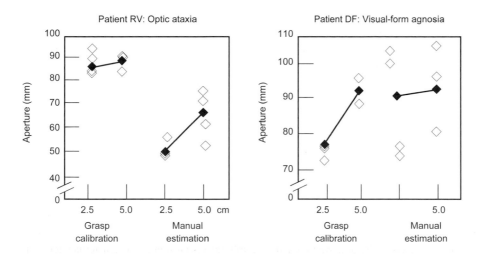

Fig. 1.4 Graphs showing the size of the aperture between the index finger and thumb during object-directed grasping and manual estimates of object width for RV, a patient with optic ataxia, and DF, a patient with visual-form agnosia. RV (left) was able to indicate the size of the objects reasonably well (individual trials marked as open diamonds), but her maximum grip aperture in flight was not well tuned. She simply opened her hand as wide as possible on every trial. In contrast, DF (right) showed excellent grip scaling, opening her hand wider for the 50mm-wide object than for the 25mm-wide object. DF's manual estimates of the width of the two objects, however, were grossly inaccurate and showed enormous variability from trial to trial. The data from DF were adapted from Goodale et al (1991).

11

grasp objects in different orientations, and she places her fingers correctly on the surface of objects with different shapes. At the same time, she is quite unable to distinguish between any of these objects when they are presented to her in simple discrimination tests. She even fails in manual 'matching' tasks in which she is asked to show how wide an object is by opening her index finger and thumb a corresponding amount (Fig. 1.4). DF's spared visuomotor skills are not limited to grasping. She can step over obstacles during locomotion as well as control subjects can, even though her perceptual judgements about the height of these obstacles are far from normal. Contrary to what would be predicted from the 'what versus where' hypothesis, then, a profound loss of form perception coexists in DF with a preserved ability to use form in guiding a broad range of actions. Such a dissociation, of course, is consistent with the idea that there are separate neural pathways for transforming incoming visual information for the perceptual representation of the world and for the control of action. Presumably, it is the former and not the latter that is compromised in DF (for more details see Goodale and Milner 2004, Milner and Goodale 2006).

Evidence from Single-cell Recording of the Monkey

A broad range of studies on the dorsal and ventral streams in the monkey lends considerable support to the distinction between perception and action. For example, monkeys with lesions of inferotemporal (IT) cortex can orientate their fingers in a precision grip to grasp morsels of food embedded in small slots placed at different orientations – even though their ability to discriminate between different orientations is profoundly impaired (Glickstein et al 1998).

Moreover, there is a long history of single-unit work showing that cells in IT and neighbouring regions of the superior temporal sulcus are tuned to specific objects and object features – with some cells maintaining their selectivity irrespective of viewpoint, retinal image size, and even colour (e.g. Gross et al 1972, Logothetis and Sheinberg 1996, Tanaka 2003). Moreover, the responses of these cells are not affected by the animal's motor behaviour but are instead sensitive to the reinforcement history and significance of the visual stimuli that drive them. It has been suggested that cells in this region might play a role in comparing current visual inputs with internal representations of recalled images (e.g. Eskandar 1992), which are themselves presumably stored in other regions, such as neighbouring regions of the medial temporal lobe and related limbic areas (Squire et al 2007). In fact, sensitivity to particular objects can be created in ensembles of IT cells simply by training the animals to discriminate between different objects. There is also evidence for a specialization within separate regions of the ventral stream for the coding of certain categories of objects, such as faces and hands, which are of particular social significance to the monkey (Logothetis et al 1995). Finally, experiments that have used a binocular rivalry paradigm, in which competing images are presented at the same time to the two eyes, have shown that cells in IT are tuned to what the monkey reports seeing on a particular trial, not simply to what is present to the two eyes (Logothetis 1998). But neurons earlier in the visual system, such as area V1, do not show these correlations. They respond in the same way, no matter what the monkey indicates that it sees. Even in intermediate areas of the ventral stream, such as area V4, the correlations are relatively weak. These results provide indirect support for the claim that the ventral stream plays a critical role in delivering the contents of our conscious percepts (in so far as activity in the monkey's inferotemporal cortex reflects what the monkey indicates that it sees). These, and other studies too numerous to cite here, lend considerable support to the suggestion that the object-based descriptions provided by the ventral stream form the basic raw material for visual perception, recognition memory, and other long-term representations of the visual world (for a detailed discussion see Milner and Goodale 2006).

In sharp contrast to the activity of cells in the ventral stream, the responses of cells in the dorsal stream are greatly dependent on the concurrent motor behaviour of the animal. Thus, separate subsets of visual cells in the posterior parietal cortex, the major terminal zone for the dorsal stream, have been shown to be implicated in visual fixation, pursuit and saccadic eye movements, visually guided reaching, and the manipulation of objects (Hyvärinen and Poranen 1974, Mountcastle et al 1975). Moreover, the motor modulation is quite specific. For example, visual cells in the posterior parietal cortex that code the location of a target for a saccadic eye movement are quite separate from cells in this region that code the location for a manual aiming movement to the same target (Snyder et al 1997, Cohen and Andersen 2002). In other experiments, cells in the anterior intraparietal region of the parietal cortex (area AIP), which fire when the monkey manipulates an object, have also been shown to be sensitive to the intrinsic object features, such as size and orientation, that determine the posture of the hand and fingers during a grasping movement (for a review see Sakata and Taira 1994). Lesions in this region of the posterior parietal cortex produce deficits in the visual control of reaching and grasping similar in many respects to those seen in humans following damage to a homologous region in the posterior parietal cortex (Glickstein et al 1998). In one study, small reversible pharmacological lesions were made in area AIP in the monkey (Gallese et al 1994). When this region was inactivated, there was a selective interference with preshaping of the hand as the monkey reached out to grasp an object. The posterior parietal cortex is also intimately linked with the premotor cortex, the superior colliculus, and pontine nuclei – brain areas that have been implicated in various aspects of the visual control of eye, limb, and body movements. In short, the networks in the dorsal stream have the functional properties and interconnections that one might expect to see in a system concerned with the moment-to-moment control of visually guided actions (for a more detailed discussion see Milner and Goodale 2006).

NEUROIMAGING STUDIES OF PERCEPTION AND ACTION
Converging evidence from a host of recent neuroimaging studies in humans has revealed that visual information from V1 is conveyed to a series of retinotopically organized visual areas (for reviews see Tootell et al 1996, Van Essen et al 2001, Milner and Goodale 2006). These areas, which include V2, V3, V3A, V4, and V5 (sometimes called area MT, for middle temporal area), typically have visual receptive fields that are much larger than those of V1 and carry out more complex analyses on the visual input, extracting higher-order information about luminance, colour, texture, simple shape, and motion. As information moves further along into the ventral stream, however, a host of functional areas emerge that appear to be 'tuned' to particular stimulus categories (for a review see Grill-Spector and Malach 2004). Functional magnetic resonance imaging (fMRI) studies in humans have revealed the existence of separate

areas dedicated to the perception of faces and places. Thus, in the fusiform gyrus, a 'face area' has been identified (Kanwisher et al 1997), which is activated much more by pictures of faces than by other pictures such as everyday objects, buildings, or even scrambled pictures of faces (see Fig. 1.5). This fusiform face area (or FFA) is quite separate from another area in the parahippocampal gyrus (the parahippocampal place area or PPA), which is activated by pictures of buildings and scenes but much less by faces (Epstein and Kanwisher 1998). Yet another area has been identified which is selectively activated by pictures of everyday objects (such as fruit and vegetables, as well as manufactured objects, such as cameras and coffee cups). This region, which has been dubbed the lateral occipital area (or area LO) because of its location on the lateral surface of the occipital lobe, can be readily seen in fMRI scans by contrasting the activation that is present when people look at pictures of intact objects and contrasting that with the activation to scrambled pictures of the same objects (Malach et al 1995). This subtraction removes the brain activation caused just by the constituent lines and edges of the objects, revealing only the activity that is related specifically to the geometric structure of the objects. As more and more fMRI studies are carried out, more and more specialized areas are being identified. For example, in addition to the FFA, other face-selective areas have been identified, such as the occipital face area (OFA), which is located in close proximity to area LO. In addition, other visual areas have been shown to be selective for pictures (or videos) of tools and still others for body parts, such as arms and legs. Although both the degree of overlap among these different areas and their functional significance remain controversial, there is no doubting their separate existence. At the same time, there is considerable debate about whether these regions really represent category-specific areas or whether they are simply nodes of higher activation in what is really a highly distributed system.

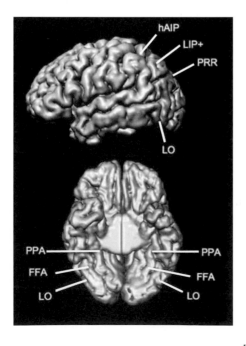

Fig. 1.5 Functional areas of the ventral and dorsal streams that have been identified with functional magnetic resonance imaging. The approximate locations of these different areas are shown on the ventral and lateral surface of the cerebral hemispheres. There is some variation in location across individuals. LO, lateral occipital area, which helps to mediate object recognition; FFA, fusiform face area, which participates in face recognition; PPA, parahippocampal place area, which plays a role in scene recognition; hAIP, human anterior intraparietal cortex, which is critical for the visual control of grasping; LIP+, the human homologue of the lateral intraparietal area in the monkey, which plays a role in the control of voluntary saccades and covert shifts of attention; PRR, the parietal reach region, which participates in the visual control of reaching.

In the human dorsal stream, a number of visuomotor areas that appear to be homologous with those in the monkey have been identified using fMRI (for reviews see Culham and Kanwisher 2001, Culham and Valyear 2006). Three of these areas are shown in Figure 1.5: LIP+, an area buried in the human intraparietal sulcus, which is involved in the visual control of saccadic eye movements as well as covert shifts of attention (Connolly et al 2000); the parietal reach region (PRR), an area in the posterior part of the human intraparietal sulcus extending into the parieto-occipital sulcus, which mediates the visual control of reaching movements (Connolly et al 2003), and hAIP, an area in the anterior part of the human intra-parietal sulcus close to the post-central sulcus, which mediates the visual control of grasping (Binkofski et al 1999, Culham et al 2003). It is perhaps important to emphasize that, although area MT has traditionally been regarded by anatomists as part of the dorsal stream, in fact this motion-sensitive area has been shown in both the monkey and the human to have strong functional relationships with both visual streams. Indeed, like area V1, from which it receives strong direct projections, MT projects heavily to areas in both the dorsal and the ventral stream. There is good reason to believe that MT plays a role not just in the guidance of movements such as visual pursuit, but also in the recognition of both moving objects and actions made by other people (for a discussion of this issue see Milner and Goodale 2006).

NEUROIMAGING STUDIES OF PATIENT DF

As described earlier, anatomical MRI conducted shortly after DF's accident showed bilateral damage in the ventrolateral regions of her occipital lobe. More recent high-resolution anatomical MRI scans of DF's brain have confirmed that this is indeed the case (James et al 2003). In fact, the damage is remarkably localized to area LO, which has been implicated in object recognition in a number of functional imaging studies (Grill-Spector and Malach 2004). It seems likely, then, that it is the lesions in area LO that are responsible for her deficit in form and shape perception. In fact, when DF was tested with fMRI, she showed no differential activation in her ventral stream (or anywhere else in her brain) to line drawings (as compared with scrambled versions of the same drawings). Neurologically intact observers, of course, showed robust activation to the same stimuli. Indeed, when a normal observer's brain was stereotactically aligned with DF's brain, the differential activation to line drawings overlapped her LO lesions.

But what brain areas are mediating DF's relatively normal visuomotor abilities? When DF was asked to grasp objects in the scanner, she showed robust activation in area hAIP, similar to that observed in neurologically intact volunteers (James et al 2003). This result, coupled with the observation that area LO is damaged bilaterally in DF, provides strong support for the idea that the visual control of object-directed grasping does not depend on object form-processing regions in the ventral stream but instead is mediated by object-driven visuomotor systems in the dorsal stream. In fact, it is worth noting that grasp-related activation in area hAIP in neurologically intact individuals is also unaccompanied by any differential activation in area LO (Culham et al 2003).

The metrics and frames of reference used by the dorsal and ventral streams

Two separate streams of visual processing evolved because perception and action require quite different transformations of the visual signals. To be able to grasp an object successfully, for example, it is essential that the brain computes the actual size of the object, and its orientation and position with respect to the observer (i.e. in egocentric coordinates). Moreover, the time at which these computations are performed is also critical. Observers and goal objects rarely stay in a static relationship with one another and, as a consequence, the egocentric coordinates of a target object can often change dramatically from moment to moment. For this reason, it is essential that the required coordinates for action be computed immediately before the movements are initiated. For the same reason, it would be counterproductive for these coordinates (or the resulting motor programmes) to be stored in memory. In short, vision-for-action works very much in an 'online' mode.

The requirements of perception are quite different, in terms of both the frames of reference used to construct the percept and the time period over which that percept (or the information it provides) can be accessed. Vision-for-perception appears not to rely on computations about the absolute size of objects or their egocentric locations. Instead, the perceptual system in the ventral stream computes the size, location, shape, and orientation of an object (and its parts) primarily in relation to other objects, object parts, and surfaces in the scene. Encoding an object in a scene-based frame of reference permits a perceptual representation of the object that preserves the relations between the object and its surroundings without requiring precise information about its absolute size or its exact position with respect to the observer. Indeed, if the perceptual machinery attempted to deliver the real size and distance of all the objects in the visual array, the computational load on the system would be astronomical.

The products of perception also need to be available over a much longer timescale than the visual information used in the control of action. It may be necessary to recognize objects seen minutes, hours, days – or even years – before. To achieve this, the coding of the visual information has to be somewhat abstract – transcending particular viewpoint and viewing conditions. By working with perceptual representations that are object or scene based, it is possible to maintain the constancies of size, shape, colour, lightness, and relative location, over time and across different viewing conditions. Although there is much debate about the way in which this information is coded, it is clear that it is the identity of the object and its location within the scene, not its disposition with respect to the observer, that is of primary concern to the perceptual system. Thus, current perception combined with stored information about previously encountered objects not only facilitates object recognition but also contributes to the control of goal-directed movements when working in offline mode, that is on the basis of memories of goal objects and their location in the world (for a detailed discussion of these issues see Goodale et al 2004).

As a consequence of these differences between the metrics and frames of reference used by vision-for-perception and vision-for-action, interesting dissociations can be observed between the ways in which the two systems deal with pictorial illusions, such as the Ebbinghaus illusion (see Fig. 1.6a). Thus, even though observers clearly perceive an object placed in the annulus of small circles as being larger than an identical object placed in the annulus of large circles, when they reach out to pick up one of the objects, the inflight opening of their hand is tuned to

16

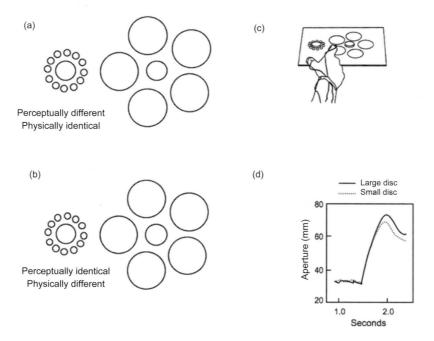

Fig. 1.6 The effect of a well-known size-contrast illusion on perception and action. (a) The traditional Ebbinghaus illusion in which the central circle in the annulus of larger circles is typically seen as smaller than the central circle in the annulus of smaller circles, even though both central circles are actually the same size. (b) The same display, except that the central circle in the annulus of larger circles has been made slightly larger. As a consequence, the two central circles now appear to be the same size. (c) A 3-D version of the Ebbinghaus illusion. Participants are instructed to pick up one of the two 3-D discs placed on either the display shown in (a) or the display shown in (b). (d) Two trials with the display shown in (b), in which the participant picked up the small disc on one trial and the large disc on another. Even though the two central discs were perceived as being the same size, the grip aperture in flight reflected the real, not the apparent, size of the discs. Adapted with permission from Aglioti et al (1995).

the real, not the perceived, size of that object. And, when the relative sizes of the objects are adjusted so that they appear to be identical in size, the grasping hand continues to be scaled to the real size of each object (see Fig. 1.6b and d). Their perceptual system might be fooled but their hand is not (for a review see Goodale and Westwood 2004).

Conclusions

Although the ventral and dorsal streams are functionally distinct, the two evolved together and play complementary roles in the control of behaviour. In some ways, the limitations of one system are the strengths of the other. Thus, although the ventral perception system delivers a rich and detailed representation of the world, the metrics of the world with respect to the organism are not well specified. In contrast, the dorsal action system delivers accurate metrical information in the required egocentric coordinates, but these computations are transient and evanescent. Both systems are required for purposeful behaviour – one system to select the goal object from the visual array, the other to carry out the required metrical computations for the goal-directed action. One of the most important questions yet to be addressed is how the two streams communicate with one another and integrate processing in the production of behaviour.

Summary

The upside-down back-to-front image of the world that is projected onto the retina (the lining at the back of the eye) is converted by the rods and cones into electrical signals that the brain can understand. These electrical signals are conveyed to nerve cells (ganglion cells) on the retinal surface, the fine single fibres of which coalesce in the optic nerve and eventually leave the eye.

The signals from the retina are carried along the optic nerve to a number of different parts of the brain, where the incoming information is processed in different ways for different purposes. Some brain structures, such as the hypothalamus, use information about daily changes in ambient light levels to synchronize the sleep-wake cycle. Other subcortical structures, such as the pretectum, use moment-to-moment information about the amount of light in the scene to control the size of the pupil, while other structures, such as the accessory optic system, use motion data from across the entire retina to help control balance. All of this happens quite unconsciously. Still other structures in the midbrain (the superior colliculus) help direct the gaze to objects that suddenly appear in the visual periphery. Other, more complex, visual information is conveyed to higher levels of the brain via the lateral geniculate bodies, which project in turn to the a region in the occipital lobes at the back of the brain known variously as striate cortex, area 17, primary visual cortex, or V1.

Beyond V1, visual information is conveyed to a bewildering number of 'extrastriate areas', but despite this complexity two principal streams can be identified: a ventral stream pathway projecting to the bottom of the brain (to the inferotemporal cortex) and a dorsal stream pathway projecting to the top of the brain at the back (to the posterior parietal cortex). Multiple sources of evidence indicate that the ventral and dorsal streams serve discrete but interconnected functions. The ventral stream serves conscious appreciation, recognition, and understanding of what is seen. The dorsal stream subconsciously assimilates incoming visual information in order to bring about moment-to-moment, immediate (on-line) visual guidance of skilled action and movement through the visual world.

Damage to the posterior parietal cortex affecting the dorsal stream leads to inaccurate visual guidance of movement (optic ataxia), despite the retention of accurate conscious visuospatial awareness and recognition of objects (afforded by the ventral stream). Such damage can also impair the ability to shift the gaze from one part of a scene to another and to attend to more than one part of a cluttered scene. Damage to the inferotemporal cortex and ventral stream pathway, on the other hand, profoundly impairs visual recognition, but visual guidance of movement remains intact, leading to the paradox that an affected person can employ subconscious dorsal stream vision to move accurately through a visual scene which is ostensibly invisible!

Perception and action need the visual signals conveyed to the brain to be processed differently. Vision for the perception of the world (and the recognition of objects within it), which is processed by the ventral stream, requires that incoming visual signals be compared to long-term detailed visual memories to facilitate understanding of what is being seen. In contrast, vision for the control of action, which is processed subconsciously by the dorsal stream, must reflect the real geometry of the outside world, which can change on a moment-to-moment basis. This means that when we are about to perform an action the dorsal stream must calculate precise and accurate 'egocentric coordinates', which relate the position of our eyes, hands, and body to the position of the goal objects in the world. Even though these two systems work in parallel, they must interact in the production of everyday behaviour. Thus, the selection of appropriate goal objects and the action to be performed depends on the perceptual machinery of the ventral stream, but the execution of a goal-directed action depends on dedicated on-line control systems in the dorsal stream.

2
CAUSES OF DAMAGE TO THE VISUAL BRAIN

2.1 COMMON AETIOLOGIES OF CEREBRAL VISUAL IMPAIRMENT

Janet Soul and Carey Matsuba

Introduction

Cerebral visual impairment (CVI) is the leading cause of visual impairment in children in developed countries. This finding probably results from increasing recognition and identification of CVI and from increased incidence of CVI related to advances in neonatal and paediatric care. CVI has many causes and presentations. The timing, location, and extent of pathology determine the severity (Jan and Groenveld 1993). This chapter describes the main causes of CVI, the neuroanatomical and neurological features, and the associated conditions.

Terminology

Children with CVI as a result of bilateral damage to the optic radiations and/or visual (calcarine) cortex rarely have total lack of sight (Whiting et al 1985, Roland et al 1986, Lambert et al 1987, Good et al 1994, Cioni et al 1996, Casteels et al 1997, Matsuba and Jan 2006) and the term 'cortical blindness' is inapplicable in most cases. Reduced visual function that tends to improve with time is most common (Roland et al 1986, Casteels et al 1997, Huo et al 1999, Matsuba and Jan 2006).

The term 'cortical' does not encompass visual impairment owing to abnormal subcortical white matter, as in, for example, periventricular leucomalacia. The term 'CVI' has been historically applied to the visual features of a range of disorders, including eye movement disorders, autism, intellectual disabilities, attention-deficit–hyperactivity disorders, visual–perceptual disorders, and others (Hoyt and Fredrick 1998, Hoyt and Good 2001). In this chapter, the term 'CVI' is limited to visual impairment owing to abnormal development of, or injury to, the optic radiations, striate cortex, and peristriate cortex regions. Elsewhere in this book, the definition also includes cognitive and perceptual visual impairment, primarily affecting the ventral and dorsal streams.

Common aetiologies

This section describes the common causes of CVI, some of which have unique clinical or anatomical features and may be associated with specific patterns of visual dysfunction.

ACQUIRED NEUROLOGICAL INJURY

Hypoxic–ischaemic brain injury

This can be divided into preterm and term hypoxic–ischaemic brain injury, because the type and location of perinatally acquired brain injury relates to gestational age at birth.

Hypoxic–ischaemic brain injury in the preterm newborn

Periventricular cerebral white matter damage, known pathologically as periventricular leuco-malacia (PVL) and radiologically as periventricular white matter injury, is the most common neurological lesion in the preterm infant. Preterm infants born at 24–34 weeks' gestation are typically affected. The pathogenesis is complex and is the subject of current research; theories relate to hypoxia–ischaemia affecting the watershed zones of the immature periventricular white matter, the vulnerability of the immature oligodendrocytes to excitotoxic and free radical injury, and a possible role of infection and inflammation. An additional neuronal–axonal component implies more diffuse cerebral injury than previously thought. The typical lesion of PVL involves at least the superior portion of the optic radiations (affecting the lower visual field) (Dutton and Jacobson 2001) and the subcortical white matter serving the visual and association cortices.

Damage to the optic radiations is particularly likely to result in CVI (Eken et al 1995, Cioni et al 1996, Hoyt 2003). Children with PVL in conjunction with CVI generally have a poorer neurodevelopmental or visual prognosis (Lambert et al 1987). The severity and extent of injury can be assessed by neuroimaging; magnetic resonance imaging (MRI) is superior to ultrasound for detecting non-cystic white matter injury. Thalamic injury has also been reported in association with CVI in the preterm infant, and affected children have poorer visual function (Ricci et al 2006). This subject is discussed in more detail in Chapter 2.2.

Retinopathy of prematurity is the most common ocular cause of visual impairment in the preterm child weighing <1.25kg, and PVL in children born at 24–28 weeks' gestation may be associated with retrograde trans-synaptic degeneration of the optic nerve, which occurs in some children with PVL. This can cause small optic nerves in those born between 24 and 28 weeks, and cupped but normal-sized optic discs in those born between 28 and 34 weeks, who usually develop better visual acuities. Nystagmus is commonly associated with PVL, and reduces visual acuity (Jacobson et al 1998a).

Hypoxic–ischaemic brain injury in the term newborn

Perinatal hypoxic–ischaemic brain injury is the most common cause of CVI (Flodmark et al 1990, Eken et al 1995, Huo et al 1999, Matsuba and Jan 2006). Brief but profound impairment of blood flow can cause mild, moderate, or severe injury, while less complete, prolonged interruption in blood flow to the brain has a more variable visual outcome (Mercuri et al 1997a,

1999). Brief, profound loss of blood flow, such as that which occurs with placental abruption or a prolapsed uterine cord, typically results in injury, predominantly affecting the subcortical nuclei of the basal ganglia, thalamus, and the nuclei of the brainstem. In mild cases, the visual pathways may be spared, but more severe and extensive injury may affect regions such as the cranial nerve nuclei of the oculomotor nerves (affecting control of eye movements) and the lateral geniculate bodies (affecting visual input to the visual cortex) (Roland et al 1986, Mercuri et al 1997b). More prolonged, partial hypoxic–ischaemic insult tends to affect the parasagittal watershed areas, including the striate cortex and underlying cerebral white matter. In these cases, the optic radiations and primary visual and association cortices may be affected to different degrees of severity and extent, causing mild to moderate CVI. Profound prolonged insult causes severe and diffuse injury to cerebral cortex, white matter, subcortical nuclei, and the brainstem. Affected children typically have problems with visual acuity, processing of visual information, and nystagmus and strabismus, although there can be some improvement in visual acuity during the first few years after birth (Lim et al 2005). Most affected children have significant cognitive and motor impairments which impede assessment and support of functional vision (Lim et al 2005).

FOCAL BRAIN LESIONS
Focal neurological lesions lead to different presentations of CVI. There is a variety of causes, but most are a result of vascular pathology such as arterial or venous stroke, or focal intra-cranial haemorrhage (deVeber et al 2000). Less commonly, lesions such as focal tumours (before or after resection) or focal cortical dysplasia may damage cerebral visual pathways or cortical regions. The nature and range of visual disability depend on the location and extent of the focal lesion. Although, initially, children may present with poor visual attention, the predominant finding is normal or near-normal visual acuity, but a visual field deficit, such as a homonymous hemianopia, is commonly identified. The visual field deficit affects the side contralateral to the cerebral lesion. A unilateral lesion behind the optic chiasm tends to cause homonymous visual field defects without loss of visual acuity. Acuity is impaired when lesions are extensive or bilateral.

Visual field deficits can be difficult to assess in the young non-verbal child, but can be inferred by observing the child's saccades to secondary targets. When the child's eyes move towards a target presented in a blind hemifield, they tend to overshoot the target. This is fol-lowed by a microsaccadic correction. When a hemifield deficit occurs early, better and more efficient scanning skills tend to develop (Meienberg et al 1981, Balliet et al 1985). Unlike in children with extensive brain injury, light-gazing tends not to occur in children with unilateral cerebral lesions (Jan et al 1990a).

Bilateral occipital infarction can, rarely, cause tunnel vision (Van Hof-van Duin and Mohn 1984). Children with central vision loss owing to a stroke tend to turn their eyes away from the field loss, which is called a gaze preference (Jan and Groenveld 1993). The fixation appears to fall eccentrically on the seeing side of the macula, which is thought to optimize use of the functional visual field.

TRAUMATIC BRAIN INJURY

Almost any type of traumatic brain injury (TBI) can lead to CVI. Child abuse from direct trauma or shaken baby syndrome is, unfortunately, a common cause, but accidental trauma is also seen in children of all ages. Contusion causes loss and injury of brain tissue. The haemorrhagic lesions often occur in a coup–contrecoup pattern, while shearing stresses cause diffuse axonal injury. Increased intracranial pressure may lead to hypoxic–ischaemic injury owing to impaired cerebral perfusion (Adelson et al 2003, Morris et al 2006). Brain displacement due to swelling or bleeding causes transtentorial herniation, resulting in unilateral or bilateral posterior cerebral artery occlusion and causing ischaemic injury of the visual brain. Thus, TBI can lead to focal, multifocal, and diffuse brain injury, resulting in a variety of types and severities of CVI.

The acute visual changes following TBI are easily observed. Interestingly, in many cases, visual recovery may be rapid (Good et al 2001). However, complete recovery is dependent upon the severity and location of injury. The presence of optic nerve atrophy, which may become evident only some time after injury, may indicate a poor visual prognosis.

Behaviourally, light-gazing tends to occur less frequently in acquired causes of CVI. When present, it often occurs shortly after the onset of brain injury (Jan et al 1990b).

Active research into the multiple mechanisms of injury, types of neuropathology, and potential treatments is currently under way (Povlishock and Jenkins 1995, Adelson et al 2003, Morris et al 2006).

INFECTIONS OF THE CENTRAL NERVOUS SYSTEM

A number of central nervous system (CNS) infections lead to damage to the visual pathways. In previous decades, meningitis was identified as a cause of CVI. Although many bacterial agents are associated with meningitis, *Haemophilus influenzae* was most commonly described (Ackroyd 1984, Newton et al 1985). The incidence of meningitis caused by *H. influenzae* has decreased significantly since the introduction of specific vaccination in the 1990s. In addition, congenital (in utero) infections with cytomegalovirus (CMV), toxoplasmosis, and rubella can all be associated with CVI (Paryani et al 1985), along with herpes encephalitis, which is, more commonly, a result of perinatal infection (El Azazi et al 1990).

These conditions may lead to optic nerve atrophy or nystagmus. Typically, congenital toxoplasmosis leads to atrophic lesions of the macula associated with cerebral calcification and cerebral destruction. Congenital rubella is associated with cataract retinopathy and CNS anomalies. Herpes encephalitis causes diffuse structural CNS disease.

Interestingly, the onset of vision loss in bacterial meningitis seems to be later in the course of the illness, typically after recovery from the acute infection. A number of possible reasons have been speculated, including thrombophlebitis or arterial occlusion (Acers and Cooper 1965, Tepperberg et al 1977, Margolis et al 1978, Ackroyd 1984). Bacterial meningitis is associated with a poorer prognosis than viral infection (Chen et al 1992, Matsuba and Jan 2006).

NEONATAL HYPOGLYCAEMIA

Neonatal hypoglycaemia is a metabolic disorder resulting from numerous aetiologies in pre-term and term newborns, and is usually transient and easily treated, and has no significant long-term consequences. When severe neonatal hypoglycaemia is present, usually resulting from hyperinsulinism or similar aetiologies, a classic pattern of bilateral posterior cerebral injury may occur, resulting in later cognitive and/or motor impairments and/or epilepsy (Barkovich et al 1998). This unique lesion may cause CVI because of the injury to much of the visual cortex, although some plasticity of this region in the newborn may result in better outcomes than expected by neuroimaging findings (Kiper et al 2002).

METABOLIC DISORDERS

There are numerous genetic metabolic diseases, such as mitochondrial, lysosomal, and peroxisomal disorders, which can result in CVI often in the context of progressive neurological deterioration. Often these inborn errors of metabolism have systemic manifestations, including health and developmental issues (Burton 1998). In the majority, there is abnormal cognitive development and/or degeneration (Whiting et al 1985). Seizures, motor impairment, and hearing loss are common. This section highlights conditions which may be associated with CVI, as either primary or secondary causes for vision loss.

Mitochondrial disorders frequently affect the eyes (particularly the retina), muscles, and brain, but other organ systems (e.g. pancreas, liver) can be involved. Although retinal and optic nerve conditions are most commonly associated with these diseases, CVI may be present when the cerebrum is involved. MELAS is the acronym for mitochondrial myopathy, encephalopathy, lactic acidosis, and stroke-like episodes, and is the mitochondrial disorder most classically resulting in CVI (Rosen et al 1990). Stroke-like events affecting the bilateral parieto-occipital areas are a cardinal feature of MELAS and affect both visual fields and visual acuity. There may also be profound cognitive and perceptual visual dysfunction. Other mito-chondrial disorders, such as Leigh syndrome, result in frequent severe and diffuse cerebral and brainstem involvement, and hence can cause a number of types and severities of CVI.

Lysosomal disorders have a wide clinical spectrum, from mild to severe. Typical features include coarse facies, neurological deterioration, hepatosplenomegaly, and skeletal dysplasia. They are typically diagnosed clinically and confirmed with studies of enzyme activity in either fibroblasts or leucocytes. Given the progressive and diffuse nature of the neuropathology in these disorders, cerebral vision centres may be affected. In addition, many of the lysosomal disorders have an ophthalmological component with deterioration of the retina or optic nerve or cornea, thereby contributing further to visual disturbances.

Sphingolipidoses are a group of conditions also associated with neurological deterioration, but there can be additional ocular disturbances. For example, in GM2 gangliosidosis a retinal cherry-red spot is a frequent finding. However, the typical presentation is of poor visual attention related to diffuse cerebral dysfunction.

Peroxisomal disorders are another group of disorders that may lead to CVI. These conditions are also neurodegenerative, presenting in early infancy or childhood with neurological features, which may lead to visual disturbances, either as a primary feature or secondary to seizures. Severe forms of peroxisomal disorders, such as Zellweger syndrome, present at birth with very severe neurological impairments because of diffuse brain dysgenesis. In some instances, the patient may have additional retinopathy or optic neuropathy which further hampers visual development (Matsuba and Jan 2006).

The visual presentation and course in metabolic diseases are variable. Although the CNS is involved in many of these conditions, retro-chiasmatic vision loss occurs relatively late, particularly for disorders with onset in childhood rather than infancy. In contrast, prominent visual impairment may present as an early manifestation in metabolic disorders such as adrenoleucodystrophy (Schaumburg et al 1975, Chen et al 1992). Specifically, X-linked adrenoleucodystrophy is a peroxisomal disorder that can present initially with relatively subtle visual findings, such as visual field deficits and reduced visual acuity. In some conditions, such as Krabbe disease, galactocerebrosidase deficiency, and GM1 gangliosidosis, there may be a rapid decline in both neurological and vision functions.

BRAIN MALFORMATIONS

A wide range of brain malformations, such as holoprosencephaly or lissencephaly, can cause CVI (Flodmark et al 1990, Barkovich et al 2005). A genetic abnormality, vascular event, or infection during embryogenesis may lead to various forms of focal and diffuse brain malformations, with resultant disruption of the normal development of the optic radiations and/ or occipital cortex (Cohen and Roessmann 1994). During the first months of embryogenesis, the neural plate forms. Anomalies in its formation may result in a cephalocele. A cephalocele refers to a defect in the skull and dura with extension of intracranial structures. There are several different types of structural defects. In Europeans and North Americans, the occipital encephalocele is most common. It can severely affect posterior visual pathways. In contrast, the ethmoid encephalocele, which is more common in south-east Asia, may not affect the posterior visual regions, although the optic nerves may be involved.

Significant brain malformations affecting the entire cerebrum (± brainstem and cerebellum) may occur at different points in embryogenesis. Holoprosencephaly is a major brain malformation that results from the failure of cleavage of the prosencephalon. There are a number of diffuse brain malformations resulting from disturbances of neuronal migration, such as lissencephaly, pachygyria, and polymicrogyria (Barkovich et al 2005). All of these severe and diffuse malformations of the brain typically result in profound visual impairment and developmental disabilities, and are often associated with severe epilepsy.

There are some brain malformations that are more focal, and thus produce less severe forms of CVI. Schizencephaly, a grey matter-lined cleft of the developing cortex, can affect visual regions of the brain. This cleft can be unilateral or bilateral. Porencephaly is a cystic area connected with the ventricle that results from focal brain injury such as that caused by in utero stroke or haemorrhage. Visual field deficits or other disturbances of cerebral visual processing may result. Notably, there is greater possibility of plasticity, or cortical reorganization, with focal brain lesions, and vision may be relatively preserved in some cases (Dumoulin et al 2007).

Most children with structural brain disease present early with poor visual attention, neurodevelopmental impairment, or seizures. Visual dysfunction can occur when the posterior pathways are directly affected. In many cases, there can be associated optic nerve anomalies. Optic nerve hypoplasia has been identified in the presence of several brain anomalies, such as schizencephaly (Brodsky and Glasier 1993). Alternatively, optic nerve atrophy may also be present. In some cases, the ocular structure may also be abnormal. Some children present with nystagmus. Like other causes of CVI, there are a number of comorbid conditions, including hydrocephalus, cognitive impairment, motor impairment, and hearing loss (Matsuba and Jan 2006). As expected, conditions in which there are significant anatomical anomalies, such as holoprosencephaly, have a poor prognosis. In addition, the presence of refractory seizures is usually associated with an unfavourable prognosis for vision (Wong 1991, Chen et al 1992, Matsuba and Jan 2006).

CHROMOSOMAL DISORDERS
There are several chromosomal disorders associated with CVI; some are associated with CVI because they result in the brain malformations described above. For example, trisomy 13 is associated with holoprosencephaly and trisomy 18 causes a number of structural brain anomalies, such as agenesis of the corpus callosum and cortical dysplasia.

Like many of the above conditions, many chromosomal disorders are associated with abnormalities of ocular structure and optic nerve. Microphthalmia and coloboma are associated with trisomy and unbalanced chromosomal translocations. Children with these disorders may have severe to profound developmental disability, although there is considerable variation. Additional multiple health issues are common to many chromosomal anomalies that affect several organ systems.

EPILEPSY
Severe, uncontrolled epilepsy may contribute to CVI and other neurodevelopmental impairments. For example, infantile spasms are a specific severe form of epilepsy often associated with CVI and other neurodevelopmental impairments. Infantile spasms and other severe epilepsy syndromes often result from diffuse brain malformations, metabolic disorders, other genetic/congenital disorders, and acquired disorders such as diffuse brain injury, congenital or postnatal infections, or trauma. When infantile spasms are present in association with structural brain disease, the prognosis for CVI is generally poor. When seizures are uncontrolled, visual attention and visual acuity are markedly impaired (Castano et al 2000). It is important to exclude the diagnosis of infantile spasms in infants with unexplained visual impairment.

Lena Jacobson and Olof Flodmark

The developing visual system is susceptible to hypoxic–ischaemic and infectious damage, both in utero and as a sequel to preterm birth. The pattern of cerebral injury found in newborn infants depends on the maturity of the brain at the time of insult. When brain damage occurs in the immature brain at 24–34 weeks' gestation, the lesions typically occur in the white matter. The four specific lesions of the myelinated tracts, or white matter, comprise germinal matrix/intraventricular haemorrhage (GMH/IVH), periventricular haemorrhagic infarction (PVHI), periventricular leucomalacia (PVL), and diffuse white matter injury (Volpe 1998, 2003). Each lesion may exist in isolation, but, more commonly, any single infant may present with multiple lesions. Abnormalities of the cortical grey matter and gyral development may accompany white matter abnormalities. The incidence of severe focal lesions in the brain's white matter has declined in the last decade, whereas diffuse white matter injury is currently emerging as the prevailing pathology occurring in preterm infants (Volpe 2003). When a child is examined with cerebral imaging in childhood, the periventricular white matter pathology may be visualized. However, at that time it may not be possible to know which acute pre- or perinatal pathologies were the cause. The end-stage lesion is described in this text as white matter damage of immaturity (WMDI).

The focal end-stage lesion may be a bilateral, fairly symmetrical loss of periventricular white matter as a result of acute PVL or an asymmetrical periventricular lesion because of PVHI. Diffuse white matter injury is believed to cause a reduction in myelinated axonal projections of neurons as the brain matures (Folkerth 2005). It is also possible that the lesion reflects a decrease in the amount of myelin per axon. Diffuse white matter injury is usually bilateral.

White matter damage of immaturity seen on magnetic resonance imaging (MRI) has been described in association with preterm birth and cerebral palsy (Bax et al 2006). Previous studies describing visual outcome in children with WMDI have focused on PVL, with the most significant impairment being found in children with cystic PVL, detected by ultrasound in the neonatal period (Scher et al 1989). However, milder forms of PVL detected by MRI are commonly associated with visual and eye movement abnormalities, and optic nerve anomalies such as optic disc cupping (Jacobson and Dutton 2000, Fazzi et al 2004).

Recent studies indicate that diffuse white matter injury and post-haemorrhagic ventricular dilatation at term correlate with reduced neurodevelopmental quotients when assessed at 18 months corrected age (Dyet et al 2006). Subtle white matter injury identified by fluid-attenuated inversion recovery (FLAIR) is associated with neurodevelopmental disorders at school age (Iwata et al 2007). The relationship between these less severe forms of diffuse white matter injury and visual outcome is still unknown, although Glass et al (2007) have found an impact on fixation and conjugate eye movements.

The following review is based on experiences of the visual, ocular, and ocular motility consequences of moderate to severe WMDI.

Cerebral imaging findings
See Chapter 3.

White matter damage of immaturity and cerebral palsy
Spastic diplegia is a well-known clinical sequel to WMDI, as this brain lesion interrupts the corticospinal tracts (Bax et al 2006). The resultant manifest functional deficit has caught the attention of paediatric neurologists. The majority of children with spastic diplegia have WMDI.

However, children with WMDI may escape cerebral palsy and exhibit only minor motor impairment despite radiologically obvious pathology and even extensive loss of brain tissue in some cases. Olsén et al (1997) showed that 9% of a population-based group of very low (<1750g) birthweight (BW) children had cerebral palsy, whereas 32% had WMDI demonstrated by MRI.

White matter damage of immaturity and intellectual disability
Bilateral extensive white matter reduction results in intellectual disability (intelligence quotient [IQ] <70) in association with cerebral palsy and visual impairment. Many children with spastic diplegia have reading and writing difficulties, even if they have fairly good verbal comprehension. Unilateral lesions may be compensated for with respect to cognitive function, and mild bilateral WMDI may not be associated with intellectual disability. Children with WMDI often have an uneven cognitive profile, with a better verbal IQ than performance IQ.

White matter damage and visual dysfunction
Several investigators have found an association between WMDI and cerebral visual impairment (Scher et al 1989, Jacobson et al 1996, Cioni et al 1997, Jacobson and Dutton 2000).

VISUAL ACUITY
In young children with severe bilateral WMDI due to cystic PVL, grating visual acuity is subnormal, although it may improve over time. These children may never be able to interpret optotypes. Children with mild or moderate WMDI may develop grating acuity within the normal range but still have subnormal but improving optotype acuity. Other children with WMDI may reach normal optotype acuity. Visual crowding is an inability to resolve linear optotypes, whereas single optotypes of the same size may be identified. This has been

described in children with cerebral visual impairment of various causes, and also in children with WMDI (Pike et al 1994, Jacobson et al 1996).

It is common that visual acuity assessed at near is lower than acuity assessed at distance, a finding that cannot be explained by problems with accommodation only, as spectacles correcting for near distance seldom normalize near acuity. Low near acuity and crowding may make reading of print difficult.

If grating acuity alone, or a single optotype acuity alone, is tested there is a risk of overestimating functional vision.

Visual Fields

When the pathology of PVL was first described in 1962, the authors noted damage to the optic radiation adjacent to the occipital horns and suggested that visual field defects would be a possible consequence of this damage (Banker and Larroche 1962). Posterior superior periventricular white matter is commonly affected by PVL. This tissue serves both the lower visual field and the dorsal stream. Dutton et al (2004) have reported lower visual field impairment demonstrated with confrontation techniques in children with cerebral visual impairment. In a multiple case study, the visual field outcome in teenagers with WMDI was studied with static computerized techniques and with kinetic Goldmann perimetry (Jacobson et al 2006). All had abnormal visual field function, more pronounced in the inferior than in the superior visual field. In participants with bilateral symmetrical WMDI the outcome varied between wide visual fields, but with very low sensitivity, and total lower altitudinal restriction, representing bilateral homonymous quadrant-dysopias (Figs 2.2.1 and 2.2.2). In children with unilateral or asymmetrical WMDI, homonymous visual field defects were found.

Many children with moderate to severe WMDI may never be able to cooperate to assess the visual fields with standardized perimetry, as it requires a developmental and attentional age of around 7 years or more. However, severe visual field restrictions may be identified with confrontation techniques.

Cognitive and Perceptual Visual Impairment

Many studies have described cognitive and perceptual visual impairment associated with WMDI (Jacobson et al 1996, Dutton 2003, Pavlova et al 2003, 2007, Stiers and Vandenbusshe 2004). Children with WMDI, even those with relatively well-developed optotype acuity, often have dorsal stream dysfunction with profound difficulties in moving through three-dimensional spaces, with difficulties judging depth. They have problems finding things on a patterned carpet or seeing things in the distance that are pointed out. Difficulties handling crowding of text are common. It may be difficult to identify someone they know in a crowd. Many children with WMDI also demonstrate ventral stream dysfunction. They may be unable to recognize people they know, when met out of context, or they may even have problems recognizing family members by only their appearance. Children with WMDI commonly have problems finding their way around. These cognitive visual problems seem to be more pronounced in children with lesions located in the right hemisphere or in both hemispheres than in children with lesions located in the left hemisphere alone. It is important to recognize that

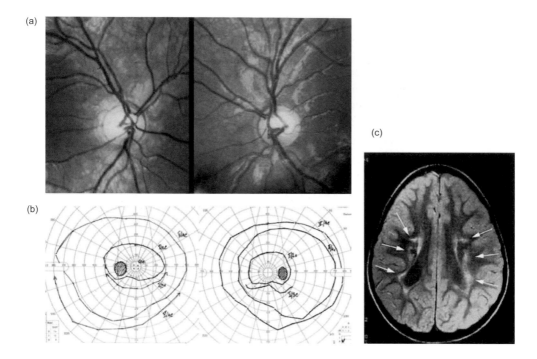

Fig. 2.2.1 Female born at gestational age 32 weeks with normal gross motor function and early-onset esotropia and latent nystagmus. At the age of 12 years she had linear optotype acuity 6/9 right eye (RE) and 6/15 left eye (LE) and single optotype acuity 6/5 RE and 6/6 LE. She has an uneven intellectual profile with very good verbal IQ but subnormal performance IQ. (a) Her optic discs have large cups. (b) Goldmann perimetry demonstrates relative altitudinal lower defects. (c) MRI using fluid-attenuated inversion recovery (FLAIR) shows abnormal signal in the periventricular white matter (white arrows). Furthermore, there is loss of white matter with compensatory symmetrical widening of the posterior horns of the lateral ventricles.

problems in daily life for a child with visual dysfunction caused by WMDI are not primarily related to visual acuity, but are dominated by cognitive visual deficiencies.

Many children have a good verbal memory, but some have problems maintaining attention. Children who have an uneven intellectual profile, with higher scores on the verbal and logical tests and a good memory, develop a battery of compensating strategies. Recognition with the help of colours is one widely used strategy. Others include recognizing people by listening to the voice or the sound of footsteps, finding things by memorizing their location and identifying objects by touch or smell – strategies which are also used by totally blind children. Finding their way around may be enhanced by memorizing sequences of landmarks. In the school setting, such children have to constantly employ strategies to handle learning situations, and this can be exhausting.

In children born extremely preterm, with diffuse white matter abnormality but no focal damage, visual acuity, visual fields, and stereo acuity may reach normal levels in those

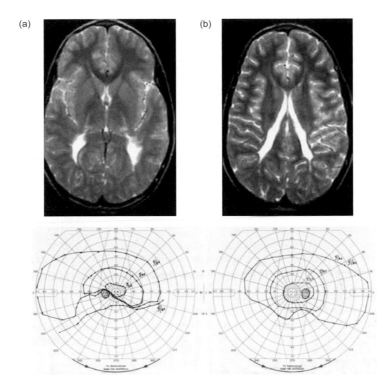

Fig. 2.2.2 Male born at gestational age 33 weeks, with a moderate spastic diplegia and early-onset eso-tropia and latent nystagmus. At 14 years of age the head was small. He had linear optotype acuity 6/12 right eye (RE) and 6/18 left eye (LE) and binocular single optotype acuity 6/6. He had normal verbal IQ and subnormal performance IQ. He has bilateral homonymous inferior quadrant dysopias, seen as an altitudinal lower visual field defect. MRI with axial T2-weighted images shows in (a), in an axial image through the inferior portions of the trigone of the lateral ventricles, abnormal signal in thalami corresponding to the location of the geniculate bodies. There is also increased signal in the posterior limbs of the internal capsule, corresponding well to the moderate spastic diplegia. The axial slice in (b) is at a level of the upper parts of both lateral ventricles. Note the almost total absence of periventricular white matter, yet normal ventricular size – a finding that has to be interpreted in the light of the small head.

individuals who escape severe retinopathy of prematurity. However, cognitive visual dysfunction frequently restricts daily life in this group of new survivors.

Ocular findings

REFRACTION AND ACCOMMODATION
In children born preterm, myopia is a common refractive error, and an association with retinopathy of prematurity (ROP) has been suggested. In addition, children with WMDI who have escaped severe ROP frequently have refractive errors, often hypermetropia and astigmatism.

The literature is sparse in describing refraction and accommodation correlated to specified lesions of the cerebral visual system. Impaired accommodation has, however, been found in a majority of a population-based group of children with cerebral palsy (McClelland et al 2006). This impairment is of multifactorial origin, and may be worsened by different medications (with anticholinergic side-effects) given to children with cerebral palsy and with epilepsy. Visual tasks in daily life, including schoolwork, such as using communication boards or computers, may be affected by inaccurate accommodation. Saunders et al (2008) demonstrated that poor near pupil response indicates accommodation impairment. Therefore, assessment of accommodative function should be performed not only in children with cerebral palsy, but also in children with cerebral visual impairment who have escaped cerebral palsy.

OPTIC DISC CHARACTERISTICS

Early WMDI, occurring before gestational week 28, may be associated with small optic discs. In WMDI, optic nerve hypoplasia probably results from trans-synaptic degeneration of optic nerve axons caused by the primary bilateral lesion in the optic radiation. Normal-sized optic discs with large cupping and a reduced neuroretinal rim area have been described as the consequence of later lesions, occurring after 28 weeks, when the supportive structures of the optic nerve have become established and have not adapted to the smaller number of nerve fibres (Jacobson et al 2003) (Fig. 2.2.1). Thus, there is a spectrum of optic disc appearances in children with WMDI, ranging from a small disc to a normal-sized disc with a large cup, whereas the optic disc appearance is normal in children with lesions after 33–34 gestational weeks.

In adults, the findings of bilateral lower visual field defects and extensive cupping of the optic discs in association with WMDI is an important differential diagnosis for glaucoma (Brodsky 2001).

NYSTAGMUS, STRABISMUS AND EYE MOTILITY

Nystagmus of different waveforms and latencies, which may be intermittent or manifest, has been described in children with WMDI (Jacobson et al 1998b, Salati et al 2002). Children with extensive WMDI and cerebral palsy may present with an oculomotor apraxia with complete disruption of ocular motor organization, including absence of fixation (and no nystagmus).

Defective smooth pursuit movements and inability to perform visually guided saccadic movements have been documented in children with WMDI (Jacobson et al 1998b, Salati et al 2002). The cause of these eye motility disorders remains unknown, but it is known that the dorsal stream pathway from occipital cortex to the parietal and frontal cortices contributes to these functions and could be disrupted by WMDI. This could be associated with impaired visual search.

Strabismus, with early-onset esotropia or exotropia, is a common finding in children with WMDI (Figs 2.2.1, 2.2.2, and 2.2.3). Although normal stereopsis is rare in children with WMDI, orthophoria with intact stereopsis has been described.

These eye motility disorders may include an inability to perform normal eye movements during reading, although some children may compensate with adaptive head movements.

Clinical implications

IDENTIFICATION OF CHILDREN WITH WHITE MATTER DAMAGE OF IMMATURITY
Children with severe WMDI usually present with abnormal fixation, delayed and limited visual maturation, and strabismus, frequently in combination with spastic diplegia and intellectual disability. In these cases, the diagnosis has often already been confirmed by ultrasound in the neonatal period, or later with computed tomography (CT) or MRI. These children with severe functional deficits are often already enrolled in neurological training programmes.

However, the diagnosis may be a challenge in milder forms of WMDI, especially if the child has escaped cerebral palsy and has normal verbal development. In these cases, the paediatric ophthalmologist may be the only physician who regularly sees the child. Such children may have presented with early-onset strabismus with latent or manifest nystagmus and with slightly subnormal acuity. At school, they have good linguistic but poor visuospatial skills. A history of preterm birth in association with strabismus should make the examiner aware of the potential for a pre-existent posterior visual pathway lesion (Figs 2.2.1 and 2.2.3). Restricted visual fields, crowding also in the better eye, and abnormal disc appearances are clues to the correct diagnosis.

A structured interview concerning visual behaviour, or a typically uneven intellectual profile, can be a useful tool to identify children with perceptual and cognitive visual impairment (Houliston et al 1999).

CONFIRMATION OF THE DIAGNOSIS
A positive ultrasound in the neonatal period can confirm the diagnosis of WMDI. If the child has already undergone neuroimaging initially reported as normal, the diagnosis may be established if the images are re-examined with special attention to the periventricular white matter. If no previous neuroimaging examinations have been performed, MRI is the method of choice for confirming the diagnosis of WMDI. Neither normal ultrasound in the neonatal period nor a normal CT performed later excludes the presence of mild WMDI.

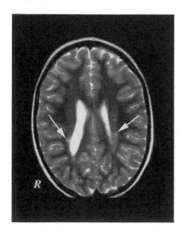

Fig. 2.2.3 Female born at gestational age 32 weeks with normal gross motor function and early-onset esotropia. At 5 years of age she had linear visual acuity 6/12 right eye and 6/15 left eye. She had normal intellectual level and was very talkative but did not like to draw. This T2-weighted magnetic resonance image shows a bright signal, representing gliosis along the posterior–superior margin of both lateral ventricles (arrows).

Occlusion Therapy and Surgery for Strabismus Associated with White Matter Damage of Immaturity

Occlusion therapy may improve visual acuity in the strabismic eye in a child with WMDI. Strabismic amblyopia superimposed on the structural abnormality seen in the optic radiations may allow such improvement. Close, periodic monitoring of visual acuity should be carried out and patching terminated if no improvement is detected. Patching should be avoided in children with low acuity in both eyes.

Spontaneous conversion from eso- to exotropia is sometimes seen in children with WMDI. In selected cases, the optimal timing of strabismus surgery may therefore be later than for early-onset esotropia as a result of other causes.

Susann Andersson

Hydrocephalus is a condition in which a disturbance of cerebrospinal fluid (CSF) circulation results in increased CSF volume, ventricular dilatation, and increased intracranial pressure. A large proportion of children with hydrocephalus have resultant visual dysfunction.

Pathogenesis and clinical features

Hydrocephalus may be of prenatal, perinatal, or postnatal origin. The most common prenatal aetiologies are malformations of the central nervous system (CNS), spina bifida, and genetic factors. Intraventricular haemorrhage and infection are the most frequent causes in the perinatal period, as are tumours, trauma, and infection during the postnatal period.

During recent decades the number of children with spina bifida (myelomeningocele) has decreased, which may be explained by improved maternal nutrition and supplements of folic acid in food, as well as the increased use of ultrasonography in early pregnancy, resulting in abortion of affected fetuses. An increasingly frequent cause of hydrocephalus is intraventricular haemorrhage in children born very preterm (Persson et al 2005) because of enhanced survival of these children.

Modern understanding of CSF dynamics includes a traditional bulk flow of CSF from the choroid plexus in the ventricles through the aqueduct of Sylvius and out through the outlets of the fourth ventricle. However, the reabsorption of the fluid is not through the Pacchionian granulations but rather directly into the capillaries of the brain and spinal cord. Obstructive hydrocephalus is caused by a block to flow of CSF somewhere in the ventricular system, for example the stenosis of the aqueduct, whereas communicating hydrocephalus is caused by decreased intracranial compliance (Greitz 2004).

Hence, 'hydrocephalus' is a generic term that needs to be defined in each case, in terms of the type (communicating or obstructive) and the cause. Two issues are important: ventriculomegaly, which is a common consequence of hydrocephalus of both types, and intracranial pressure, which may be raised to a greater or lesser degree in children with hydrocephalus. Ventriculomegaly is often more pronounced in the posterior horns of the lateral ventricles (colpocephaly) and, if marked, is thought to have a local adverse effect on the ventricular wall and the immediate periventricular white matter, whereas raised intracranial pressure may cause herniation of brain tissue with a secondary risk of arterial obstruction, particularly of the posterior cerebral arteries, and cerebral infarction.

The clinical symptoms of hydrocephalus are a consequence of raised intracranial pressure, decreased intracranial compliance and the expansion of intracranial CSF-filled spaces, particularly the ventricular system.

Raised intracranial pressure in communicating hydrocephalus is a consequence of decreased intracranial compliance compressing the capacitance vessels and increasing the vascular resistance. The clinical expression of this condition depends on the age of the child. In small infants, a rapidly increasing head size is the most important clinical marker of hydrocephalus. The cranial sutures widen, allowing for an increased volume of the intracranial cavity, and thus accommodating the dilating ventricular system. Expansion of the soft skull allows the absolute value of the intracranial pressure to be only slightly elevated or just at the upper limit of normal. In preterm birth infants, the extracerebral CSF-containing spaces are wide and become occupied by brain tissue first, before an increase in head circumference becomes obvious. Hence, ventriculomegaly, even when a result of hydrocephalus, can initially be clinically silent.

The classical symptoms of raised intracranial pressure include headaches, nausea and vomiting, and visual disturbances, and require a rigid skull for their expression. These symptoms are therefore present in older children and adults, in whom the sutures do not readily widen or split when the intracranial pressure increases. Children up to the age of 4–6 years can still accommodate a gradual increase in intracranial pressure by separation of sutures. Other frequently described findings are a prominent forehead and the 'sun-setting' phenomenon of the eyes, with impaired upgaze.

INCIDENCE

The incidence of hydrocephalus varies in different parts of the world. For example, in Western parts of the world the incidence is 0.7 per 1000 live births, compared with 1.6 per 1000 live births in Saudi Arabia (Murshid et al 2000, Persson et al 2005).

TREATMENT

The primary aim of the treatment in acute obstructive hydrocephalus is to decrease the size of the ventricles and restore a normal intraventricular pressure. Inserting a CSF shunt diverts the excess volume of CSF trapped within the ventricles, restoring anatomy and normalizing CSF pressure. The most commonly employed strategy, irrespective of aetiology, is to shunt the flow of CSF from a lateral ventricle to the peritoneal cavity. There are many different kinds of shunt systems, but they all have the same principal parts. The intraventricular tubing is usually located in one of the two lateral ventricles. The ventricular catheter exits the cranial cavity through a burr hole and is then connected to a shunt mechanism. This mechanism has two main functions – it provides resistance with counterpressure to CSF flow and it prevents back-flow in the shunt system. An anti-siphon device may sometimes be added to the shunt. Treatment by shunting has reduced the mortality rate from 50% to 5–10% (Hadenius et al 1962, Fernell et al 1986, Persson et al 2005). Another treatment that has been more commonly used during the last 10–15 years is ventriculostomy, where a stoma is made in the lower end of the third ventricle, leading the CSF to the subarachnoid spaces, where it can be reabsorbed. Both procedures have advantages as well as disadvantages, and the aetiology and age of the patient determine the course of treatment. Delayed intervention may result in profound damage to the brain, including loss of vision.

Shunt complications are common. Blockage and infection are the most common. In a child who remains dependent upon the shunt to normalize intracranial pressure, shunt failure is manifested by headache, nausea, and vomiting as a result of raised intracranial pressure, which requires urgent surgical intervention.

Shunt failure has a number of causes. Outgrowth of the shunt system, blockage, and infections are the most common. One of the most severe complications of shunt failure is transtentorial herniation. The posterior cerebral arteries come around the brainstem and are in the tentorial slit found over the edge of the tentorium. The herniating cerebrum will move inferiorly with a forceful downward movement into the tentorial slit and will push the brainstem and its associated vessels downwards. Pinching and occlusion of the posterior cerebral arteries causes bilateral infarction of the territories supplied by these arteries, most importantly the visual cortex, and may lead to cortical blindness.

Hydrocephalus and neurological outcome
Children with hydrocephalus constitute a heterogeneous group. Some manifest subtle neurological and/or visual symptoms, while others have severe disability. Motor impairment is common and is found in about 60% of cases (Hoppe-Hirsch et al 1998, Heinsbergen et al 2002), whereas epilepsy affects about 30% (Fernell et al 1988a,b, Persson et al 2005, 2007). The aetiology, gestational age, and abnormalities in the brain parenchyma are important in relation to the severity of the motor disability and the occurrence of epilepsy. Children born preterm with a perinatal cerebral haemorrhage, as a cause of the hydrocephalus, are most severely affected (Fernell et al 1988a,b). In children with spina bifida, the motor function is dependent on the extent of the spinal pathology; about one-half of affected children learn to walk by themselves, some with aid (Bowman et al 2001).

Visual Outcome and Ocular Abnormality
Refractive error, especially hypermetropia and astigmatism, is more common in children with hydrocephalus than in the general population (Biglan 1990, Andersson et al 2006).

Raised intracranial pressure leads to raised pressure within the optic nerve sheath with subsequent atrophy. Enlargement of the optic nerve sheath is an early feature of acutely raised intracranial pressure in hydrocephalus and can be detected by ultrasound examination. This can provide a rapid and efficient means of detecting acutely raised intracranial pressure (Newman et al 2002). The optic chiasm is closely related to the anterior wall of the third ventricle and can be damaged by distension of the third ventricle. In the acute stage, treatment by shunting has been shown to improve visual acuity in a number of cases (Gaston 1985, Connolly et al 1991, Aoki et al 1997). The majority of children with hydrocephalus have some visual deficits despite treatment. Delayed visual maturation is common in affected infants. The optic radiations are situated close to the lateral ventricles and may be damaged by ventricular dilatation. The dorsal stream and ventral stream pathways may be damaged in many cases, with one-half of affected children being found to have evidence of perceptual and cognitive visual dysfunction by structured history-taking. Children whose hydrocephalus is associated with spina bifida are less likely to be affected in this way (Houliston et al 1999, Andersson et al 2006).

Some of the children who have been shunted for their hydrocephalus may develop acutely raised intracranial pressure because of a blocked shunt. The associated brain swelling can result in the posterior cerebral arteries being pressed against the tentorium cerebelli, resulting in loss of vision because of ischaemia. Reversal can occur with prompt treatment, but loss of vision may otherwise be permanent. Untreated chronic papilloedema can also result in loss of vision due to optic nerve damage. In the past, before shunting procedures were carried out, stretching of the optic nerves was the attributed cause of loss of vision (Harcourt and Jay 1968).

VISUAL ACUITY
Most children with treated hydrocephalus have a good visual acuity. About one-third have mildly reduced vision, while 10–15% are significantly visually impaired with a visual acuity of <0.3 (Heinsbergen et al 2002, Andersson et al 2006). Visual crowding is common. The visual acuity measured with single symbols may be significantly better than that measured with a linear letter chart, which may be indicative of visual crowding on account of dorsal stream dysfunction.

OCULAR MOTILITY
Strabismus occurs in between 40% and 70% of children with hydrocephalus, and there is a wide variety of patterns of eye movement disturbance (Mankinen-Heikkinen et al 1987, Biglan 1990, Heinsbergen et al 2002, Aring et al 2007). Nystagmus is common and may lead to a head posture to optimize vision by placing the eyes in the position in which there is least movement (the null position) (Mankinen-Heikkinen et al 1987, Aring et al 2007). Acute blockage of a shunt can give rise to impaired upgaze and poor convergence of the eyes, associated with a tendency of the eyes to converge on attempted upgaze, which may persist.

VISUAL FIELDS
Any part of the visual field may be affected in children with hydrocephalus. Between 5% and 17% of affected children have been reported to have visual field defects (Rabinowitz 1974, Andersson et al 2006). However, visual field examination is difficult to carry out in children with disabilities, and the frequency of visual defects is likely to be underestimated. Typical visual field defects include homonymous hemianopia (in cases where the optic radiation on one side has been significantly disrupted) and lower visual field impairment in those cases in which the superior posterior periventricular white matter has been damaged.

Detailed structured clinical history-taking of parents of children with hydrocephalus has shown that more than half have perceptual and cognitive visual difficulties. These are more frequently found in children with low visual acuities but have also been identified in about one-third of children with normal visual acuities. Children with additional diagnoses such as cerebral palsy and epilepsy have high frequencies of cognitive and perceptual visual dysfunction with increasing problems as the severity of the overall condition increases. The visual difficulties described include those relating to dorsal stream dysfunction (problems with visual crowding and impaired visual guidance of movement) and problems with ventral stream dysfunction (problems with recognition and orientation). Difficulties with seeing moving targets have also been described by parents (Houliston et al 1999, Andersson et al 2006).

The relationship between brain function and behaviour is traditionally tested by neuropsychologists with investigations such as the WISC-III (Wechsler Intelligence Scale for Children, constructed for ages 6–16 years), and the WPPSI-R (Wechsler Pre-school and Primary Scale of Intelligence, for ages 3–7 years). These investigations, which measure a range of cognitive abilities, may show an uneven pattern, with low scores in areas related to vision.

Children with hydrocephalus constitute a heterogeneous group with a wide range of neurological visual and perceptual/cognitive dysfunction. The majority of these children have ocular and/or visual functional problems including strabismus, ocular motility dysfunction, refractive error, and difficulties interpreting visual information. These problems are most common among children with additional problems such as cerebral palsy and epilepsy. However, children without additional neurological or cognitive diagnoses, and with good visual acuities, may manifest evidence of visual–perceptual dysfunction.

Summary

The two halves of the brain, or cerebral hemispheres, have an outer mantle of grey matter (or cortex), mainly made up of cell bodies, and inner white matter, containing myriad interconnecting nerve fibres. The white matter surrounds two inner water spaces in the brain called lateral ventricles.

A large proportion of the brain is devoted to vision. Cerebral visual impairment (CVI) is the most common cause of low vision in childhood in developed countries, but it is rarely completely blinding. Additional cerebral palsy and intellectual disability are common. Damage to one side of the brain causes impaired vision on the opposite side (homonymous hemianopia). Damage to both sides also reduces visual acuity. Visual perceptual disorders are common.

The most frequent cause of cerebral damage is lack of oxygen or blood supply to the developing visual brain shortly before or around the time of birth (hypoxic ischaemic encephalopathy). Before birth, this tends to damage the developing white matter surrounding the lateral ventricles (white matter damage of immaturity [WMDI]), which can cause nystagmus, impair visual acuities and visual fields (most commonly inferiorly), and lead to perceptual visual problems, in any combination or degree. In the term infant, the severity and nature of the resultant CVI depends on the location, degree, and extent of brain injury and whether eye movements are impaired.

Lack of blood and oxygen delivery to the brain during or after birth tends to cause generalized or multiple foci of brain damage, which range considerably in severity. The visual system is commonly damaged, and, when there is additional damage to the deeper structures of the brain, vision is more likely to be profoundly impaired. Hydrocephalus results from expansion of the water spaces in the brain due to blockage of flow of cerebrospinal fluid. This damages white matter and leads to similar visual problems to WMDI. Recurrence of hydrocephalus due to a blocked shunt can distort the brain and block the blood vessels to the back of the brain on one or both of the sides, with loss of vision.

If a distinct part of the visual brain has focal damage, lack of vision in one part of the visual field with the same distribution in both eyes (homonymous visual field impairment) tends to result. Causes include impaired blood flow, or haemorrhage causing an early onset stroke, and focal brain malformations.

Head injury, which may be accidental or non-accidental, infection with a range of infective agents, and low blood sugar shortly after birth are additional acquired causes.

There are a number of metabolic disorders in which there is progressive failure of brain function. As a large proportion of the brain is devoted to vision, and the optic nerves are ostensibly an extension of the brain, progressive visual impairment owing to combined optic nerve and brain dysfunction is a common consequence of these rare conditions.

The overall structure of the brain can also be malformed, and this may be a result of chromosomal disorders, in which impairment of vision is common. There can also be associated maldevelopment of the optic nerves, such as the small nerves found in optic nerve hypoplasia.

Epilepsy of early onset (as infantile spasms) or later onset may occur in isolation, or may accompany any of the disorders described in this summary. When seizures are uncontrolled, visual attention and visual acuity can be markedly impaired, and effective treatment can be accompanied by gradual improvement in visual function.

3
CLINICAL FEATURES AND DIAGNOSTIC IMAGING OF DAMAGE TO THE VISUAL BRAIN

3.1 CLINICAL MANIFESTATIONS OF CEREBRAL VISUAL IMPAIRMENT

Carey Matsuba and Janet Soul

Introduction

The visual function of children with cerebral visual impairment (CVI; as defined in the introduction to Chapter 2), who present early in the first year of life, is often described as being poor to non-existent, although some are able to respond to targets from greater than 10 feet (3.05 metres) away (Jan et al 1987). As visual function matures in the first months after birth, it becomes easier for caregivers to identify their child's visual responses. In many cases, the development of visual function follows a trajectory. Initially, children with severe CVI may tend to gaze at light. This is followed by the ability to identify simple, familiar, colourful toys. Some children may look at their caregiver's face, while others may not. Children typically tend to respond to near objects before responding to more distant ones.

With time, almost all children gain some vision (Baker-Nobles and Rutherford 1995). The extent of impairment of visual acuity and visual fields is often correlated with the extent of damage to the central nervous system (CNS). There are a number of visual features commonly considered in the context of CVI. In addition to visual acuity and visual field deficits, many children with CVI have additional visual dysfunction, including abnormalities of contrast sensitivity, impairment in visual processing, and disorders of ocular motility.

VISUAL FUNCTION
Physiologically, vision is divided into five constructs: light, contrast, colour, movement, and stereopsis. Traditionally, impairments of both visual acuity and visual fields are used to define visual impairment.

VISUAL ACUITY
Impairment in visual acuity compared with age-matched healthy control individuals is the standard measure defining visual impairment. Typically, reduction in visual acuity is the result

of bilateral damage to the occipital cortex or optic radiations ranging from no light perception to near normal. Where possible, standardized matching visual acuity is measured. Typically, the child with CVI will have the ability to consistently and accurately match shapes at developmental age 3 years. But acuity testing is challenging in children with CVI as behaviour, ability, changes in the environment, variable visual attention, and eye movement disorders complicate the assessment.

Measurement of visual acuity

Visual acuity is a quantitative measure of the ability to identify black symbols on a white background at a standardized distance as the size of the symbols is varied. It is the most common clinical measurement of visual function. Where possible, a standardized matching visual acuity provides the most accurate measure of visual acuity. There is a variety of different types of visual acuity tests.

In young non-verbal children, visual acuity is difficult to measure behaviourally. In addition, acuity testing can be challenging in children with CVI as changes in the environment, variability in visual attention, and extraneous movements can complicate the assessment. In this population, visual acuity can be measured behaviourally using forced-choice preferential looking (FCPL) tests. Although the visual function using FCPL tests may not reflect the degree of neurological insult, it probably demonstrates dysfunction of pathways subserving saccadic (fast) eye movements (Hoyt et al 1982). Nonetheless, it can provide a measure of visual function, which can be used to understand the visual adaptations needed for a child. When testing visual acuity, assessors get an opportunity to observe additional visual functions, such as visual attention, gaze palsies, and visual field deficits.

An alternative means to assess visual function is through the visual evoked potential (VEP). The simplest form, the flash VEP, may not accurately assess higher order visual functions or visual acuity. However, it has been shown that a normal response accords a better prognosis (Clarke et al 1997). The VEP provides information about geniculocalcarine function and occipital cortical responses to photic stimuli. Serial pattern VEPs are probably more useful than flash VEPs to follow visual function, but the test has some limitations (Taylor and McCulloch 1991). Children require enough visual attention and eye stability to fixate on the pattern. Thus, responses can be variable because of non-visual causes.

There are other non-specific means of assessing visual function. The electroencephalogram (EEG) is one such measure. Although it does not measure visual acuity, an EEG is useful in the diagnosis of CVI. When used in combination with a VEP, the presence of normal alpha rhythm superimposed on a normal background in an EEG essentially rules out CVI in children (Jan and Wong 1988).

VISUAL FIELD

Visual field deficits are a frequent component of CVI. The visual field is the spatial array of visual sensations available for observation. As with visual acuity, standard visual field measurements are difficult to make in children with CVI. Visual field tests require children to respond to stimuli within a short time-frame. Thus, comorbid conditions such as motor, communication, or cognitive impairments may hamper standard testing. To identify a visual field deficit, functional testing can be used, such as kinetic perimetry (van Hof-van Duin and Mohn 1984). Observation of children's responses to environmental objects may yield useful information about their visual impairments.

Large field deficits, such as a homonymous hemianopia, are easily identified. With striate cortex involvement, the visual field deficit is readily apparent as a complete inability to identify visual information on the contralateral side. However, subtle visual field deficits can be difficult to identify, for example inferior or relative visual field deficits. Children with severe neurological injury to the visual cortex may present with severe tunnel vision (Jan and Groenveld 1993).

OTHER VISUAL FUNCTION CONSIDERATIONS

Contrast sensitivity is the ability to discern between luminosities of different levels in a static image. Often, children with CVI respond better to high-contrast (black and white) patterns. However, their visual acuity may be best determined under low luminance conditions (Good et al 2001). There are several different contrast acuity charts to estimate contrast acuity; however, they all rely on ambient lighting. In practice, varying the environmental lighting conditions can be used to identify the light level, which accords the better responses.

Colour vision is an important visual function served by a number of brain areas (Gegenfurtner and Kiper 2003). For most children, colour vision, which is a quality constructed by the visual brain and not a property of objects as such, leads to the better discrimination of surfaces and edges through visual processing. Children with CVI appear to use this feature, and often demonstrate colour preferences even when there is limited functional visual ability to identify shape and form. Some children appear to engage better for some colours than others, with reds and yellows being a common preference (Groenveld et al 1990).

Higher order (cognitive) visual functioning may also be impaired in children with CVI (Cioni et al 1997). Visual disturbances include agnosias, akinetopsia (the inability to perceive motion), simultanagnosia (the inability to focus on more than one item), and optic ataxia (impaired visual guidance of movement [see Chapter 1]).

Many children with CVI have impairment of ocular motility, such as dyskinetic eye movements, leading to interference with visual function. Moreover, optokinetic nystagmus may be absent in CVI (Lambert et al 1987).

VISUAL BEHAVIOURS

Children with CVI have a unique set of behavioural characteristics. Some may initially present with roving eye movements. As their visual function improves, their visual attention and curiosity also progresses, as if vision 'starts to make sense'. This improvement may be linked to better organization of visual information, which takes time to develop in the context of static occipital cortical injury. In contrast to children with ocular or optic nerve causes of visual impairment, most children with CVI do not appear to be blind. However, when engaged in visual activities, many may not show typical visual social behaviours (Jan and Groenveld 1993). They often have poor visual attention and a lack of visual curiosity (Jan et al 1987) and may manifest an expressionless response to some visual stimuli.

43

Even with improvement in visual interests, children with CVI may show variability in visual function, even during the course of the day. Spontaneous visual activity often occurs in short duration. Visual function may diminish depending on environmental and health conditions, such as a noisy room or an intercurrent illness. Children often respond better in familiar environments or when cued to focus on specific targets. Sometimes visual learning in its own right can be fatiguing. Although children may be able to visualize distant objects, they may have difficulty identifying them. In general, visual interests and activities are better for nearer objects, even for children who lack significant refractive errors. This mechanism appears to reduce the crowding effect. So, when several toys are presented, children may be able to focus on only one. Those with limited visual interests may choose not to use their vision, preferring to close their eyes to focus on listening. Others regularly choose to explore visual objects through touch.

When reaching for objects, some children with CVI may use their vision to recognize objects; however, when they attempt to reach for them they may look away. This may give the appearance of using their peripheral vision for reaching – 'retinal reach'. This phenomenon is seen in as many as one-third of children with CVI (Lambert et al 1987, Good et al 1994). Other children with CVI appear to look past objects (Porro et al 1998a). In certain instances, children appear to avoid looking at objects, either by turning their head away or occasionally by demonstrating withdrawal from the object (Porro et al 1998a).

Those children with more severe CVI will overlook their caregivers or toys to look instead towards light sources – light gazing. Light gazing is more common with congenital causes of CVI. It can be a compulsive behaviour which becomes evident in infancy (Jan et al 1990a). Interestingly, concentrated light sources are preferred over diffuse lighting, yet there may also be concomitant photophobia. As vision improves, light gazing may evolve into more meaningful visual behaviours.

Many children with CVI, regardless of aetiology, have photophobia. Typically, children with CVI present with narrowing of their eyelids, or bowing of their heads in bright lighting. Some appear more comfortable in low lighting conditions or prefer a visor or a hat. The range of photophobia varies. In more severe cases, children may close their eyes, while others may cry (Jan et al 1993). Fortunately, in many cases photophobia tends to improve with age and improving visual acuity. Although it may be a common feature in a number of acute neuro-logical disorders such as meningitis or subarachnoid haemorrhage, it rarely persists after the acute illness. Some animal studies suggest that when cortical areas 17, 18, and 19 are damaged, animals shun bright areas (Denny-Brown and Chambers 1976). Recently, reduced luminance was found to improve visual acuity thresholds in some children with CVI (Good and Hou 2006). This may be another reason for apparent photophobia.

Other self-stimulatory visual features include flicking fingers in front of their eyes against a light source. Alternatively, some children with CVI may demonstrate eye pressing or eye poking. These behaviours tend to manifest in those with more severe developmental impair-ments (Jan and Groenveld 1993), similar to the rocking movements observed in some children with profound developmental disabilities.

Abnormalities of eye movements are common, such as apraxias, gaze palsies, and poor smooth pursuit (Jan and Groenveld 1993), but such disorders are rarely seen in children with pure CVI (striate cortex) unless there is also widespread brain injury. Typically, children prefer to use head rather than eye movements to follow moving objects (Porro et al 1998a).

Some children with CVI appear to exhibit a striking ability to detect movement, possibly as a result of preservation of secondary visual pathways (Dutton et al 2004). Perception of movement is subserved bilaterally in the middle temporal lobes. Therefore, movement of visual targets may reinforce visual identification.

Cerebral visual impairment is rarely an isolated disorder, as it is often the result of injury to multiple areas of the brain. Several different visual and cognitive processing centres may be affected in children with CVI. As described in Chapter 1, visual information is processed along two principal pathways, the dorsal and the ventral streams (Goodale 1998). The dorsal stream runs between the occipital and parietal areas. This area serves visual attention and visual guidance of movement. The ventral stream runs between the occipital and temporal areas. Injury to these areas may lead to impaired visual perception (Dutton et al 1996).

COMORBID CONDITIONS
Children with CVI may have multiple associated neurological and developmental conditions. In the context of hypoxic–ischaemic brain injury, many present with a variety of additional health and developmental conditions. Health problems are commonly the result of the under-lying aetiological conditions, and severe brain malformations or injuries cause coexisting neurological disorders such as epilepsy, microcephaly, hydrocephalus (Whiting et al 1985), and developmental disabilities (Matsuba and Jan 2006).

OPHTHALMIC CONDITIONS
Children with CVI need to be examined for additional causes of vision loss and ophthal-mic problems (Flodmark et al 1990), which may be present in up to 65% of patients (Huo et al 1999). Common ocular and optic nerve disorders include impaired accommodation and refractive error (Chapter 6), cataract (Guzzetta et al 2001), ocular structural problems, retinal diseases, optic nerve hypoplasia, optic nerve atrophy, and nystagmus (Whiting et al 1985, Matsuba and Jan 2006). While optic nerve diseases and nystagmus are most commonly asso-ciated with CVI, other structural ocular conditions, such as coloboma, retinal disorders, and optic nerve hypoplasia, may occur with various aetiologies of CVI. Optic nerve atrophy is often found when there is diffuse CNS injury and/or in severe cases of CVI. Although the optic nerve is resistant to asphyxia, it can be injured in the setting of profound hypoxia–ischaemia (Good et al 1987), leading to problems with visual function. In addition, increased intracranial pressure can result in optic nerve atrophy as well as injury to the oculomotor nerves. Similarly, nystagmus is a common feature in CVI. It is associated with periventricular leucomalacia, optic nerve anomalies, and ocular structural diseases.

Eye misalignment is common. Since many children with CVI do not have stereopsis and fusional vergence, they can present with strabismus. In the presence of poor visual attention, children with CVI may have an exotropia. With better visual attention, esotropia is more common. Estimation of the amount of surgical correction required for strabismus in this group tends to be less accurate than for children without cerebral damage.

Health and development

Children with CVI have a high prevalence of such comorbidities as non-ambulatory cerebral palsy, cognitive impairment, seizure disorders, and hearing impairment (Whiting et al 1985, Huo et al 1999, Matsuba and Jan 2006).

Children with CVI may initially present with variable tone, depending on age and aetiology. Genetic metabolic disease may present with diffuse hypotonia, whereas children with periventricular leucomalacia are likely to develop spastic diplegia. Tone can vary in the first year of life, so it may take more than a year for motor posture, tone, and movements to become stable. Some children with CVI initially present with poor head control. As a result, many experience head and eye movement difficulties (Jan and Groenveld 1993), which may prevent a child from gaining and maintaining visual fixation on targets.

Medical management

The early identification of CVI plays a key role in management. CVI can be missed if the diagnosis is not considered. Once diagnosed, the manner in which the parents are informed can positively or adversely affect them and their child for years to come. The diagnosis should be given with patience, understanding, compassion, and optimism for progressive improvement in visual function, without giving hope for unrealistic levels of visual recovery (Jan et al 1990b).

When vision is reduced or absent, it can influence body tone (Jan et al 1975), eye movements (Jan et al 1986), primitive reflexes (Sherman and Keller 1986), and circadian rhythm (Krieger and Rizzo 1971). Therefore, management requires a multidisciplinary approach, involving optimal medical (ophthalmology, neurology, and paediatrics), habilitation (physical, occupational, speech, and psychology), and educational strategies. In order for vision to develop, a constant visual experience which accords meaning is ideally needed, which can be accomplished through deliberate intervention. With experience, children may learn to use their vision better (Wiesel 1982). Initially, support for children with CVI is based on community-based therapies and early vision support service providers, working alongside healthcare providers. The ophthalmologist plays a role in performing regular refraction, identifying, characterizing, and monitoring the visual manifestations, and initiating vision support services.

Neurological health plays a key role. For example, good control of seizure disorder, hydrocephalus, metabolic diseases, and infection optimizes visual function. Some anticonvulsants cause sedation, particularly in combination, reducing the time for visual interaction, and some anticonvulsant medications can cause retinopathy, necessitating careful choice of medication to optimize health, visual function, and development.

Children with CVI are at high risk of hearing impairment (Matsuba and Jan 2006), which needs to be identified and optimally managed, especially as hearing contributes significantly to development.

The majority of children with CVI, as described in this chapter, have some form of motor impairment. Most commonly, they are grouped under the term 'cerebral palsy'. This umbrella term comprises a group of non-progressive, neurological disorders that cause motor disability that requires long-term management. The potential for muscle contracture, and consequent joint subluxation and dislocation, requires surveillance and management through therapists, paediatricians, and orthopaedic surgeons.

Feeding problems can be a result of impaired mastication and swallowing. Gastro-oesophageal reflux can cause aspiration. Both must be sought as they can affect growth and development.

Impaired sleep may be a result of gastro-oesophageal discomfort and orthopaedic pain. Careful assessment is required. If sleep problems persist, management using mild sedatives or melatonin warrants consideration (Jan et al 1999).

Habilitation and rehabilitation
The goal of vision habilitation/rehabilitation is to maximize visual and developmental function. Late identification of CVI delays remediation and can lead to adverse developmental sequelae (Sonksen 1993a). Early intervention is vital to improving visual function and general neurodevelopment (Groenveld et al 1990). Appropriate environments and activities that promote vision, acuity, and visual attention may lead to improvement in visual function (Malkowicz et al 2006).

Children with CVI are a diverse population and there is no uniform approach to assessment and rehabilitation. Typically, a holistic multidisciplinary approach that addresses not only vision but also the overall health and development of the child is needed.

Vision is important in early development. Motor skills, such as reaching and walking, employ visual guidance (Moller 1993). Typical vision strategies focus on providing a simplified environment which highlights the material of interest (Groenveld et al 1990, Baker-Nobles and Rutherford 1995). Emphasis on high-contrast and brightly coloured objects is combined with the use of motion, touch, and sound to reinforce vision. Consistent environments and schedules help to organize visual information. As visual function improves, visual strategies employ progressively more complex scenarios with fewer reinforcements.

Posture plays an important role in vision rehabilitation. There is a relationship between vision and neck control (Groenveld et al 1990). Poor positioning of the child may impede visual function, and proactive positioning and seating is required to optimize visual function. Appropriate head support must be considered, as it will allow the child to position the eyes and head to identify with visual information in their surroundings. As cerebral palsy (CP) with weakness and/or dyskinetic movements is common in children with CVI (Huo et al 1999, Matsuba and Jan 2006), trunk instability and dyskinetic movements may hamper visual fixation combined with reaching. Thus, trunk support may be needed to ensure positional stability during visual motor-based activities.

Limited mobility as a result of CP is common. Since vision motivates exploration, reduced vision may further limit development of reaching, rolling, crawling, and walking. Impaired vision can limit opportunities for language interaction because vision assists with labelling items in the environment, and children with CVI may miss out on language reinforcement. Early intervention with compensatory approaches is needed to develop skills and to motivate exploration and development.

Children with CVI usually have impairments of higher order visual perception skills. In part, this may be because of cognitive limitations, which are common in children with CVI (Matsuba and Jan 2006). For example, some children may have independent challenges with selecting items from an array. This may be because of a 'crowding' effect. Crowding occurs when children have difficulties in viewing symbols or objects that are flanked by other symbols or items. Enlargement of the material, decreasing 'visual clutter', or directing the child's visual attention towards the item of interest may assist (Jan and Groenveld 1993). Assessing the abilities of children with CVI requires skill and understanding of the unique features that accompany the condition to ensure that the skills of children with CVI are not underestimated.

A fuller account of habitation/rehabilitation can be found in chapters 14–16.

Prognosis

In the majority of cases, CVI diminishes with time, even with severe brain injury (Huo et al 1999, Lim et al 2005, Matsuba and Jan 2006). However, most do not develop normal visual acuity (Groenendaal and van Hof-van Duin 1992). The rate of visual development may also be slower than in children without CVI (Lim et al 2005).

There is considerable variation in visual progress, which may depend on the severity of neurological insult, although imaging findings do not always predict visual outcome (van Hof-van Duin et al 1998). In some instances, visual acuity may improve dramatically but, more typically, improvement is gradual.

The reasons for generalized improvement over time are unclear. Some have suggested that it is a normal maturational process (Hoyt et al 1982). Most believe that children have plasticity in the brain, which leads to improvement in, or 'recovery' of, visual and other neurological functions (Lambert et al 1987, Good et al 1994).

There are a number of predictors of visual prognosis. Children with better abilities and health tend to have better visual function, whereas children with deteriorating neurological conditions may not progress in their visual skills (Matsuba and Jan 2006). Electrophysiological studies can yield information on prognosis. Children with better EEG recordings are more likely to have visual recovery (Robertson et al 1986). A normal flash VEP is generally associated with better outcome (Taylor and McCulloch 1991, Clarke et al 1997). Mapped VEPs are generally abnormal in permanent CVI (Whiting et al 1985). Computed tomography (CT) or magnetic resonance imaging (MRI) of the brain can also assist with prognosis, since neuroimaging can define the extent and location of brain lesions or injury. For example, multicystic encephalomalacia caused by hypoxic–ischaemic injury is typically associated with a poor visual outcome, and imaging studies early in life can assist in distinguishing between the less severe focal schizencephaly and a more severe brain malformation such as lissencephaly, and help to predict visual (and neurodevelopmental) outcome. However, for most children, the precise prediction of the type and severity of CVI is not possible in infancy, and careful sequential assessment of visual function, along with other developmental milestones, is the best way to identify and guide management of visual impairment in children at risk for CVI.

Summary

Cerebral visual impairment, as defined in Chapter 2, first manifests in infancy and ranges in severity from delayed visual maturation with good but incomplete improvement to profound permanent visual impairment. Assessment methods are matched to the age of the child and the degree of visual disability. All aspects of visual function can be impaired. Low visual acuity and visual field deficits are characteristic. Visual field deficits are usually similar in both eyes (homonymous) and most frequently affect one or other side, or the lower visual field.

Visual crowding is common. The more elements there are within a visual scene, the harder it becomes to identify one of them. This may account for difficulty seeing items in the distance, where the scene tends to be more crowded. Objects may be reached for while looking to the side, and people may not be looked at while having a conversation. This could relate to difficulties in splitting attention. Children with more profound visual difficulties may show evidence of compulsive light gazing. On the other hand, there are those whose visual function may be enhanced under reduced illumination. Variable visual function is commonly seen, with reduced performance when tired.

Children who develop good acuities may go on to exhibit features of cognitive and perceptual visual impairment.

Accompanying disorders include cerebral palsy, seizures, hearing dysfunction, and strabismus and other eye movement problems.

Early diagnosis of cerebral visual impairment, with early implementation of habilitative strategies, is ideal.

3.2 PATHOGENESIS AND IMAGING OF DISORDERS AFFECTING THE VISUAL BRAIN

Olof Flodmark and Lena Jacobson

Introduction

Cerebral visual impairment (CVI) can be caused by many different pathological entities. The aim of this chapter is to provide an overview of such pathologies and their imaging characteristics.

The development and maturation of the fetal and infant brain includes organizational changes over time. Insults affecting the developing human brain may cause brain damage, the patterns of which are dependent on three factors: the stage of brain development at insult, the severity of the insult, and the duration of the insult. The most important of these three factors is the timing of the insult in relation to the developmental stage of the brain.

The processes involved in brain maturation during the first and second trimester are cell proliferation, neuronal migration, and cortical organization. Brain pathology caused by an insult during this period in time will cause maldevelopment, recognized as cerebral malformations on neuroradiology. Although a large and increasing number of cerebral malformations are found to have a genetic basis, the morphology as seen by imaging can be used for classification of cerebral malformations and provides a framework for timing of the insult involved in cerebral malformations caused by extrinsic insults (Barkovich et al 2001, Krageloh-Mann 2004).

Organogenesis has been concluded in the third trimester and the gross architecture of the brain has been established. This is the time when the processes of growth and differentiation start. This extends into post-natal life. Important features of this period are myelinization and also formation of synapses and the proliferation of dendrites and axons.

Insults affecting the brain during this period of development cause destructive or clastic lesions. The location of these lesions is determined by the vulnerability of the various parts of the developing brain and this turns out to be different at varying developmental stages.

Periventricular leucomalacia (PVL), intraventricular haemorrhage (IVH), and periventricular haemorrhagic infarctions (PVHIs) are all well-recognized forms of white matter damage of immaturity (WMDI). More recently, focus has shifted to diffuse white matter injury, which recently has been defined (Dyet et al 2006) and is found to have a correlation to neurodevelopmental disorders at school age (Iwata et al 2007).

The parts of the brain most susceptible to injury shift from white matter to grey matter structures towards the end of the third trimester. Thus, in general, two patterns of damage to grey matter can be recognized at term: damage to central grey matter, thalamus and basal ganglia, and damage to cortical structures in a parasagittal distribution. These patterns of damage are considered to be caused by hypoxia–ischaemia with different degrees of severity and duration. The developmental stage at which this transition from white to grey matter damage occurs is around 34 gestational weeks. Other factors causing recognizable patterns of damage to grey matter includes kernicterus, hypoglycaemia, and deep venous thrombosis (Triulzi et al 2006).

Some of the patterns of damage, particularly white matter damage, appear to relate very well to clinical motor symptoms whereas the plasticity of the brain will have a profound effect on the ensuing symptoms following damage to grey matter.

The patterns of brain damage are now well studied and reported, and it is established that neuroradiological imaging provides invaluable information about brain damage in children with cerebral palsy, with or without coexisting CVI (Krageloh-Mann 2004, Bax et al 2006). The efficacy of neuroradiological imaging is now so great that it is generally recommended that magnetic resonance imaging (MRI) of the brain should be included as an obligatory component in the assessment of children with cerebral palsy (Ashwal et al 2004).

By recognizing the pattern of damage in an individual case and classifying the damage into one of the patterns recognized, it is possible to estimate the timing of the lesion and hence to suggest the mechanism behind the damage. Although it is not possible to determine the cause of the injury, the facility to limit the insult to a certain time window is a major step in the direction of determining the cause of brain injury in children with CVI.

The most common cause of post-natal damage to the developing visual brain is trauma, with abusive head trauma to small children resulting in the most severe brain damage and visual impairment. The pattern of damage is much more dependent on the nature of the insult than on the timing of the insult in relation to the developmental stage of the brain. Other causes of post-natal damage to the developing brain include such entities as meningitis; neonatal meningitis, whether bacterial or viral, is particularly destructive to immature brain structures, which offer little resistance to the spread of infection.

Hydrocephalus causing raised intracranial pressure is another cause of brain damage in small children. The extent of damage is dependent on the ability of the child's skull to compensate for the increasing pressure by widening of the skull sutures. Hence, focal stretching of periventricular white matter may be at most risk in the very young infant whereas herniations and their consequences for vessels and cranial nerves may be a more realistic course of events in the older child, who may develop high pressure inside a less pliable skull.

First- and second-trimester patterns – congenital brain malformations

Classifications
It is difficult to classify cerebral malformations because most structures of the brain form at the same time. Hence, it is common that events leading to malformations result in anomalies

of more than one structure. Furthermore, not one malformation is exactly the same as another. Malformation of cortical development is the only group in which the presumed embryology of the lesions can be used to formulate three distinct groups of malformation. When discussing the various brain anomalies, the concept of timing becomes important. An insult of any type to the brain at the time when a certain structure is formed will result in an anomaly of that structure. However, genetic disorders can cause identical anomalies if they are involved in the formation of that structure. Hence, it is not possible, on the basis of neuroimaging alone, to determine whether an anomaly is caused by a defective gene or is the result of an in utero injury. This chapter is not a complete review of cerebral malformations, but focuses on those involving the 'visual brain'.

Cerebral malformations can be classified in many ways. The nomenclature for these disorders is not uniform and no standard system has been established. In this chapter we give a short review of major cerebral malformations according to their MRI appearance in relationship to the embryological timing of normal development. The earliest malformations to appear are related to the formation of the neuronal tube, i.e. abnormalities of dorsal induction or cranial dysraphism (3–4 weeks of gestation). The event following the formation of the neural tube is called ventral induction, when the two separate cerebral hemispheres are formed (5–8 weeks of gestation). The structures in the posterior fossa are also formed during this period. When the basal structures of the brain are established, the development is characterized by proliferation of glial and neuronal precursors and histogenetic expression of cells into different functions (2–4 months of gestation). This period overlaps with the developmental stages which follow – neuronal migration and the formation of cerebral cortex (2–5 months of gestation).

Malformations of *dorsal induction* include *cephalocele*, an extracranial extension or protrusion of intracranial structures through a congenital defect of the skull and the dura mater. For ophthalmologists, it is important to know that a nasopharyngeal encephalocele of the base of the skull will have an association with such midline malformations as anomalies of the cerebral commissures (80%) and dysplasia of the optic nerves. Contained in the encephalocele will be parts of not only the third ventricle and major vessels but also the optic chiasm (Naidich et al 1992). The most common malformation in this group is Chiari II malformation, which is a congenital malformation of the hindbrain in a posterior fossa that is too small. The impact on the visual system is minimal, unless poor control over hydrocephalus with ventriculomegaly and high intracranial pressure gives rise to impaired blood flow to the visual cortex.

Malformations of *ventral induction* include a spectrum of malformations with holoprosencephaly at one end and *septo-optic hypoplasia* at the other. Septo-optic dysplasia, or de Morsier syndrome, includes the triad of hypopituitarism, hypoplasia of the optic nerves, and, often, but not always, absence of the septum pellucidum. The syndrome is not uncommon and the clinical manifestations are variable. This syndrome is characterized by two findings – optic nerve hypoplasia and absence, total or partial, of the septum pellucidum. Two-thirds of these patients also have hypothalamic–pituitary dysfunction. The diagnosis is established when optic disc hypoplasia is seen in conjunction with absence of the septum pellucidum. The small optic nerves in this group may be secondary to trans-synaptic degeneration of the optic nerves secondary to in utero destruction and hypoplasia of the optic radiation (Brodsky and

Glasier 1993). The clinical presentation ranges from total blindness to delayed and limited visual maturation, often with strabismus and nystagmus.

Malformations of cerebral cortical development
The classification of these malformations has developed significantly as a result of recent discoveries about the biological basis for malformations of cortical development and the discovery of new such malformations, which have rendered previous classifications out of date (Barkovich et al 2001). Three main groups of these malformations are now recognized:

1 malformations secondary to abnormal stem cell proliferation or apoptosis;
2 malformations secondary to abnormal neuronal migration; and
3 malformations secondary to abnormal cortical organization and late migration.

Although patients with anomalies classified in the first two groups may have visual problems, the most important types of malformation to consider in this context are those of abnormal cortical organization.

Malformations secondary to abnormal cortical organization and late migration
The most important feature of this group is polymicrogyria. Polymicrogyria can be an isolated anomaly of the cortex but is often seen as one component of a more complex malformation with other morphological features added. In polymicrogyria, cortical development is interrupted during the later stages of neuronal migration when the cortex is organized. The deeper layers of cortex develop abnormally and the result is the formation of multiple small gyri. The histology of polymicrogyria, although variable, has derangement of the normal six-layer cortex and subsequent sulcation as common features. There are no normal sulci in areas of polymicrogyria. The malformation may be focal, multifocal, or generalized. Polymicrogyria can manifest in any distribution – uni- or bilateral, symmetrical or asymmetrical. It is most commonly seen around the Sylvian fissure, but any part of the brain may be affected.

Patients with polymicrogyria will present clinically with a variety of focal neurological signs and symptoms depending on the location of the malformation and the parts of brain involved. It is usually not possible to predict the clinical symptoms from knowledge of the extent and location of the anomaly. Polymicrogyria can be caused by chromosomal mutations, hypoxia, or congenital infections, and the clinical presentations do not differ depending on cause. The areas involved are often bilateral and symmetrical (Barkovich et al 1999). Psychomotor delay and various neurological deficits are seen but also eye motility problems, particularly in cases of bilateral symmetrical frontoparietal polymicrogyria. Perisylvian syndrome is a term used to describe bilateral more or less symmetrical involvement of cortex adjacent to the Sylvian fissures. Patients with large unilateral areas of polymicrogyria may present with epilepsy and hemiplegia. Normal visual field function examined with computerized perimetry has been described in adults with bilateral occipital parasagittal polymicrogyria (Dumoulin et al 2007). It has been demonstrated with functional MRI (fMRI) and electrophysiological studies that dysplastic neural tissue in malformations of cortical development

53

may participate in task performance (Vitali et al 2008). Thus, fMRI may add important information when planning epilepsy surgery.

Polymicrogyria is a constant feature of *schizencephaly*, which is an anomaly difficult to classify in the scheme above. The malformation can be the result of both genetic and acquired causes. Some of these malformations occur during cell proliferation, some during cell migration, and some during cortical organization. Hence, these malformations are difficult to classify and, in particular, difficult to time correctly. Some cases of schizencephaly are obviously caused by in utero transmantle injury during the midportion of the second trimester. The injury is thought to be a vascular catastrophe with an early infarction into vessels supplying the fetal brain. Hence, schizencephaly is a defect that involves the complete cerebral mantle and connects the superficial subarachnoid space over the outer surface of the brain with the lateral ventricles. There is sometimes a thin membrane overlying the cleft, separating the ventricular cerebrospinal fluid (CSF) within the cleft from that of the overlying subarachnoid space (Hayashi et al 2002). The defective cleft is lined by grey matter with leptomeninges, differentiating it from a transmantle infarction, which manifests after formation of the cortical mantle in which the defect is lined by white matter.

It is useful to divide the cases of schizencephaly into those with unilateral and bilateral clefts, the latter being slightly less common. The schizencephaly may have open lips with an open cleft, or it may have closed lips, in which case the cleft is closed but lined with grey matter entirely into the ventricle. The gyral pattern of the cortex adjacent to the clefts comprises polymicrogyria and is abnormal (Fig. 3.2.1).

The clinical correlate is quite variable, depending on size and location of the cleft. Severe seizure disorder is quite common, as is spasticity. Children with bilateral clefts tend to have a more severe cognitive and psychomotor developmental delay. Wide clefts are usually associated with moderate to severe developmental delay, while children with narrow or closed lips may have only hemiplegia and/or seizures. However, one should exercise caution in predicting neurodevelopmental deficits from neuroimaging studies. The location is typically central involving the pre- and post-central gyri. However, the clefts may be found parasagittally, frontally, or occipitally. The clinical manifestations are often mild in these cases. If the cleft involves the parts of the brain including the optic radiation, it may cause visual impairment and the optic nerves can become hypoplastic because of trans-synaptic degeneration. CVI and optic nerve hypoplasia are reported to be common in patients with bilateral open clefts (Barkovich and Kjos 1992).

The diagnosis of schizencephaly is best made with MRI. Closed lips are best detected with coronal T1-weighted images. MRI also shows the abnormal appearance of the cortical mantle along the cleft. The cortex looks thicker than normal because of the presence of polymicrogyria. There may also be polymicrogyria in the contralateral hemisphere, subependymal heterotopias and absence of the septum pellucidum (in 70%). The septum pellucidum is always absent in cases of bilateral clefts. CT may, in many cases, show calcifications subependymally or in the parenchyma. This is taken as an indication that the cause of schizencephaly was an intrauterine infection, possibly with cytomegalovirus (CMV).

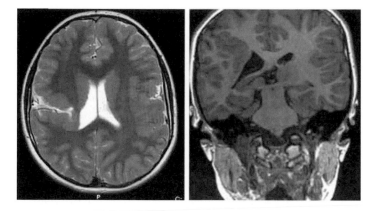

Fig 3.2.1 This 9-year-old female was born at gestational age 36+5. She had early-onset right esotropia and was found to have a left hemiplegia during the first year of life. She attends regular school but she has difficulties reading. Structured history taking revealed problems with depth and simultaneous perception. Her linear visual acuity was 6/7.5 in both eyes. Goldmann perimetry was normal. MRI reveals right-sided schizencephaly involving the posterior temporal and parietal lobes. Abnormal cortex with polymicrogyria is seen to extend down to and abut the ventricular wall. The malformation involves the usual location of the optic radiation. Considering the normal visual fields, it is clear that the function of the right optic radiation must have been transferred to another, unknown, location.

Early third-trimester patterns

DISEASES OF THE IMMATURE BRAIN

During the early parts of the third trimester, insults cause destructive damage, manifesting different pathologies depending on the timing and intensity of the insult rather than the type. Thus, the same insult will cause different pathologies if the insult occurs in, for instance, the 24th or the 36th gestational week. Similarly, insults of different types, for example infection or hypoxia, will cause the same type of pathology if the insults occur during the same stage of brain development. The intensity, and thus duration, of the insult will also have effects on the pathology, as various parts of the brain may express different degrees of vulnerability to certain insults.

Thus, the resulting pathology, as seen by neuroradiology, will inform about the timing of an insult and, in most situations, the intensity. However, at our present stage of knowledge, it is, with single exceptions, not possible to say anything specific about the nature of the insult.

Damage to the brain occurring during the third trimester, before 34 gestational weeks, is referred to as white matter damage of immaturity (WMDI). This is an umbrella term for periventricular leucomalacia (PVL) and intraventricular haemorrhage (IVH) with or without associated periventricular haemorrhagic infarction (PVH), both pathologies involving periventricular white matter but with different pathophysiologies.

Current research into the cause of PVL focuses on inflammatory reactions in the fetal brain as a response to external factors that may be responsible for not only the brain injury but also preterm birth (Nelson et al 2003). Cytokines, circulating in the infant's bloodstream, have, in animal studies, been shown to cause damage to certain parts of the brain more vulnerable to these substances than others. Damage such as that seen in PVL has been demonstrated in these experiments. It is not fully known what factors play a role in causing elevated levels of cytokines, but infection and hypoxia–ischaemia may be such factors. Damage through a high level of cytokines may be the 'final common path', causing tissue destruction, whatever the nature of the insult. Maternal infection was the only clinical factor shown to have a significant correlation with cerebral palsy in a large multinational study (Bax et al 2006).

Periventricular leucomalacia is an ischaemic brain injury that tends to be more or less symmetrical in distribution and involves the periventricular white matter, most often adjacent to the trigone or the foramina of Monro of the lateral ventricles. The true incidence of PVL in all preterm children is not known, but recent studies of an entire population in northern Finland found that about one-third (32%) of all children born preterm had MR evidence of end-stage PVL at 8 years of age (Olsen et al 1997). This is far more frequent than suggested by studies in which neonatal neurosonography was used in the diagnosis of PVL (Claris et al 1996).

Whatever the pathophysiological mechanism behind PVL, there is a window in time when the focal vulnerability of the immature brain is such that an injury will cause damage known as PVL. This window is not thought to extend much beyond the end of the 34th gestational week. Similar windows exist for other types of destructive damage to the more mature but still developing brain. The physiological conditions necessary for the development of PVL are thought to be present from 24 to 34 gestational weeks. This window in time is usually considered quite reliable. Therefore, if diagnosed in a child born before or at 34 weeks of gestation, PVL is usually considered to have a strong association with preterm birth, possibly caused by the same insult causing the preterm birth (Krageloh-Mann 2004). The imaging pattern of brain injury seen in those infants who have suffered in utero damage is identical to that found in neonates who have been damaged post-natally during the same stage of development (Barkovich and Truwit 1990). Thus, PVL found in an infant born at term should be considered a sequel to a prenatal insult (Krageloh-Mann et al 1995).

Neuroradiological diagnosis of PVL in neonates is not easy. The principal mode of imaging is ultrasonography. CT has no role to play. MRI does not play a major role in the early diagnosis of PVL, but is occasionally used early in life on preterm neonates. Later stages show development of cysts, which eventually become incorporated into the lateral ventricles and show the typical features of end-stage PVL. The lateral ventricles remain normal in size and shape in mild cases but become dilated in more severe cases in which the periventricular white matter may be locally absent and grey matter abuts the ventricular wall directly. The lateral ventricles become irregular in shape, with cortical structures at the deepest reaches of the sulci, particularly the posterior Sylvian fissures, indenting the walls of the lateral ventricles. The deep portions of the Sylvian fissures often show focal dilatation; when present, this provides quite specific proof that PVL is indeed the cause of the reduced amounts of periventricular white matter. The corpus callosum is thinner than usual. Both CT and MRI will establish the diagnosis of end-stage PVL, but MRI is clearly the preferred technique as it is harmless and shows all components of the damage to best advantage (Flodmark et al 1987, 1989) (Fig. 3.2.2).

The common clinical sequel of PVL is spastic diplegia or, in more severe cases, spastic quadriplegia. CVI is common, particularly if PVL is predominantly posteriorly located. Such visual impairment may manifest as a short visual attention span. Intellectual disability is usually mild, except in very severe cases. Epilepsy is not a common feature of PVL, but has been described in cases of severe brain damage.

Periventricular leucomalacia is a lesion more or less symmetrical in its distribution. However, there are cases with brain damage that is limited to one hemisphere, and these children may or may not have hemiplegia, which may be accompanied by hemianopia. In fact, when children with hemiplegia are studied with MRI, WMDI is the most common finding, explaining the motor disability of a patient with hemiplegia (Bax et al 2006). In most cases,

(a)

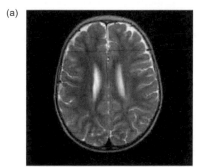

(b)

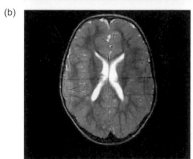

(c)

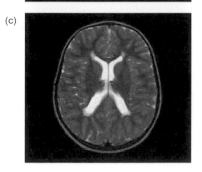

Fig 3.2.2 White matter damage of immaturity. Three separate children with white matter damage of immaturity of different severity, in this case caused by periventricular leucomalacia. Note in (a) the increased signal in the periventricular white matter representing gliosis. The damage in (b) is associated with loss of volume of white matter seen as the direct abutting of deep grey matter to the ventricular wall in the region of the trigones. The damage in (c) is severe, with almost total loss of white matter. The lateral ventricles, particularly posteriorly, have an irregular outline conforming to the deep portions of the gyri. Gliosis (high signal) is also seen in remaining small amounts of white matter around both the anterior and posterior horns.

there are bilateral abnormalities, but in an uneven distribution, explaining the hemiplegia. Careful clinical examination of such a child will often demonstrate subtle contralateral symptoms from the least damaged hemisphere.

Intraventricular haemorrhage is common in the immature neonate but is also, like PVL, seen in the unborn fetus. The cause of IVH is thought to be systemic hypertension and subsequent hyperperfusion of the brain. Cerebral circulation in the immature fetus or neonate is dependent on maintenance of systemic blood pressure. Hence, the causes of IVH, like PVL, are thought to be mediated through excessive variations in the systemic blood pressure causing secondary fluctuations in cerebral perfusion in a fetus or neonate with poor autoregulation of cerebral perfusion. The origin of this haemorrhage is found in the germinal zone, the part of the brain in which the cells that constitute the brain are generated (Hambleton and Wigglesworth 1976, Wigglesworth and Pape 1978). The germinal zones show most activity during the period between 8 and 28 weeks of gestation. The germinal matrix diminishes in activity towards the end of the second trimester and begins to involute. In IVH, the fragile blood vessels in the involuting germinal matrix break open and a haemorrhage occurs in the lateral ventricle. The frequency of haemorrhage decreases with increasing maturity, and germinal matrix haemorrhage is unusual after 34 weeks of gestation.

Thus, the aetiology behind PVL is related to, but different from, that of IVH. Although IVH and PVL often occur together in the same individual, the two lesions are different, and indeed often unrelated. IVH is, by itself, not associated with any clinical sequelae, but may cause ventricular dilatation because of hydrocephalus. This hydrocephalus is transient and, when left without treatment, resolves without permanent cerebral damage. However, mild and general ventricular dilatation is a common residual finding in children who have had IVH as neonates or as a fetus in utero. Such mild ventricular dilatation may persist for a long time without coexistence of other signs of hydrocephalus, such as increased head circumference. IVH occurs, like PVL, before 34 weeks of gestation, but is more common in the more immature brain and thus more frequent before 28 weeks of gestation.

Periventricular haemorrhagic infarction (PVH) is a common complication of IVH. The mechanism is thought to relate to venous congestion in the periventricular veins. This congestion is secondary to ventricular dilatation caused by IVH. Such venous congestion can cause brain damage, and when the cerebral perfusion is restored, there is a secondary haemorrhage into the damaged periventricular white matter. PVH is typically located adjacent the foramen of Monro and is seen to affect the central parts of the brain.

Like PVL, the mechanisms behind IVH and PVH are not well understood. Serial ultrasound studies in the neonatal period can demonstrate the development of severe lesions despite the fact that no obvious cause can be determined.

Maturity at the time of injury is a very important – but not the only – factor, influencing the location and extent of damage. It is usually thought that the presence of gliosis in remaining white matter is indicative of a lesion occurring later within the interval of 25–34 gestational weeks, as formation of gliosis is a process requiring a certain degree of maturity to operate.

End-stage WMDI is today the most common cause of CVI (Gronqvist et al 2001). It may result in subnormal visual acuity, visual field defects, strabismus, nystagmus, and ocular motor problems and cognitive and perceptual visual impairment.

Systematic MRI of surviving very immature neonates has identified another lesion in white matter. A large proportion of these infants have been shown to have, as an independent finding but also in addition to focal lesions described above, a diffuse white matter abnormality described as diffuse excessive high signal intensity (DEHSI). This observation has been apparent in MR studies performed at a time when the infant has reached maturity at term. This abnormality is not associated with any significant loss of brain tissue and is defined as high signal on T2-weighted images in periventricular white matter. The distribution is diffuse, as opposed to focal in PVL, and is, in mild cases, limited to periventricular white matter, but in more severe cases it is seen to involve subcortical white matter also. The finding of DEHSI has been associated with decreased neurodevelopmental scores at follow-up but has not been found to be associated with cerebral palsy. The exact nature of this finding is still unknown, and much has to be learned before we know the significance of this finding in terms of prognostic value. Children with DEHSI may develop normal visual acuity and visual fields, but they often suffer from cognitive visual problems (Dyet et al 2006, Iwata et al 2007).

Late third-trimester patterns

Hypoxic–Ischaemic Injury in the Term Neonate

Severe brain damage caused by a partial hypoxic–ischaemic insult to the neonatal brain of 35 weeks' gestation or more may cause neuronal cell death. Neuronal cell death will cause accumulation of toxic substances in damaged tissue, resulting in cytotoxic cerebral oedema. With time, usually after 5–7 days, the oedema will subside and the damaged brain undergoes destruction with reduction in brain volume, the degree of which depends upon the severity of the damage. This type of hypoxic–ischaemic damage first manifests in the border zones between vascular territories. Thus, in cases of less severe damage, the most severely damaged tissue is found in the watershed regions between the territories supplied by the different major arteries supplying the brain with oxygen. The most obvious watershed regions are found in the parasagittal cortical areas corresponding to the watershed zones between the anterior, posterior, and middle cerebral arteries. In the most severe damage, brain tissue disappears and is replaced with liquid-filled spaces. In less severe damage, some tissue remains and organizes into scar tissue. Destruction of neonatal brain leads to volume loss and cystic spaces, which lead to multicystic encephalomalacia in the most severe cases. These cysts may collapse, culminating in cerebral atrophy.

The pathophysiological mechanism behind multicystic encephalomalacia is usually described as *partial hypoxia/asphyxia*, indicating a reduction in, but not total, cessation of oxygen supply to the brain. An insult such as partial hypoxia/asphyxia is thought to act under a period of time of several hours or even days, often but not always during the final days and hours of pregnancy. The clinical outcome of this type of injury is commonly microcephaly with severe intellectual disability, CVI, and spastic quadriplegia (Triulzi et al 2006).

The other mechanism known to cause severe damage in the neonatal term brain is usually described as *profound asphyxia*. In this situation, there is complete or near-complete cessation of blood flow to the fetal or neonatal brain. Complete asphyxia causes damage to those parts of the brain with the highest rates of metabolism at the time of injury, which in the term infant are the putamen, thalami, hippocampi, and cortex adjacent to the central sulcus. It is usually recognized that profound asphyxia lasting more than 20–25 minutes causes complete brain damage with a slim possibility for survival. Profound asphyxia lasting less than 10 minutes, in an otherwise healthy neonate, is not thought to cause any permanent brain damage. In late follow-up after such an injury, the neuroradiological findings, as shown by MRI, are typical, with tissue loss and signal changes more or less limited to the brain structures mentioned previously. The clinical sequel from this pattern of brain injury is usually that of severe cranial nerve dysfunction and athetoid or dyskinetic cerebral palsy (Krageloh-Mann et al 2002).

It is obvious from the above discussion that the maturity of the brain at the time of injury is by far the most important factor determining the type of brain injury. PVL and DEHSI are the dominant pathologies before 34 weeks' gestation, while cortical damage and damage to central grey matter occur closer to term.

LOCALIZED INFARCTIONS

Stroke in children is not an uncommon disease, with a long list of causes. As many as one-half of focal brain infarctions in children are idiopathic, and no cause for the infarct can be found. Known causes include a central source of an embolus, perhaps from a congenital heart defect, trauma with or without vascular dissection, or other vasculopathies secondary to infection or inflammation. Coagulation defects associated with a high risk of intravascular thrombosis and metabolic diseases are further causes. The causes of stroke in children are very different from those of an adult population. Hence, the clinical work-up of the child is very different. However, the clinical effect of a stroke in a child is quite similar to that of an adult. In the mature child's brain, the effect of an infarct is predictable.

The situation is quite different in neonatal strokes, or focal infarcts of adult appearance in the neonate. These events are, in most cases, clinically silent, associated with a single seizure or hypotonia, and become evident only when the child starts to move around and an early hand preference is detected. Thus, most of these children are not diagnosed until their second year of life and most often first by their parents and only later by the paediatrician. The reason for neonatal stroke is rarely known. Again, cardiac problems must be excluded as well as coagulation defects. Factor V Leiden is not an uncommon finding in these children. It is thought that most cases of neonatal stroke occur during or very near the time of delivery. It is known that infarction is almost twice as common in the left hemisphere than it is in the right. This is thought to have an anatomical explanation as an embolus from the placenta could pass into the child's arterial circulation through an open oval foramen in the heart and further through a patent duct (ductus arteriosus) into the descending aorta. Fluctuating flow in the briefly persistent fetal circulation into the aorta may predispose to bidirectional flow, allowing the embolus to enter the left common carotid and the left cerebral circulation (De Vries et al 1997, Lynch et al 2002, Nelson and Lynch 2004, Nelson 2006) (Fig. 3.2.3).

The prognosis of children with focal infarction and no identified cause is dependent on the location of the infarct and the maturity of the brain at the time of insult. Not surprisingly, extensive infarcts involving critical areas of the cortex and central structures of the brain carry a more severe prognosis than limited infarcts in less vital areas of the brain. With infarcts of

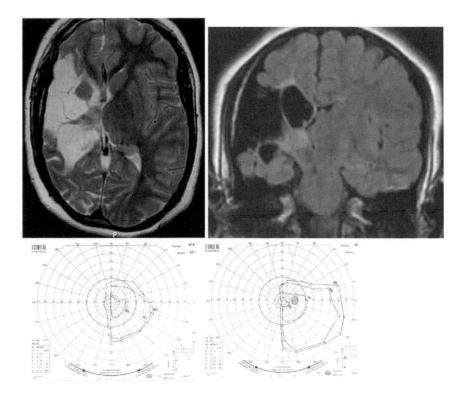

Fig 3.2.3 Focal cortical damage – infarction. This 14-year-old female was born at term but was small for her gestational age. She developed left-sided hemiplegia during her first year of life. She has a diagnosis of having Asperger syndrome and attends a special school. The girl developed left esotropia when she was 4 years old, and she is hyperopic +4D. She has reading difficulties. Structured history-taking revealed problems with orientation. Linear visual acuity was 6/9 in both eyes. Goldmann perimetry revealed total homonymous hemianopia to the left but when tested she demonstrated, as a compensatory mechanism, automatic scanning into the visual field defect. Her tendency to scan with her eyes during perimetry can provide a false impression that she has near-normal visual fields. The MRIs show destruction within the territory of brain tissue supplied by the right middle cerebral artery. Note compensatory widening of the right lateral ventricle and scar tissue (bright signal on T2-weighted magnetic resonance image) replacing most of the temporal lobe. The right cerebral hemisphere, and hemicranium, is significantly smaller than the left. This insult, which took place close to term, involves the optic radiation. Although there is early damage, brain plasticity has not compensated for this brain injury.

similar extent or location, more immature children have less severe deficits than older children. Children in whom the cause of infarct cannot be established have a lesser risk of another insult. The plasticity of the child's brain is much greater than that of the adult brain as other regions of the brain can take over functions. The vessel involved in the infarct is of great significance in predicting CVI. The visual outcome may include strabismus and homonymous hemianopia, whereas visual acuity is less affected and nystagmus is rarely seen. A majority of children with middle cerebral artery infarct have relative or total homonymous visual field defects.

61

Post-natal conditions

INFECTIONS

Both congenital and acquired infections can cause brain damage and symptoms in the neonate.

Congenital cytomegalovirus

Congenital cytomegalovirus (CMV) disease is the most common serious viral infection among newborns in the USA (Alford et al 1990). Congenital CMV infection occurs in approximately 1% of all births. Of these, 10% have the various haematological, neurological, and developmental symptoms and signs that define the disease. These include hepatosplenomegaly, microcephaly, impaired hearing, and small head size. Severe, permanent neurological conditions were found in 55%, including intracranial calcifications (43%), microcephaly (27%), chorioretinitis (15%), and seizures (10%).

Findings on cross-sectional imaging examinations are variable depending upon the degree of brain destruction and the timing of the injury. On CT and MRI, some patients, presumably infected during the first half of the second trimester, have complete lissencephaly with a thin cortex, a hypoplastic cerebellum, delayed myelination, marked ventriculomegaly, and significant periventricular calcification. Those injured later, presumably in the middle of the second trimester, have more typical polymicrogyria, whereas patients infected near the end of gestation have normal gyral patterns, mild ventricular and sulcal prominence, and scattered periventricular calcification or haemorrhage (Barkovich and Lindan 1994). Cortical dysplasia is far more common in CMV than in other causes of cerebral calcification. When these four findings are present in a child with developmental delay or seizures, a diagnosis of congenital CMV is likely.

Congenital toxoplasmosis

Toxoplasmosis is caused by the protozoan *Toxoplasma gondii*. Pregnant women usually acquire the infection by ingestion of oocysts in uncooked meat (Desmonts and Couvreur 1974). The infection in the fetus may be generalized or primarily concentrated in the nervous system or, most frequently, it may be latent, only manifesting as retinochoroiditis and diagnosed many years later. The principal CNS findings are retinochoroiditis (bilateral in 85% of affected patients), abnormal cerebrospinal fluid, hydrocephalus, and seizures.

A diffuse inflammatory infiltration of the meninges is found and hydrocephalus is frequent, most often caused by ependymitis causing occlusion of the aqueduct. It is important to note that, in contrast to congenital CMV, malformations of cortical developments, such as polymicrogyria, are not a common feature of congenital toxoplasmosis.

The findings on cross-sectional imaging studies reflect the pathological findings of meningeal infiltration. Calcifications are common; they usually involve the basal ganglia, periventricular region, and cerebral cortex. Large ventricles are common and may be the result of hydrocephalus, brain destruction, or both.

Congenital rubella

Congenital rubella is now extremely rare in Western countries because of immunization and screening of pregnant women. This virus affects the fetus more commonly during the first and second trimester; ocular, cardiac, and neurological defects are most common when infection occurs in the first and second post-natal months. In fact, rubella infection is nearly benign when occurring during the third trimester (Miller et al 1982).

The appearance of the brain on imaging studies varies depending upon the time of the in utero infection. Early infection will result in congenital anomalies whereas late infection will result in a non-specific generalized oedema or loss of brain tissue. CT typically shows multifocal regions of hypodensity throughout the cerebral white matter, often in association with calcification. In addition, calcification may be seen in the basal ganglia and cortex. In severe cases, nearly total brain destruction and microcephaly are present.

The ocular manifestations (cataract and retinal disease) render it difficult to determine the degree and nature of superadded CVI.

Neonatal herpes simplex encephalitis

Infection of the fetus with herpes simplex virus (HSV) may result in a fatal generalized disease. Most cases of HSV infection result from exposure of the infant to maternal type 2 herpetic genital lesions as he or she passes through the birth canal. The incidence of neonatal herpes simplex infections is estimated to be 1 per 2000–5000 deliveries per year. The brain is involved in approximately 30% of infected infants.

Imaging studies of patients with neonatal herpes encephalitis show patchy, widespread areas of abnormal signal (prolonged T1 and T2 on MR) in the grey and white matter, which rapidly progress in prominence and area of involvement during the course of the disease. Loss of brain substance occurs rapidly, often as early as the second week. Eventually, severe diffuse cerebral atrophy evolves, with profound cortical thinning, leucomalacia (often multicystic in nature), and punctate or gyriform calcification. Profound CVI is the most frequent visual outcome.

Neonatal meningitis

Bacterial meningitis can cause severe brain damage to the neonatal brain as a result of accompanying vasculitis and ventriculitis. *Arteritis* accompanying meningitis can be reliably diagnosed by CT or MR because of the resulting infarcts, which tend to be sharply delineated and confined to a specific arterial vascular territory. Large and small vessels can be affected. When major vessels such as the middle or anterior cerebral arteries are involved, large, usually cortical, infarctions result. Cerebritis and abscesses develop when the infectious process travels through thrombosed venules into the cerebral parenchyma. The only differences between cerebritis/abscess in neonates and in older children are the speed at which brain destruction occurs and the amount of reactive astrogliosis that occurs. Because of the reduced immune response of the neonate, brain destruction is rapid, resulting in cystic encephalomalacia with large cysts and a relatively minimal astroglial response. Destruction caused by infarcts or abscesses can occur anywhere in the brain and the location of the damage will influence the resulting neurological deficit and degree of visual impairment.

Head injury in the small infant is not uncommon, and falls from a bed or changing table are the common explanations. However, in a classical study of infants <1 year of age admitted to a large children's hospital, 64% of all head injuries (excluding uncomplicated skull fractures) and 95% of all severe brain injuries were inflicted (Billmire and Myers 1985). In the UK it is estimated that 1 in 1000 children <1 year of age sustain physical abuse, and about one-half of these will have brain injury. Population studies in Scotland (Barlow and Minns 2000), the USA (Keenan et al 2003), and Estonia (Talvik et al 2006) confirm these numbers. Of small infants who are abused, shaking injury is most common. The majority of infants who have been shaken are between 3 and 5 months old, most of them <6 months and almost all <1 year of age. The long-term outcome of abuse of infants is poor. Mortality is between 20% and 25% and, of those surviving, only about 10% are considered normal and more than 80% in one study were in need of multidisciplinary care for the rest of their lives (King et al 2003).

Shaking injury to the brain includes subdural haemorrhages, tearing injuries in brain tissue, and hypoxic brain damage. The subdural haemorrhages are caused by tearing of bridging veins. When shaken, the infant's brain, supported only by thin membranes and vessels bridging over from the meninges, moves inside the skull. This results in contusions and tearing of the brain substance. Disruption of nerve tracts in the brainstem can result in unconsciousness and respiratory arrest. This may culminate in hypoxic injury to the brain, as a secondary effect of the shaking.

Retinal haemorrhages are commonly seen if the infant has been shaken. In one study (Morad 2002), 83% of children aged <3 years who had subdural haemorrhages because of abuse also had retinal haemorrhages. Low vision is a common sequel to inflicted brain injury. The most common cause of low vision is CVI directly related to the child's brain injury and not to any damage in the eye (Kivlin et al 2000).

HYDROCEPHALUS

The word hydrocephalus means abnormal accumulation of fluid in the brain or cranial vault and the term is thus applicable to such disparate conditions as cerebral atrophy and obstruction to flow of cerebrospinal fluid (CSF) because of a blockage of the interventricular foramen of Monro. Hence, any discussion using the term hydrocephalus must include a definition clearly stating the context in which the term is used.

In this chapter, hydrocephalus is used, in analogy with ventriculomegaly, to describe the result of obstruction to CSF flow within the ventricular system, causing accumulation of CSF upstream of the obstruction. Hydrocephalus is also used to describe the condition caused by a disturbance in the hydrodynamic balance within the intracranial cavity, usually known as communicating hydrocephalus. 'Ventriculomegaly' is a purely descriptive term implying a larger than normal ventricular system without any reference to the cause of such dilatation. 'Colpocephaly' is sometimes used to describe a condition in which the occipital horns of the lateral ventricles are dilated out of proportion to other parts of the ventricular system.

Except in small infants, in whom the open fontanelle can be palpated, no non-invasive method to measure the intracranial pressure is available. However, there is evidence that measurement of the optic nerve diameter 4mm behind the globe elicits the dilated optic nerve sheath behind the eye, which is seen in acute raised intracranial pressure following shunt blockage (Newman et al 2002). Evaluation of the fundi for possible papilloedema is difficult for the inexperienced and is of no use in the smaller children and infants who do not develop a high enough intracranial pressure to cause papilloedema. The most important information comprises head circumference charts, in which head growth is observed by serial measurement. Most children's heads grow at a normal pace and are known to follow their own growth 'channel'. Infants with large heads will often maintain a large head through infancy and may follow the normal growth pattern in the 97th centile or even higher. This is not a pattern suggesting the presence of hydrocephalus. Much more suspicious is a growth chart illustrating crossing of centiles, particularly at a steep angle, even though the absolute head size may be within normal limits for age. It is not uncommon that this is the only clinical sign of developing hydrocephalus. Thus, it is not the absolute measurement of head size that is most relevant but the pattern of growth over time. Frequent use of a tape measure is a far more efficient tool in the diagnosis of hydrocephalus than a single or even repeated neuroradiological investigation. Thus, macrocephaly is a common but not obligatory finding in hydrocephalic children. By the same token, hydrocephalus is an uncommon association with microcephaly, but the combination is not impossible.

The neuroradiological work-up of infants and children suspected of suffering from hydrocephalus should focus on two issues that may require different strategies or may be solved concurrently. First, the clinical suspicion of hydrocephalus must be confirmed or disproved. This task may be the most challenging, requiring sophisticated investigations. Once the diagnosis is established, further investigations must concentrate on finding the cause of the hydrocephalus.

The clinical presentation to the ophthalmologist can vary greatly from completely normal findings to CVI with subnormal acuity, strabismus, and nystagmus, as well as ventral and dorsal stream dysfunction. The group of children with most visual problems is that with Arnold–Chiari II malformations. The relative contributions of the ventriculomegaly itself are difficult to establish. Persistent papilloedema is well known to cause optic atrophy, although this is not a neuroradiological diagnosis. The most threatening situation for the child's vision is associated with shunt failure and subsequent transtentorial herniation.

Summary

The pattern of damage to the developing visual brain depends on the timing and stage of brain development at the time, and the severity and duration of injury. The patterns seen on MRI often indicate the mechanism and timing of injury.

Injury in the first two trimesters causes congenital malformations that may impair vision. Small optic nerves (optic nerve hypoplasia) can accompany impaired development of the structures between the lateral ventricles. The result is septo-optic dysplasia, often associated with lack of pituitary hormones. The visual outcome varies from total blindness to delayed and limited visual maturation, often with strabismus and nystagmus. Malformation of cerebral cortex results from disturbed brain cell growth, impaired movement of brain cells to the right location, or disordered final modelling or

65

cortical organization. Polymicrogyria is the most common form. Clefting of the brain (schizencephaly) has multiple causes and is accompanied by adjacent polymicrogyria. Vision may be affected, but in many cases the visual field function is relatively spared, possibly by brain plasticity.

Injury at 24–34 weeks' gestation tends to cause periventricular white matter damage of immaturity (WMDI). Lack of oxygen (hypoxia) and blood supply (ischaemia) are the most common causes, however, often in combination with infection. WMDI almost always affects vision, with an outcome varying from severe visual impairment with low visual acuity, ocular motility dysfunction, altitudinal inferior visual field defects, and severe cognitive visual problems to early-onset esotropia or slightly subnormal visual acuity only.

Blockage or rupture of a blood vessel in the brain (or stroke) has many causes and often occurs near term. It leads to focal damage, or infarction. The extent of damage determines the severity; the location dictates whether and how vision is affected. Middle cerebral artery infarction often results in homonymous visual field defects.

Infection of the brain tissue can be congenital or acquired. Congenital cytomegalovirus, toxoplasmosis, rubella (German measles) and herpes simplex show a range of patterns of damage on brain imaging, and all impair visual development, often profoundly. Neonatal bacterial meningitis inflames arteries, which then block and cause circumscribed focal damage on imaging. Focal infection inside the brain causes abscess formation and destructive cyst formation. The overall and visual outcome again depends upon the extent and severity of the damage.

Progressive, sight-threatening hydrocephalus leads to more rapid and greater head growth than normal, detected by serial measurements of head circumference. Brain imaging is required to make the diagnosis and determine the cause, and guide management. In hydrocephalus, vision may be affected because of optic nerve atrophy, by periventricular white matter damage and, and in shunt failure, by occipital infarction. Besides visual field defects, subnormal visual acuity and strabismus, cognitive visual dysfunction is commonly found when looked for.

Low sugar (hypoglycaemia) in the neonatal period tends to damage grey matter. After birth, the most common cause of brain damage is non-accidental head injury. MRI shows a range of patterns. One-quarter of patients do not survive, and vision is impaired in a majority of the survivors.

Brain imaging, primarily by MRI, facilitates making a diagnosis, and predicting and estimating morbidity in this wide range of disorders.

3.3 VISUAL DYSFUNCTION IN INFANTS WITH DAMAGE TO THE BRAIN AND ITS RELATIONSHIP TO BRAIN IMAGING

Eugenio Mercuri, Andrea Guzzetta, Daniela Ricci, and Giovanni Cioni

Introduction

Over the last 20 years, the combination of behavioural tests, neuroimaging, and electrophysiological techniques has helped to elucidate the correlations between different aspects of visual function and different brain areas. Visual function is served by the 'classic' visual pathway (from the retina and optic nerves to the occipital cortex via the optic radiation) and the complex network of cortical and subcortical areas such as the parietal, temporal, and frontal lobes as well as the basal ganglia, serving visual attention, visual guidance, recognition, and other functions (de Vries et al 1987, Cioni et al 1996, 1997, 1998, Mercuri et al 1997b).

Longitudinal studies of visual acuity, visual fields, or visual attention during the neonatal period and through the first years of life have provided age-dependent normative data for their onset and development (Dubowitz et al 1983, Atkinson et al 1992, van Hof-van Duin et al 1992, Allen et al 1996). Other such studies in infants with focal or generalized lesions of cortical and subcortical areas have provided evidence of their role in processing specific aspects of visual information. 'Congenital' lesions occurring prenatally or in the neonatal period do not always produce an equivalent degree of visual impairment to that observed in adults or older children with similar acquired lesions, indicative of the greater plasticity of the developing brain.

This chapter reviews the tests available to assess visual function in newborns and infants, and their application in preterm and term infants with brain lesions, and reports our experience and reviews the literature on the correlations between visual function and the extent and timing of neonatal brain lesions occurring in preterm and term infants.

How early is early?

We have recently proposed a simple and short protocol that includes nine items exploring various aspects of visual function ranging from ocular motility and the ability to fix and follow a target to more complex aspects of visual abilities such as reaction to a coloured contrast target, discrimination of black and white stripes with increasing spatial frequency, and attention at distance (Ricci et al 2008a).

Figure 3.3.1 shows the items included in the battery, the targets used, and the instructions for each item. This protocol has proved feasible in term-born infants as young as 48

No.	Assessment					Intermittent		Continuous	
			Mainly conjugated	Occasional strabismus	Occasional/ lateral nystagmus	strabismus	nystagmus	strabismus	nystagmus
1.	**Spontaneous ocular motility:** note spontaneous oular movements before presenting a target		R L	R L	R L	R L	R L	R L	R L
			Mainly conjugated	Occasional strabismus	Occasional/ lateral nystagmus	Intermittent strabismus	nystagmus	Continuous strabismus	nystagmus
2.	**Ocular movements with a target:** note ocular movements while presenting the target	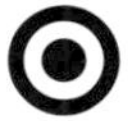	R L	R L	R L	R L	R L	R L	R L
3.	**Fixation:** with the target in front of the infant at 25cm, note the ability of the infant to fix on the target	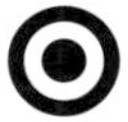	Stable (> 3s)	Unstable (< 3s)	Absent				

Tracking – black/white target

No.	Assessment		Complete	Incomplete	Brief	Absent
	Tracking: note the infant's eye movement in response to the target's movements 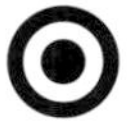					
4.	**Horizon:** with the target at 25cm and starting in the midline, move it slowly to both left and right		Complete R L	Incomplete R L	Brief R L	Absent
5.	**Vertical:** with the target at 25cm and starting in the midline, move it slowly upwards and downwards		Complete U D	Incomplete U D	Brief U D	Absent
6.	**Arc:** with the target at 25cm, move it slowly tracing an arc		Complete R L	Incomplete R L	Brief R L	Absent

Colour/discrimination/attention

No.	Assessment			
7.	**Tracking coloured stimulus:** note the infant's eye movement in response to the target movements, starting from the midline towards the lateral	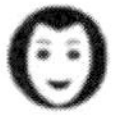	Present	Absent
8.	**Stripes discrimination:** note the infant's ability to fixate on a series of targets of decreasing stripe widths held at a distance of 38cm starting with the widest stripe; note the narrowest stripe width on which the infant fixates	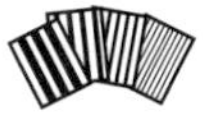	Last card identified	
9.	**Attention at distance:** after eliciting central fixation move the target slowly away and a few cm laterally from the infant and note the maximal distance at which focusing is maintained	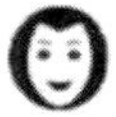	.........cm	

Fig. 3.3.1 Proforma with instructions for the assessment of visual functions in the first days of life.

and 72 hours from birth. It is easy to perform, and has good interobserver reliability (Ricci et al 2008b). The assessment has been validated in 124 infants assessed at 48 hours. Fifty of the 124 were re-assessed at 72 hours. Around 90% of the infants are able to complete the assessment if assessed at the optimal time – between feeds – with the newborns propped up at 30° in a quiet environment with low background lighting which affords good eye-opening (Brazelton 1973, Ricci et al 2008a).

Spontaneous occasional abnormal ocular movements were present in 32% of infants, and this increased in response to fixing/tracking a target. All infants were able to horizontally track a target moving in a complete arc to both sides and to track the target moving vertically and in a circle but not always completely, especially for the circle.

We also assessed discrimination of stripes and attention at distance that have not previously been systematically assessed in newborns soon after birth. All but one infant were able to discriminate at least the first four Teller cards (up to 0.86 cycles/degree), with the highest spatial frequency ranging from card 4 to card 8 (0.86–3.2 cycles/degree), and all were able to keep attention for at least 30cm, with a maximal distance ranging between 30 and >70cm. By 72 hours from birth, vertical and horizontal arc tracking, stripe discrimination, and attention at distance were the functions which improved significantly.

This battery has also been used in preterm infants assessed between 35 and 40 weeks postmenstrual age. All the infants were able to complete the test battery in one session without interruption. The responses at 35 weeks were less mature than at 40 weeks, but with minimal differences (less than 10%) for six of the nine items, but with significant differences for tracking a coloured contrast target, attention at distance, and stripe discrimination responses (Ricci et al 2008c).

The value of the battery in identifying normal or abnormal early visual function has also been suggested by a recent study combining clinical assessment and brain magnetic resonance imaging (MRI) performed during the same day in 37 preterm infants. Twenty-seven of the 37 had a normal scan or only minimal changes while the other 10 had major lesions on conventional brain MRI. Diffusion tensor imaging (DTI) with probabilistic diffusion tractography was used to delineate the optic radiations at term-equivalent age and to compare the fractional anisotropy (FA) to a contemporaneous evaluation of visual function (Bassi et al 2008). The results of this study showed that visual assessment independently correlated with FA values in the optic radiations, whereas gestational age at birth, post-menstrual age at scan, or the presence of lesions on conventional MRI did not appear to be equally correlated to the visual findings, suggesting that, in preterm infants, at term-equivalent age, visual function is directly related to the development of white matter in the optic radiations.

These data confirm that it is possible to perform a structured assessment exploring different aspects of visual function at very early ages. The data recently collected in both term-born and preterm cohorts may be used as a reference when examining newborns with brain lesions or clinical neurological problems, or in infants known to be at risk of visual impairment, in both clinical and research settings.

Assessment of visual function in the first years of life

In the first years of life, the combined use of behavioural and electrophysiological techniques allows a detailed assessment of many different aspects of visual function and of their maturation.

BEHAVIOURAL TECHNIQUES

Behavioural techniques are based on the observation and assessment of spontaneous or elicited visual behaviours. A number of methods designed or modified for the assessment of young infants and uncooperative patients are presented.

Oculomotor behaviour can be assessed by testing fixation, following reactions and saccadic movements, that is the rapid eye movement to shift fixation from one stimulus to another. A short period of fixation on a target can be observed by 30 weeks' post-menstrual age (PMA). Following reactions are better observed from 34 weeks' PMA. At term age, newborns are generally able to follow a target, such as a red ball, in a full arc (Dubowitz et al 1998). Saccadic movements for short distances can be elicited from birth, but they have high latency and little accuracy. A more mature pattern is reached at around 3 months post term. Strabismus and eye alignment can be tested by commonly used orthoptic techniques, such as the cover test, in which covering the eye which appears to be looking leads to discernible movement of the deviated eye. The presence of abnormal eye movements, such as spontaneous nystagmus, can also be noted.

Acuity can be tested from the first weeks of life by using forced-choice preferential looking (FCPL). The infant is presented at eye level on one side of the midline with a target consisting of black and white stripes paired with a uniform grey background on the other side. The level of acuity is measured as the finest grating (i.e. width of black and white stripes) for which the infant shows a consistent preference (in cycles/degree), and compared with age-specific normative data (Teller et al 1986). As a rule of thumb, visual acuity shows a maturation of one cycle per degree per month in the first year of life. Other measures of acuity can be obtained by means of visual evoked potentials (see below).

Contrast sensitivity is tested with grating patterns in which the stripes are not sharp but have a sine-wave distribution of light intensity. Contrast is defined as the intensity difference between the brightest and the darkest points of the grating, divided by the sum of these intensities, and it can vary from 0 to 100%. A rapid increment in contrast sensitivity has been found over the first 2–3 months of life, and at 4 weeks post term peak contrast sensitivity is about a factor of 5 to 6 lower than that of adults (Norcia et al 1990). By 33 weeks post term, adult levels are reached. The contrast sensitivity function is useful in showing pathological visual losses (e.g. amblyopia, glaucoma, and demyelinating diseases) which are not adequately revealed by acuity measure alone.

Visual fields can be assessed using kinetic perimetry. The apparatus consists of two perpendicular black metal strips bent to form two arcs, each with a radius of 40cm. The infant is held in the centre of the arc perimeter. During central fixation of a white ball, an identical target is moved from the periphery towards the fixation point along one of the arcs of the perimeter. Eye and head movements towards the peripheral ball are used to estimate the outline of the visual fields. Normative data for full-term and preterm infants are available (Mohn and van Hof-van Duin 1986, van Hof-van Duin et al 1992). The fields are quite narrow in the first months of life (approximately 30°) and become progressively wider (approximately 60° at 6 months and 80–90° at 1 year of age).

Optokinetic nystagmus (OKN) can be elicited by using a large piece of paper or a computer-generated random dot pattern in front of the infant's face. The examiner observes the infant's eye movements, recording the presence and the symmetry of the OKN in response to the movement of the pattern in either direction. Normally, binocular OKN is symmetrical from birth onwards, whereas monocular OKN shows a better response to stimulation in a temporonasal direction up to about 3–6 months of corrected age (Atkinson and Braddick 1981).

Fixation shift is a test of visual attention evaluating the direction and the latency of saccadic eye movements in response to a peripheral target in the lateral field. A central target is used as a fixation stimulus before the appearance of the peripheral target. While in some trials the central target disappears simultaneously with the appearance of the peripheral target (non-competition), in others the central target remains visible, generating a situation of competition between the two stimuli. Normal children can reliably shift their attention in a situation of non-competition during the first weeks after birth, but prompt refixation in a situation of competition is found only after 6–8 weeks post term and reliably by 12–18 weeks post term. Absent or delayed (a latency of more than 1.2s) refixation at 5 months of age is considered abnormal (Atkinson et al 1992).

ELECTROPHYSIOLOGICAL TECHNIQUES
Different types of visual evoked potentials (VEPs) can be used for the early assessment of visual functions.

Flash VEPs can be used to follow the normal or abnormal maturation of the visual pathway, although their contribution to the assessment of infants at risk of CVI is quite limited (Hrbek et al 1973, Taylor et al 1987, Eken et al 1996, Tsuneushi and Casaer 1997).

Steady-state VEPs can be recorded by using orientation-reversal and phase-reversal stimuli, and are used to assess the maturation of visual cortical processing (Mercuri et al 1995a). For phase-reversal VEPs the orientation of the black and white stripes is fixed but the contrast reversed periodically. For orientation reversal VEPs, stimuli periodically change orientation between 45° and 135°. The phase-reversal response is already present at term, whereas the orientation reversal response is consistently elicited only at 10 weeks post term for slow changes (four reversals per second) and after 12 weeks for faster changes (eight reversals per second) (Braddick et al 1986).

The sweep VEP is an alternative technique for the estimations of grating acuity. In the steady-state sweep VEP, the spatial frequency of a high-contrast grating is systematically varied, and acuity is measured by extrapolating the VEP amplitude versus the spatial frequency. Grating acuity measured by this technique develops from around 5 cycles/degree at 1 month to around 15–20 cycles/degree by 8 months (Allen et al 1996, Auestad et al 1997, Birch et al 1998). Figure 3.3.2 shows the profile of development of different aspects of visual function.

	First month	3 months	5 months	12 months
Acuity	1 cycle/degree	3 cycles/degree	5 cycles/degree	12 cycles/degree
Visual fields	30°	40°	50°	90°
Fixation shift Non-competition	Not always present	Always present	→	
Fixation shift Non-competition	Absent	Not always present	Always present	→
VEP PhR	Significant responses at 4r/s	Significant responses at 8r/s	→	
VEP OR		Significant responses at 4r/s	Significant responses at 8r/s	→

Fig. 3.3.2 Profile of development of different aspects of visual function in the first year of life. OR, orientation reversal; PhR, phase reversal; VEPs, visual evoked potentials; r/s, reversals per second.

Other aspects of visual functions, of both higher and lower levels of processing, are obviously present from the first months of life, but we limited our review to the functions that can be assessed by standardized tests, available for the clinical setting. Other tools are available for older children.

Visual disorders in children with brain lesions
The significant improvement in neonatal intensive care and in the early assessment of brain lesions by means of neuroimaging has allowed a detailed evaluation of the type and extent of brain damage right after birth. This new scenario has made it possible to explore the correlation between development of visual functions and brain damage. Because of the complexity of the visual system, most of the more common types of brain disorder are associated with a significant risk of impairment of different aspects of visual function, in relation to the brain areas involved. The main types of congenital brain lesions and the associated disorders of visual function are presented.

PERIVENTRICULAR LEUCOMALACIA
Recent studies have reported that approximately 10% of very low birthweight infants develop cerebral palsy, which is caused by periventricular leucomalacia (PVL) in nearly 90% (Shevell et al 2003). The lesion often involves the axons in the optic radiations and there is, therefore, a high risk of impaired visual function. Indeed, using a combined clinical and imaging approach, it was shown that the presence and the severity of visual abnormalities are related to the severity and the extent of the lesion. Infants with 'prolonged flares', persisting for more than 7 days or evolving into small localized frontoparietal cysts, generally have normal acuity (Eken et al 1995, Cioni et al 1997). Isolated abnormalities of ocular movements, usually strabismus (50%), or of other aspects of visual function, such as visual fields (22%) or OKN (35%), could, however, be found occasionally in infants with such lesions (Eken et al 1995, Uggetti et al 1996, Cioni et al 1997). In contrast, infants with PVL grades 3 and 4 almost invariably show marked impairment of multiple aspects of visual function including strabismus, acuity,

visual fields, and OKN (Scher et al 1989, Gibson et al 1990, Eken et al 1994, Cioni et al 1997, Lanzi et al 1998). The presence of reduced visual acuity, and other visual functions, has been related to lesions in the peritrigonal white matter and in the optic radiations, as well as with the extent of involvement of the occipital cortex (Eken et al 1995, Uggetti et al 1996, Cioni et al 1997). Concomitant involvement of the thalami is associated with a greater degree of visual impairment (Fig. 3.3.3) (Ricci et al 2006).

The early diagnosis of visual impairment in infants with PVL is important because of the relation between visual function and neurodevelopment (Eken et al 1995, Cioni et al 2000). In particular, in our series, multivariate analysis indicated that visual impairment was the principal variable in determining the neurodevelopmental scores in affected infants, more than the severity of motor disability or the extent of lesions on MRI (Cioni et al 2000).

INTRAVENTRICULAR HAEMORRHAGE
Abnormalities of visual function are frequent among preterm infants with intraventricular haemorrhages (IVH), but they are less common and generally less severe than in infants with PVL. Although visual field defects are usually transient, persisting until 1 year of age, the reduction in visual acuity can persist beyond the fourth year of age (Harvey et al 1997a). Transient anomalies of visual function may be due to the effect of IVH on the thalamus or the tectal area, or to bleeding of the germinal matrix at the origin of the optic radiations and the posterior thalami. On the other hand, permanent effects may be present in cases of deeper tissue involvement, as demonstrated by the positive association between visual deficit and neuromotor impairment (Harvey et al 1997a). However, not all infants with parenchymal involvement (grade IV lesions) show a deficit of visual function, as the lesion is more often located in the midanterior parietal lobe and not in the posterior parietal and occipital lobes.

NEONATAL CEREBRAL INFARCTION
Ischaemic brain stroke in adults, and in children, commonly impairs vision. Lesions affecting the occipital striate cortex and the optic radiations cause contralateral hemianopia while

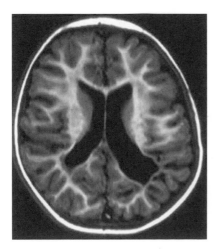

Fig. 3.3.3 MRI of a child with periventricular leucomalacia. Note the concomitant involvement of optic radiations and thalami. The child has reduced acuity and asymmetrical visual fields at school age.

lesions affecting the parietal lobe tend to cause contralateral impairment of visual attention or visual neglect. Conversely, in infants with neonatal infarction, the correlation between neurobehavioural visual tests and neonatal MRI does not show the same consistency (Mercuri et al 1996). We demonstrated that, although acuity and ocular movements are usually normal, other aspects of visual function, such as visual fields and visual attention, can be impaired. When the same infants are tested at school age, the proportion of children with visual abnormalities is lower (Mercuri et al 1996a). Thus, the prognosis for visual field defects detected in infancy is that of spontaneous resolution in the majority of cases (Fig. 3.3.4).

The low incidence of abnormal visual functions following cortical infarction, in comparison with adults with similar lesions, is indicative of effective mechanisms of plasticity of the brain structures serving vision. In our experience, however, the risk of developing visual dysfunction following neonatal infarction is higher in those who develop hemiplegia than in those with a normal outcome. This reflects the extent of the underlying lesion, as visual abnormalities are a more frequent sequel to lesions involving the middle cerebral artery than those involving its cortical branches.

NEONATAL ENCEPHALOPATHY/HYPOXIC–ISCHAEMIC ENCEPHALOPATHY
Neonatal encephalopathy and hypoxic–ischaemic encephalopathy commonly cause visual dysfunction (de Vries and Dubowitz 1985, Groenendaal et al 1989, Cioni et al 1996). The severity of hypoxic–ischaemic encephalopathy at birth cannot always predict the severity of visual impairment (Mercuri et al 1997a,b), but the degree of visual impairment is greater if the basal ganglia and thalami are involved.

Predictive value for outcome
In term-born infants with asphyxia, both the pattern of brain lesions observed on neonatal MRI and the results of visual assessment performed in the first year predict visual abilities at school age. As a rule of thumb, patients with normal MRI or isolated white matter changes,

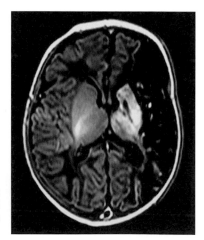

Fig. 3.3.4 MRI of a child with neonatal infarction involving the main branch of the left middle cerebral artery. The child has normal symmetrical fields at school age, even though the lesion involves the homolateral optic radiation.

even when diffuse, develop normal visual function when assessed in the first year and at school age. In contrast, the children with diffuse lesions involving the basal ganglia have persistent abnormalities of vision throughout the first year of life, which persist at school age, with the exception being children with minimal lesions in the basal ganglia, in whom visual function is abnormal in the first few months but tends to normalize by the end of the first year, and remains normal at follow-up (Mercuri et al 1997c). These infants can therefore be labelled as having 'delayed visual maturation' (DVM), a term used to describe infants with reduced vision at birth, which improves by the end of the first year of life (Tresidder et al 1990).

Insults occurring antenatally often produce a higher risk of persistent abnormal visual function, with less plasticity being observed than in patients with similar lesions of perinatal origin. These findings are consistent with similar findings reported for motor outcome. Brain plasticity is often proposed as an explanation for the usually better than expected outcome found in many neonates with perinatal brain injury, with the implication that the neonatal brain is able to relocate functions to unaffected areas or to maintain connections that would have been lost in the course of normal maturation and development (Lomber and Payne 2001, Eyre 2003, Hensch 2005, Seghier et al 2006, Poo and Isaacson 2007).

Combined clinical and imaging studies have also suggested that other clinical variables should be considered in the search for early markers of plasticity. The role of early epilepsy as an additional risk factor for abnormal neurodevelopmental outcome has been reported for both preterm and term infants. In term infants with encephalopathy, the presence of epilepsy in the first 2 years was always associated with an abnormal visual outcome, irrespective of the extent of the lesion (Mercuri *et al* 1999). There are similar findings in full-term and preterm infants with antenatal post-haemorrhagic ventricular dilatation (Ricci et al 2007), in whom the severity of the outcome was worse in those with seizures in the first year of life.

Conclusions

Visual function in infants with brain lesions is related to several distinct factors. The type and extent of lesion is one of the most important prognostic indicators, with early brain MRI being able to identify early markers of plasticity of the brain. In our experience, even relatively large lesions involving the visual pathway have a chance of being associated with a relatively good outcome if sustained around term age and when there is little or no concomitant involvement of subcortical structures. On the other hand, additional early-onset epilepsy, and subcortical damage accord a poorer prognosis for vision. The development of newer techniques such as functional MRI (fMRI), tractography and magnetoencephalography (MEG), and their increasing application in young infants, may allow a better understanding of the mechanisms underlying the association between lesions and function.

Summary

Observation of an infant's visual behaviour and eye movements, in response to a variety of visual stimuli, allows visual function to be estimated from as young as 48–72 hours. Optokinetic nystagmus (in which to and fro movements of the eyes are caused by moving black and white stripes), the ability to shift visual fixation from one target to another, and electrophysiological measurement using visual evoked potentials provide additional information. These methods provide effective ways of estimating the degree of visual dysfunction when the visual system has been affected by damage to the brain, for example in periventricular leucomalacia causing impaired vision, which is most marked when the thalamus of the brain is also affected.

Neonatal cerebral infarction is rarely associated with the development of poor vision, but when this does occur impaired movement of one side of the body, or hemiplegia, is often seen as well.

Neonatal encephalopathy and hypoxic–ischaemic encephalopathy are common causes of visual dysfunction, the severity of which is difficult to predict. However, the outcome is worse if the basal ganglia and the thalami are damaged.

Bleeding into the lateral ventricles posteriorly in the brain tends to cause early visual impairment, which resolves spontaneously unless deep tissues of the brain are also involved.

Spontaneous resolution of visual dysfunction, which is detected at an early stage, is probably a result of the considerable powers of healing and regeneration (or plasticity) in the developing brain.

Impairment of vision is the main variable leading to a poor neurodevelopmental outcome in children with early-onset damage to the brain.

Acknowledgement

The authors of this chapter were partially supported by the Mariani Foundation, Italy.

4
IMPAIRMENTS OF CENTRAL VISUAL FUNCTION AND ITS MEASUREMENT

William V. Good and Anne B. Fulton

Introduction and background

Optotype acuity is the most commonly measured visual function and is mediated by the central retina and visual cortex. In this chapter, we discuss visual acuity and other visual functions that are mediated by the central retina and that dominate the central visual field. The other visual functions are Vernier acuity and colour vision, each of which is likely to be subserved by different processing mechanisms and anatomical locations in the brain. Thus, these different types of visual functions may be disproportionately affected in cerebral visual impairment (CVI). Each of these visual functions normally develops during infancy and childhood. Procedures that have been devised to study these visual functions in healthy infants have been extended to measurements in paediatric patients with CVI. This chapter concentrates on such measurements. Older patients with CVI may be capable of participation in conventional, clinical tests of vision.

The visual functions

Visual Acuity

Visual acuity, literally clarity of vision, is formally defined by the finest detail (minimal angle of resolution) that is visually detectable (Westheimer 1975, 1979, Hamer and Mayer 1994). For optotype acuity, a convention is used to indicate the distance at which a symbol of a specific size and stroke can be seen, for example 20/20 (or 6/6; 1.0; 0.0) indicates that a symbol can be seen 20 feet (6 metres) away. The specific size is one that subtends 5 minutes of arc visual angle and stroke width of 1 minute of arc visual angle. If seven or eight block letters were written equally spaced across a thumbnail, and the thumb were held at arm's length, each letter would subtend approximately 5 minutes of arc. Symbols for 20/200 symbols are 10 times larger. Letter acuity of 20/200 is often used as a criterion for legal blindness and thus eligibility for vision support services.

The acuity in healthy adults and older children is measured by having them read letters or by following particular instructions, such as matching to kind. Because such responses cannot be obtained in infants and young children, or in those whose repertoire of responses is limited by cognitive, or a combination of motor and cognitive, impairments, electrophysiological procedures (visual evoked potentials, VEPs) and psychophysical (behavioural) procedures (preferential looking, PL) have been adopted by many for measuring acuity in paediatric patients with visual impairment resulting from brain injury (Fig. 4.1a and b). For both the electrophysiological and psychophysical procedures, the individual's response is under stimulus control, and the stimuli are specified in precise physical terms.

The stimuli used in VEP and PL tests of acuity are simple patterns (Fig. 4.2), usually black and white stripes (gratings), rather than letters or pictures, which are complex symbols. The width and contrast of the stripes specify these stimuli. In the VEP test, the child's electrical response to the gratings is recorded at the scalp over the occipital cortex. In the PL test, an adult observer judges the right–left position of the stimulus grating based on the child's looking behaviour. Thus, the VEP and PL responses depend on different sets of processes in the child's visual system (Good 2001, Lim et al 2005). The grating acuities obtained using the sweep visual evoked potential (SVEP) (Norcia and Tyler 1985) and PL are expressed in cycles per degree and are compared with normal values for age (Gwiazda et al 1989a, Mayer et al 1995). Although both VEP and PL are valid and reliable measures of acuity in children with visual impairment secondary to brain injury, neither PL nor VEP measures assess exactly the same visual processes as those assessed by tests of acuity using complex symbols such as numbers or letters (Good 2001, Lim et al 2005).

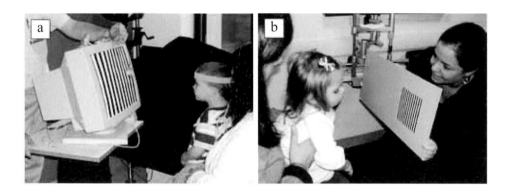

Fig. 4.1 Children with CVI being tested with sweep visual evoked potential (VEP) and preferential looking (PL) procedures. (a) VEP. The child is seated on the parent's lap and shown the stimuli – black and white stripes – on the video monitor. Temporal changes in the black and white stripes evoke a mass electrical response that is recorded by disc electrodes placed on the surface of the posterior scalp over the visual cortex. The amplitude of the response varies with strength of stimulus, such as the width of the black and white stripes. In the sweep VEP procedures, the stimulus is 'swept' rapidly through the parameter of interest, such as width of the stripe. Acuity is estimated by using reliable analytical techniques to extrapolate to a zero microvolt response (Good and Hou 2006). (b) PL. The child is seated on her parent's lap. The examiner, who is unaware of the right–left position of the black and white stripes (grating) on the hand-held grey Teller acuity card test (McDonald et al 1985), observes the child's looking response. In the acuity cards (McDonald et al 1985) the examiner shows the child a series of gratings, from coarse to fine, and judges whether each grating is detected by a child. The finest grating that the examiner judges that the infant detects gives the child's acuity. Normal values for monocular acuities are given in Mayer et al (1995) and for binocular acuities by Salomao and Ventura (1995).

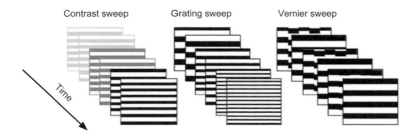

Fig. 4.2 For visual evoked potential and preferential looking measures of grating acuity and Vernier acuity, simple patterns, such as shown here, are used. To determine grating acuity (centre), the width of the black and white stripes is varied, usually from wide (more easily seen) to narrow. Contrast sensitivity can be determined by varying the contrast (left) of the black and white stripes. Vernier acuity is determined by varying the amount of offset in a line (right).

Through infancy and early childhood, grating acuity in developmentally healthy children gradually improves. That is, with increasing age, narrower and narrower stripes produce a threshold response. This trend of improving acuity as normal development goes forward holds, whether measured using VEP or PL procedures (Norcia and Tyler 1985, Norcia et al 1988, Mayer et al 1995). Developmental decreases in the spatial grain of the fovea in early infancy and then continued development of the brain constrain development of normal acuity (Banks and Bennett 1988, Blakemore 1990). Criteria for legal blindness based on grating acuities, obtained by PL or VEP, are not established.

The smallest detectable, high-contrast, black and white stimulus ordinarily defines acuity. If the stimuli are lower contrast, the element must be larger to be detected. Developmental changes in contrast sensitivity have been demonstrated using both VEP and PL procedures. (Norcia et al 1990, Gwiazda et al 1997). Besides grating acuity and contrast sensitivity, VEP and PL procedures have also been used to assess Vernier acuity and colour vision.

Attractive line drawings of high-pass visual stimuli (Harris et al 1984, 1986, Adoh et al 1992, Woodhouse et al 1992, Adoh and Woodhouse 1994) have been designed for measuring acuity in infants (Harris et al 1984) and young children (Harris et al 1986, Adoh et al 1992, Woodhouse et al 1992, Adoh and Woodhouse 1994). One of the motivations for creating these stimuli was to maintain the attention of notoriously restless 1- to 3-year-olds (Adoh et al 1992, Woodhouse et al 1992, Adoh and Woodhouse 1994). The harlequinned line drawings, in which a white line is bordered by thinner black lines, are presented on a grey background. The space-averaged luminance of the lines of the drawings is equal to that of the grey background. Altogether, the white line and the black lines constitute one grating cycle by which the stimulus is specified. These stimuli are designed to disappear at threshold. It is somewhat difficult to design these drawings to be free of artefacts, perhaps especially at high frequencies. Indeed, results of spectral analysis of the spatial content indicate that the drawings have multiple spatial frequencies rather than the single frequency present in grating stimuli (Charman

2006). Nonetheless, the most widely used of the picture stimuli, the Cardiff cards (Adoh et al 1992, Woodhouse et al 1992, Adoh and Woodhouse 1994), have been evaluated by empirical comparison of Cardiff acuity and grating acuity. Acuities obtained using both types of stimuli are similar in healthy participants with normal eyes (Harris et al 1986, Sharma et al 2003) as well as in those with visual and cognitive impairments (Mackie et al 1998, Johnson et al 2009). Feasibility, time to complete the test, and test–retest reliability are also similar (Johnson et al 2009). Thus, the Cardiff cards add to the clinical armamentarium of acuity tests for young and disabled patients.

VERNIER ACUITY

Vernier acuity (Fig. 4.2, right) is defined as the ability to detect discontinuity in a line (Westheimer 1975, 1979). Mature individuals with healthy visual systems can detect 5 arc seconds (Westheimer 1979). Vernier acuity depends on central visual processing, not just the retinal photoreceptors and receptive fields (Hou et al 2007). Compared with grating acuity, Vernier acuity (Fig. 4.2), and also stereopsis, develops rapidly during infancy followed by continued slower development during childhood (Gwiazda et al 1989b, Skoczenski and Norcia 1999). Vernier acuity is relatively resistant to defocus, motion, and luminance, but it is subject to practice effects and attention. One appealing attribute for Vernier acuity is its close approximation to Snellen acuity. Adult observers measured psychophysically on a Vernier task and optotype task demonstrate a nearly one-to-one correlation for these acuity types (McKee et al 2003). In the case of CVI, there is evidence that Vernier acuity is more negatively affected than grating acuity (Skoczenski and Good 2004). The possibility that Vernier acuity in infants with CVI can predict future Snellen acuity is appealing, but as yet unproven. Vernier measures in infants and non-verbal children must be performed using electrophysiology techniques because behavioural techniques have not been developed for clinical application. Questions as to whether VEP Vernier acuity is really a measure of Vernier thresholds, and not simply a surrogate for motion or other acuity types, have largely been answered (Hou et al 2007).

COLOUR VISION

Colour vision depends primarily on the three categories of cone photoreceptors in the retina. Short (blue), medium (green), and long (red) wavelength-sensitive cones have separable, but overlapping, spectral sensitivities. Beyond capture of light by the cones and opponent processes in the retina, colour sensation and colour vision involve further pathways and higher level processes in the brain. Psychophysical and electrophysiological procedures have been used to assess colour vision in mature individuals and also infants. Although immaturities of colour vision are demonstrable in healthy, term-born infants, colour vision capabilities become established in early infancy (Bieber et al 1995, Knoblauch and Maloney 1996, Teller and Palmer 1996, Teller et al 1997, Zemach et al 2007).

Structural substrate for central vision

The fovea in the central retina projects to a large area of the visual cortex (V1) – the striate cortex. This magnification factor is related to visual acuity in healthy adults (Cowey and

Rolls 1974). An analogous relationship may be present in paediatric patients and subject to disruption by disease. The striate cortex (V1) serves as a relay to extrastriate visual areas that may be considered regions for specialized processing. Traditionally, the dorsal stream processes motion, and the ventral stream processes form, but both dorsal and ventral streams feed into further regions of the brain with diverse functions such as those involved in attention and emotion. Paediatric brain injuries and abnormalities that cause impairment of acuity are sometimes circumscribed, but often involve many areas of the brain and thus affect diverse, but inter-related, functions. Furthermore, there is a range of severity for each abnormality.

The paediatric disorders that are frequently associated with acuity deficits are white matter damage of prematurity and hypoxic–ischaemic encephalopathy. Also well represented among paediatric patients with CVI are disorders of neuronal migration in the developing brain. In a few of these, the molecular basis has been identified, or the condition is specified by structure of the brain (schizencephaly, porencephaly, lissencephaly, polymicrogyria, heterotopias) or a constellation of features defines a syndrome, such as Aicardi or the tuberous sclerosis complexes. Some of the conditions have ocular components but often the ocular abnormalities are not sufficient to explain the child's visual acuity. Brain tumours and their treatment may alter the brain substrate for vision. Even in the absence of conspicuous structural abnormalities, metabolic disorders, such as the mitochondrial encephalopathies, or seizure disorders may affect visual processing and produce low acuity and clinical signs of CVI in children (Roman-Lantzy 2007).

Visual functions in children with cerebral visual impairment

GRATING ACUITY

Grating acuity has been measured electrophysiologically (using VEP) and behaviourally (using PL) in children with CVI (Birch and Bane 1991, Good 2001).

Thresholds are elevated (worse) in both methods, and signal amplitudes are substantially diminished on the VEP. The finding that amplitudes are diminished is interesting, as signal amplitudes are actually increased in healthy, extremely low-birthweight infants (Mirabella et al 2006). In the case of intraventricular haemorrhage, amplitudes are diminished, even for grades I and II, where the risk for CVI is very low (Good et al 2008). This suggests that signal amplitudes, perhaps more so than traditional threshold measures, may indicate subclinical damage, or injury on a more favourable end of the CVI continuum. Certainly, in CVI, signal amplitudes are diminished, most likely because of neuronal loss (Good 2001).

Another characteristic of children with CVI is their response to environmental light. Clinically, this is manifest as light gazing or, conversely, light sensitivity approaching photophobia. Good and Huo (2006) explored this phenomenon in the laboratory by measuring grating acuity under low- and normal-luminance conditions. A luminance level that would normally degrade grating acuity was chosen for comparison. Surprisingly, children with CVI paradoxically have improved acuity in the low-luminance condition. Meanwhile, healthy age-matched comparison children show the expected reduction in acuity in low luminance.

This finding could have ramifications for rehabilitation efforts for children with CVI (Good and Hou 2006). Possibly the responses to low and high luminances map to different parts of the visual cortex as rod-driven responses and cone-driven responses have distinct cortical representations (Hamer and Mayer 1994).

Longitudinal measures of grating acuity

Several groups have made serial measurements of visual acuity, using either VEP or PL, or both (Groenveld et al 1999, Huo et al 1999, Lim et al 2005, Matsuba and Jan 2006, Khetpal and Donahue 2007, Watson et al 2007). These studies present ample evidence that many of the young children with acuity deficits associated with a variety of brain abnormalities show developmental increments in acuity. Despite improvement, almost always the child's acuity is significantly below normal for his or her age. Furthermore, the acuity deficits, by both PL and VEP, do not appear to reflect the visual impairment manifest by the child's behaviour and visual–perceptual disabilities. Processes in extrastriate brain, beyond V1, are not completely assessed by these acuity tests in which the stimuli are simple patterns. Thus, other tests of processes in extrastriate visual regions are needed to characterize the visual functions of children with visual impairment associated with brain abnormalities (Weiss et al 2001, Dalen et al 2006, Lavery et al 2006, Ricci et al 2006, Atkinson et al 2008).

VERNIER ACUITY

Good and colleagues found that Vernier acuity was relatively lower than grating acuity in children with CVI (Good and Hou 2004, Skoczenski and Good 2004). This result is consistent with the theory that Vernier acuity is cortically mediated and dependent on higher order visual processes. Thus, Vernier acuity appears to be a more sensitive measure than grating acuity for quantifying vision deficits in patients with CVI.

COLOUR VISION

In adults with acquired central achromatopsia, the areas of brain vulnerable to ischaemia (V1, V2, and also V4) are implicated (Girkin and Miller 2001). Classically, the ventromedial surface of the occipitotemporal region of the brain is damaged. Affected adults complain of washed-out or absent colour sensation, prosopagnosia (faces), agnosia (objects), and visual field defects corresponding to the region of brain that is injured. Although thresholds for detection and discrimination of colours are much elevated, at higher luminances, moving, high-contrast, suprathreshold colour stimuli are readily detected (Cavanagh et al 1998). These results imply that the colour vision pathway is quite complex.

Colour vision has been evaluated in children with CVI and appears to be relatively well preserved, perhaps because the brain locations for representation of colour vision are relatively less vulnerable to hypoxia and ischaemia (Dutton 1994, Dowdeswell et al 1995). Theoretically, shrewd selection of stimuli could be paired with efficient psychophysical or electrophysiological procedures to assess the central colour vision system in children with brain injury, and so learn more about the pathobiology of their condition. We are unaware of any researcher accepting this challenge.

Summary and recommendations

In current practice, clinicians generally rely on non-quantitative measures such as visual fixation responses, presence or absence of nystagmus, and parental history for the child's visual behaviour in different environments. However, reliable quantitative measurement of acuities in young children with CVI is feasible. Such measures of acuity can track a child's visual function over time. Direct service providers may consider this information as one guide to selection of learning media as they design the child's programme for success and continued developmental advances. Fortunately, there are clinical centres dedicated to this work as CVI is the most common diagnosis for permanent bilateral visual impairment. But limitations are recognized. For instance, measures of acuity do not provide valid estimates of the child's visual–perceptual status. Also, the circumstances in which early measures are predictive of future performance have yet to be defined.

Even today there are practical matters that deserve the attention of the community dedicated to serving these children. Potentially, measures of acuity, the most commonly performed test of visual function, would be one of the criteria for determining eligibility for vision services. For adults, optotype (letter) acuity of 20/200 is the most common definition of legal blindness and eligibility for services. There is no corresponding cut-off for grating acuities, which normally change with age. Possibly an acuity below normal for age, say by two octaves, would be one of the criteria. However, one must caution against over-reliance on grating acuity as a criterion for eligibility for services because acuity does not necessarily capture the severity of the child's visual impairment, and other aspects of the child's visual performance should be taken into consideration. An algorithm for a simply stated, vision-based prescription for services would, ideally, include measurements of the central vision (acuity), but also incorporate assessments of other aspects of visual performance. Such a prescription would be a great addition to the care of children with CVI.

Ideally, ophthalmologists would learn to assess children with complicated neurological-based vision problems. Even though the ophthalmologist may not have assessment tools at his or her disposal, an understanding of community and medical resources for these assessments is invaluable.

Summary

The visual acuity is an index of the clarity of central vision, measured as the smallest high-contrast black and white stimulus which can be distinguished (or resolved). (If the contrast is reduced by not being black and white, the stimulus needs to be larger to be seen.) The appendix of this book provides a conversion table for the different measures which are used internationally. Methods of measurement include the following:

- Visual evoked potentials for pattern are visual brain signals detected in response to viewing black and white stripes. As the stripes become narrower, the signal detected gets smaller until it disappears. This gives an estimate of acuity, but this type of test does not assess ability to interpret what is seen.
- Preferential looking entails watching visual behaviour as a child is presented with either black and white stripes (Teller cards) or images (as in Cardiff cards). The stripes and Cardiff card images are constructed so that when the child's acuity is insufficient for the target to be seen it blends imperceptibly into the background grey, as the target image reflects the same amount of light as the background.
- Snellen acuity requires the child to match or recognize progressively smaller images, and therefore requires greater ability and cooperation, but provides more information as it also assesses recognition and understanding.
- Vernier acuity measures ability to detect a discontinuity (or offset) in a line. In children with cerebral visual impairment (CVI), this may be more affected than other measures.
- Colour vision develops early in infancy, and is relatively well preserved in CVI.
- CVI reduces visual acuity. In some children, the acuity is better in dim lighting conditions. The cause is unknown. Vision progressively improves with age in many children.

5
IMPAIRMENT OF PERIPHERAL VISION AND ITS MEASUREMENT

Giorgio Porro and Dienke Wittebol-Post

Introduction

Peripheral vision is that part of vision peripheral to the centre of gaze. It is the area simultaneously visible to an eye when the eye does not move (Stedman 1984).

Recording peripheral vision results in a 'visual field map' of the field of vision as the patient sees it (Walsh 1990). Visual field testing can be performed with confrontational methods, keeping the individual's gaze fixed while presenting objects at various places in their visual field, but can also be done by perimetry, either manually with a tangent screen or (semi-) automatically with a perimeter. With perimetry the visual field can be more carefully mapped and quantified than by confrontation methods.

The function of perimetry is to indicate the site and extent of lesions of the visual pathways (Walsh 1990). It is a subjective assessment and requires cooperation (Lachenmayr and Vivell 1993). Examination of peripheral vision in children is difficult and is not routinely performed.

Anatomy of peripheral vision: from the eye to the cerebral cortex

Vision begins in the retinae, the stimulation of which initiates the visual signal along the optic nerve fibres. At the optic chiasm, all fibres from the opposite nasal halves of the retina cross and join the fibres from the temporal retina of the same side, to form the optic tracts, which carry information from the opposite field of vision to the lateral geniculate nucleus (LGN). From the LGN the signal goes through the optic radiation and ends in the visual area 1 (V1), which is also known as area 17 of Brodmann, or primary visual cortex, and is located in the calcarine fissure of the occipital lobe. V1 is connected to several cortical and subcortical (collicular) areas (Balcer 2001).

For clinical purposes, the LGN, the optic radiation, and V1 are called retrochiasmatic visual pathways (Hubel 1998). The method of choice for visualization of the retrochiasmatic visual pathways, and the detection, localization, and characterization of their abnormalities, is magnetic resonance imaging (MRI) of the head (Cioni et al 1996).

Topography of the visual field

Interpretation of the visual field forms a key part of ophthalmic and neurological examinations. If the visual field is not intact, something is wrong in the retina or in the visual pathways (Walsh 1990).

Each part of the retina is connected, via the entire lower portion of the brain, to the primary visual cortex (V1), which contains a topographic representation of the contralateral hemifield of vision (Horton 2006). The right V1 receives projections from the right temporal retina and the left nasal retina, and thus registers events in the left (contralateral) hemifield view, and vice versa (Fig. 5.1).

In each V1, the upper retinal quadrants, which register events in the lower field of view, are represented in the upper lip of the calcarine cortex, while the lower retinal quadrants, which register events in the upper field of view, are represented in the lower lip (Horton 2006). The fovea is represented at the posterior pole, with the paracentral and more peripherally situated parts of the retina being represented more frontally. The temporal crescent, the most temporal part of the visual field that does not overlap with the visual field of the other eye,

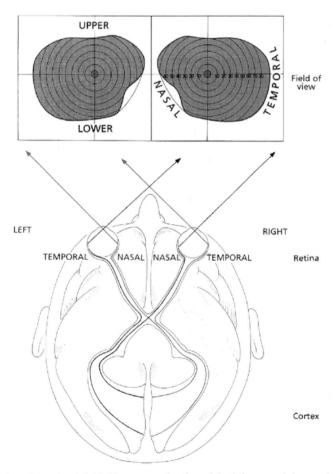

Fig. 5.1 Topography of the visual field. The temporal retina of the left eye and the nasal retina of the right eye (shown in black), which look at the right side of the field of view, project the image to the left hemisphere where the left primary visual cortex (V1) is located. Consequently, the left V1 'looks' at the right half of the field of view. Reproduced, with permission, from Zeki S (1993) *A Vision of the Brain.* Oxford: Blackwell Scientific Publications.

is represented only contralaterally and farthest frontally in the calcarine fissure (Lachenmayr and Vivell 1993, Horton 2006).

Branches of the middle cerebral and of the posterior cerebral arteries supply the retro-chiasmatic visual pathways. Both vascular systems anastomose so that the occipital pole of the cortex is well vascularized and relatively spared in ischaemic conditions (Lachenmayr and Vivell 1993), but the only triple watershed areas are the parieto-occipital areas and the area of the body of the caudate nucleus. These are particularly susceptible to hypoxic–ischaemic brain injury (Brodsky et al 1996).

The manner in which the retina connects with the visual cortex dictates the topographical position of a visual field defect, or scotoma. In general, retinal and optic nerve defects produce defects of the visual field of one eye, damage to the chiasmal part of the visual pathways produces defects of the temporal visual fields of both eyes, and damage to the retrochiasmal part of the visual pathways produces defects of the contralateral visual field of both eyes, as a homonymous quadrantopia, or hemianopia.

The fibres from the LGN, serving the upper visual fields, course through the anterior temporal lobes, where lesions cause contralateral homonymous superior quadrantanopia (Kline and Bajandas 2004). Those serving the lower visual fields pass through the parietal lobes, where lesions tend to cause contralateral inferior homonymous quadrantanopia (Kline and Bajandas 2004).

The types of field defects seen in lesions of the occipital radiation or the striate cortex are congruous quadrantanopia, homonymous hemianopia, altitudinal hemianopia, and chequer-board quadrantanopia. Chequerboard quadrantanopia is actually a bilateral hemianopia with relative sparing of two quadrants (Kline and Bajandas 2004). Another field defect, peculiar to the visual cortex, is the homonymous paramacular scotoma (Walsh 1990).

Homonymous field defects can be congruous (exactly alike) or incongruous. The closer the lesion to the chiasm, the greater the incongruency; congruency increases with proximity to the cortex. This is caused by the fact that the spatial separation of the nerve fibres of both eyes belonging to corresponding retinal elements is relatively great in the tract, but decreases towards the cortex, where the corresponding nerve fibres lie close to each other and intertwine. This explains why lesions in the tract or the lateral geniculate body will produce nerve fibre bundle defects in different areas in the two eyes. Therefore, the resulting field defects are incongruous (Lachenmayr and Vivell 1993).

As a result of the spatial separation of central and peripheral projections, the macula may be spared in cases of homonymous field defects. Splitting of the macula occurs if a homony-mous defect goes through the centre of the visual field. Central acuity is usually decreased, but acuity for distance is often remarkably good. Reading, however, will always be poor because at least 2° of intact visual field to both sides is necessary for easy reading. Sparing of the macula is small or absent in lesions close to the chiasm; sparing increases towards the cortex (Lachenmayr and Vivell 1993).

Examining peripheral vision

INTRODUCTION

Standard clinical perimetry tests the distribution of light difference sensitivity in the visual field. This sensitivity reflects the capability of the eye to perceive a brightness difference between a test target and its background. From the centre, this sensitivity decreases quickly towards the periphery, leading Traquair to coin the descriptive term 'hill of vision'. The two principal methods of measuring the hill of vision are kinetic perimetry with moving targets of constant luminance and static perimetry with stationary targets of varying luminance (Lachenmayr and Vivell 1993).

Conventional perimetry is a subjective examination technique, in which discrete light targets are projected onto the inner surface of a grey hemisphere. The patient fixates a point at its centre. Small spots of light are flashed (static or automatic perimetry) or moved (kinetic perimetry or manual perimetry) in different positions and the patient is asked to report a sensation of light. In adults, the peripheral visual field extends approximately 60° nasally, 90° temporally, 50° superiorly, and 70° inferiorly. The areas where the patient is not able to report a light sensation are documented and constitute the scotomatous region. The position and extent of a scotoma often makes it possible to predict the site of causative lesion.

Conventional perimetry requires cooperation, alertness, and a firm posture. This can be very difficult for infants and children, especially those with a neurological impairment or those confined to a wheelchair because of motor problems.

PERIMETRY IN HEALTHY CHILDREN

Many authors have tried to assess visual fields in healthy children using conventional or slightly modified devices, such as the Goldmann perimeter (Quinn et al 1991), the Tübinger perimeter (Matsuo et al 1974), the Octopus perimeter (Safran et al 1996), the Humphrey perimeter (Stiebel et al 2004), the automated peripheral isoptometer (Suzumura et al 1995), the fundus photoperimeter (Fausset and Enoch 1987), the Ophthimus high-pass resolution ring perimeter (Frisen 1991), the computer-assisted moving eye campimeter (Mutlukan and Damato 1993), the pupil perimeter (Matsui et al 1995), and the frequency doubling technology (FDT) (Blumenthal et al 2004, Quinn et al 2006). Moreover, the multifocal visual evoked potential (mVEP) has recently been introduced as an objective laboratory evaluation of the visual field in children (Klistorner et al 2005).

Data from the above-mentioned studies show that manual perimetry can give reliable results in children older than 4–6 years (Tschopp et al 1995), whereas automatic perimetry can be performed only in children older than 7 years of age (Bowering et al 1993).

PERIMETRY IN CHILDREN WITH NEUROLOGICAL IMPAIRMENT

In children with neurological impairment, these techniques are usually not applicable. This may explain the delay in diagnosing visual field defects in children with cerebral visual impairment (CVI) (Lowery et al 2006). Recognition of visual field defects in children with cerebral insults is, however, very important because homonymous hemianopia may interfere with learning, reading, and rehabilitation therapies (Kedar et al 2006).

Accurate visual field measurement in children is important for several reasons. Vigabatrin, an antiepileptic drug that can cause a permanent constriction of the visual field (Werth and Schadler 2006, Wild et al 2007), requires visual field testing before prescription and periodically during use; vigabatrin should be used with great caution when a pre-existing visual field defect is demonstrated (Russell-Eggitt et al 2000).

Follow-up of children with hydrocephalus treated by a shunting procedure is important (Ramadan et al 1997) because deterioration of visual functions is often associated with shunt failure, when ophthalmological signs may precede neurological symptoms.

Epilepsy surgery often causes visual field defects (Nagata et al 2006, Powell et al 2006), and visual field measurement assists evaluation of the child's subsequent quality of life.

Behavioural techniques to assess and quantify the visual field in children under the age of 4 years and in children with neurological impairment have therefore become important. The most commonly used techniques are described below.

History-taking: what do we ask the parents?
One can obtain the first indication for the presence of a visual field defect from history-taking (see Chapter 8.1).

Confrontation method and binocular directional preference
The confrontation method consists of jiggling fingers in the four quadrants of the field of view and registering the child's reactions (Good et al 1994, Buckley 1995). Instead of fingers, Stycar balls (van Hof-van Duin and Mohn 1987, Good 1993) or toys (Mercuri et al 1996b) are also used.

The peripheral vision test, also called binocular directional preference (Groenendaal et al 1988), easily determines the side of preference (Fig. 5.2). The child sits on either a chair or the parent's lap while an observer in front of the child attracts attention to a central target. When the child is fixating steadily, the examiner, standing behind the child, moves two white balls mounted on thin black sticks simultaneously and at the same speed right and left from behind the child. The movement is made along the horizontal meridian and is interrupted as soon as the child has shown the side of preference. Any orientating reactions, such as eye movements or eye and head movements in the direction of one of the balls, are considered a response. Five consecutive trials are necessary to test a directional preference for the left or the right side (Hermans et al 1994). This technique detects homonymous visual field defects, but is not accurate for follow-up.

The kinetic double-arc perimeter
The kinetic double-arc perimeter can be used to assess the horizontal or diagonal meridians of the visual field. The child is held with the head at the centre of the perimeter (Fig. 5.3). A white ball at a distance of 36cm is brought to the attention of the child, while a second identical ball mounted on a thin black stick is slowly moved from the periphery towards the centre

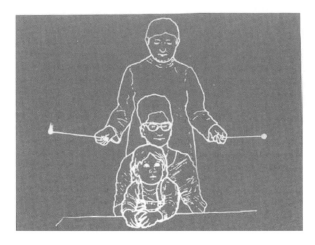

Fig. 5.2 The binocular directional preference test. Reproduced, with permission, from Sheridan MD (1976) *Stycar Vision*. Windsor: NferNelson Publishing Co. Ltd.

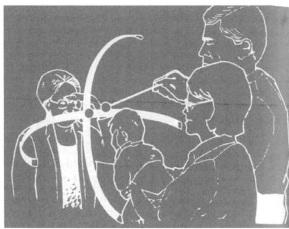

Fig. 5.3 The kinetic double-arc perimeter. Reproduced, with permission, from Schwartz TL (1987) *Vision Research*, Vol. 27, no. 12. Elsevier Science Ltd.

along one of the four arms of the perimeter. An examiner, hidden behind a large uniform black screen, observes the child's reactions. Reflex eye or head movement towards the peripheral ball is used to estimate the borders of the visual field.

By using this technique, several authors have shown that this attentional visual field reaches adult values around the age of 2 years (Heersema et al 1989, Buncic 1991, Wilson et al 1991, Pott 1992, Sireteanu 1996).

The double-arc perimeter has widely been used for testing peripheral vision in healthy and sick children (Groenendaal and van Hof-van Duin 1990, Quinn et al 1991, Fetter et al 1992, Lewis et al 1992, van Hof-van Duin et al 1992, Schiefer et al 1993, Weisglas-Kuperus et al 1993, Good et al 1994, Hermans et al 1994, Berezowsky et al 1995, Fea et al 1995, Hermans 1995, Luna et al 1995, Harvey et al 1997b, Delaney et al 2005). However, it is difficult to keep the child's head centred in the double-arc perimeter, and young children may be frightened by the black curtain.

The translucent sphere perimeter

The translucent sphere perimeter consists of a white translucent hemisphere (diameter 68cm), on the back of which are painted concentric and radial lines at 20° and 30° intervals respectively (Pott 1992, Fea et al 1995). While the child is fixating a point at the centre of the hemisphere, small spots of light are flashed or moved. Any reflex eye or head movement towards the light is used to estimate the borders of the visual field. Similar apparatus, but with yellow light-emitting diodes (LEDs) instead of painted lines distributed over the surface of the hemisphere, has also been described (Cummings et al 1987, Mayer et al 1988, Harvey et al 1997a, Delaney et al 2000). Like conventional perimetry, the translucent perimeter requires cooperation, alertness, and firm posture, which is difficult for children with neurological impairment.

BEFIE test

The BEFIE test (acronym of <u>be</u>havioural visual <u>fie</u>ld screening), conceived at the Department of Ophthalmology at the Utrecht University Hospital, Utrecht, the Netherlands, is a simple behavioural test to assess peripheral vision in children in a clinical setting (Porro et al 1998b). A uniform background is not necessary.

The child sits either on the parent's lap or in a (wheel)chair (see Fig. 5.4). The examiner stands behind the child and with one hand rotates an arc with a ball attached to its tip around the child's head, from the periphery towards the centre of the visual field. The angle at which the child first detects the presence of the stimulus (in this case the ball) determines the size of the visual field. The angle is determined by a thin straight black metal stick with a level fastened onto it at an angle of 45°, held in the examiner's other hand.

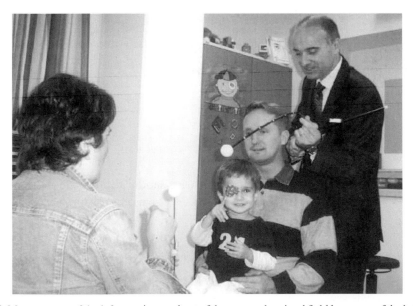

Fig. 5.4 Measurement of the left superior quadrant of the monocular visual field by means of the behavioural visual field screening (BEFIE) test. The child, who was first gazing at the fixation target, suddenly looks at the peripheral stimulus moved by the examiner.

If the child is not able to maintain a fixed head position, the parent is asked to support the chin so that the child is looking straight at the fixation target, but is allowed free movement towards the peripheral stimulus. One eye is occluded with an orthoptic eye patch for monocular testing, which, for example, is indicated in children with horizontal strabismus. An observer sits in front of the child, holding the fixation target and watching the child through a tube. This allows the observer to see the face but not the peripheral stimulus. The observer attracts the attention of the child to the fixation target. Once fixation is steady on the target, the examiner presents the peripheral stimulus by moving it along one of the four virtual diagonal meridians or the horizontal meridians from the periphery towards the fixation target.

Reactions, such as eye movements, eye and head movements, eye and hand movements, or a verbal response, are accepted. When the child reacts, the examiner stops moving the peripheral stimulus and places the thin black metal stick parallel to the child's forehead at first, and then perpendicular to the graded semicircular stick. The point indicated by the thin black metal stick on the graded semicircular stick is considered the measure in degrees of visual field extension along that meridian. Figures 5.5 and 5.6 illustrate the visual field defects that have been identified.

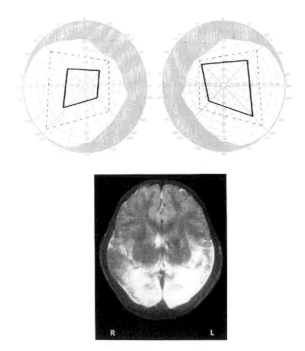

Fig. 5.5 Bilateral infarctions (left more than right) in the occipital and parietal areas. At the top is shown the patient's corresponding visual field as measured with the behavioural visual field screening (BEFIE) test; the right visual field is on the right side and the left on the left side. This child showed a constricted visual field (continuous black lines which join the diagonal meridians). The dashed lines represent the suggested normal reference values of the visual field for the age group.

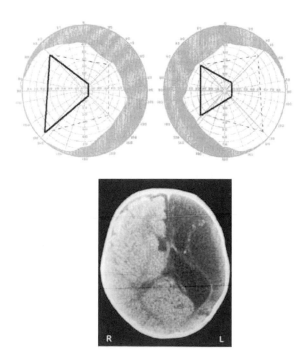

Fig. 5.6 Infarctions in the territory of the anterior and middle cerebral artery with severe ventricle dilatation on the left side. At the top is shown the patient's corresponding visual field as measured with the behavioural visual field screening (BEFIE) test; the right visual field is on the right side and the left on the left side. This child showed a right homonymous hemianopia (continuous black lines which join the diagonal meridians). The dashed lines represent the suggested normal reference values of the visual field for the age group.

The BEFIE test is accepted by very young children or children with neurological impairment as friendly play. It is relatively cheap, portable, suitable for children who have abnormal posture or are confined to a wheelchair, and excellent in a clinical setting. However, it takes time to learn.

Visual field defects in children with cerebral visual impairment
Most cases of CVI arise from hypoxic–ischaemic injury to watershed areas of the brain. In the preterm infant the watershed areas are in the subcortex around the ventricles (Keeney et al 1991, Barkovich et al 1995, Edmond and Foroozan 2006), whereas in the term infant the watershed areas are between the major arteries with injury to the subcortex and cortex (Uggetti et al 1996, Casteels et al 1997, Hoyt 2003, Edmond and Foroozan 2006, Lowery et al 2006).

On magnetic resonance imaging (MRI), different patterns of damage along the retrochiasmatic visual pathways are observed, such as infarctions, periventricular leucomalacia (PVL), and ventricular dilatation.

In children with very low birth weight, and in those who sustained perinatal hypoxia, restriction of the visual fields has been described with partial recovery in time, probably representing delayed visual maturation (Groenendaal and van Hof-van Duin 1990, Jacobson and Dutton 2000). In many cases of PVL, both hemifields are affected (bilateral lesions) and the defect is often more pronounced in the inferior field (Jacobson et al 2006).

The optic radiations that serve the lower visual field lie above and adjacent to the occipital horns of the lateral ventricles, where they are susceptible to damage by PVL. The greater the degree of PVL, the greater the extent of the lower visual field loss. This suggests that the fibres serving the lowermost visual field are closest to the lateral ventricles. The optic radiations serving the upper visual field follow a sigmoid course through the temporal lobes and are less likely to be damaged by PVL (Dutton et al 2004).

Brain ischaemia in term-born infants tends to cause 'watershed' infarcts of cerebral cortex in the boundary zones between major vascular territories (Uggetti et al 1996, Casteels et al 1997, Hoyt 2003, Lowery et al 2006). Ischaemic lesions most commonly involve either the frontal or parieto-occipital regions at the posterior parasagittal area, and the visual cortex is particularly susceptible (Brodsky et al 1996). Occipital infarction or ischaemia may cause partial or complete quadrantanopia or hemianopia, chequerboard quadrantanopia, temporal field constriction, or homonymous scotomata (Walsh 1990).

Multiple widespread small hypoxic–ischaemic lesions in the retrochiasmatic visual pathways can cause multiple homonymous scotomata, resulting in islands of vision in homonymous hemianopia (Kasten et al 1999) or in a Swiss-cheese visual field (Good et al 1994). This may, in turn, explain certain visual behaviours as 'overlooking' and 'avoiding'.

Visual dysfunction in the scotomatous or hemianopic field is commonly incomplete (e.g. for motion but not form perception, or for stationary targets but not for moving or flickering targets) (Kupersmith 1993).

Interestingly, some children with CVI may detect and localize targets within a blind region of their visual field. This phenomenon, called 'blindsight', could be due to small areas of functioning visual cortex (Kasten et al 1999), intact function in the motion detection brain (see Chapter 1), or extrageniculate (subcortical or collicular) visual potential (Lim and Siatkowski 2004, Boyle et al 2005).

Ventricular dilatation can be caused by intraventricular haemorrhage or hydrocephalus, or both (Brodsky et al 1996, Dyet et al 2006). In hydrocephalus, or shunt malfunction, damage to the posterior visual pathway presumably results from compression of the posterior cerebral arteries against the tentorium (Arroyo et al 1985, Brodsky et al 1996). This is thought to produce laminar necrosis of the visual cortex (Brodsky et al 1996). Patients with hydrocephalus may show a spectrum of visual impairment with a variety of visual field defects, including homonymous hemianopia (Brodsky et al 1996). CVI as a result of hydrocephalus may be transient or episodic, presumably because of vascular dysfunction mediated by intracranial hypertension (Brodsky et al 1996).

Brain plasticity and visual field loss in children with cerebral visual impairment: result of a retrospective clinical study

The authors have retrospectively analysed the files of 313 children with neurological impairment tested in the last decade at the Paediatric Neuro-Ophthalmological Center of the Utrecht University Hospital, Utrecht, the Netherlands. The ages of the children varied from 8 months to 16 years (range 6y; SD 3y 3mo). Brain imaging (MRI and CT) showed that 139 (44%) were suffering from CVI.

In 266 (85%) of the 313 children, the BEFIE test could successfully be performed, either monocularly or binocularly; the other 47 children could not be tested because of a lack of fixation. Conventional static (Peritest or Humphrey) or kinetic (Goldmann) perimetry was possible in only 13 cases.

Of the 139 children with CVI, 28% had a normal peripheral field. A visual field defect was found in the other 72%; in 31% this was a homonymous hemianopia, in 20% a concentric loss, in 11% an inferior quadrantanopia, and in 10% a temporal defect. In most of the children with CVI the defect was correlated with the neuroradiological defect of the retrochiasmatic visual pathways.

In accordance with the literature, roughly half of the 83 children with spastic hemiplegia had homonymous hemianopia in addition to the hemiparesis and hemisensory loss (Porro et al 1999, Prayson and Hannahoe 2004, Kedar et al 2006, Zhang et al 2006).

Several signs of neuronal plasticity of the visual system were evident, probably because of functional reorganization or (subcortical) re-routing of neuronal axons through non-damaged parts of the visual pathways, a phenomenon that seems to occur frequently after early brain damage (Hertz-Pannier 1999, Lachenmayr 2006). For instance, visual field defects diminished with time in 10 children (7%), varying between decrease in the defect size (seven children) and complete normalization (three children). This amelioration occurred at a mean age of 64 months. Three children with extensive visual cortical damage had developed normal visual fields by a mean age of 6 years.

Interestingly, 34 children with a homonymous hemianopia or quadrantanopia showed several types of ocular motor adaptations, such as exotropia or torticollis towards the side of the homonymous field defect. These ocular motor adaptations, probably based on activation of primitive reflexes (Brodsky 2002), are supposedly developed to achieve a better vision of the surrounding world (panoramic vision). According to several authors, the beneficial effect of such a compensational posture of the eyes and the neck should not be discouraged because correction of divergent strabismus or torticollis could, for example, diminish the binocular visual field (Herzau et al 1988, Fielder 1993, Gote et al 1993, Quah and Kaye 2004). On the other hand, one can imagine that inferior oblique muscle overaction could exacerbate the effect of a homolateral inferior temporal quadrantanopia and could warrant treatment (G. Porro, personal communication, 2005). Amelioration of a visual field defect and ocular motor adaptations are indicative of plasticity of the visual system.

Future developments: objective diagnosis of visual field defects and plasticity of the visual system

The newer neuroimaging techniques, such as functional MRI (fMRI), high-resolution fMRI, diffusion tensor imaging (DTI), and white matter fibre tracking (WMFT), have recently provided insights into the topography and functional organization of the visual pathways and make possible in vivo reconstruction of white matter fibre pathways (Hoon et al 2002, Clark et al 2003, Hüppi and Dubois 2006, Mori and Zhang 2006).

Event-related fMRI can facilitate retinotopic mapping of the human cortex. A rotating chequerboard visual stimulus of all quadrants of the field of view creates a travelling wave of neuronal activity within retinotopically organized visual areas. The fMRI signal caused by this stimulus is measured and the results are denoted by colour images of the flattened cortical sheet. In this way, the cortical representations of discrete visual stimuli can be identified within V1 and the extent of tissue serving the visual field can be determined objectively (Tootell et al 1998, Conner et al 2004).

Study of functional neuronal reorganization after (early) brain damage could be helpful to gain more insight into the cortical plasticity of the visual system in children (Watts et al 2003, Matthews et al 2006). This could lead, in turn, to the development of a rehabilitation programme with probable beneficial effects when introduced during the first years of life (Sonksen et al 1991). Unfortunately, fMRI requires cooperation, steady fixation, and body control, which is problematic for children with neurological impairment.

Many authors describe saccadic training as a means of improving a visual field defect (Hyvarinen 2002, Sabel et al 2004, Poggel et al 2006, Pelak et al 2007). However, cooperation is a prerequisite and the results are controversial (Horton 2005, Reinhard 2005).

Concluding remarks

Although the effect of training of visual functions after (early) brain damage is not known and is controversial, we commend parents to encourage visual search by presenting, for example, toys and food in the impaired field of view. When the child is able to ride a bicycle, we suggest attaching a mirror to bring the defective field into view. In order to naturally bring about saccades towards the blind (hemi)field, we advise placing the car seat on the side of the field defect.

We instruct schoolteachers on positioning of the child in the classroom and during reading tasks. In fact, reading seems to be more difficult when left-sided homonymous hemianopia or quadrantanopia is present because of difficulties in finding the beginning of the next line. However, recent studies have shown that reading speed is lower with right hemifield disorders (Safran and Landis 1996).

Measuring and quantifying visual field defects in children with neurological impairment is a fascinating task that is, however, possible only with sufficient cooperation of the child, at a time when the child is capable of stable fixation, and with the use of appropriate devices.

Preliminary data seem to point to the existence of plasticity of the field of view. Further studies are necessary to conceive of more reliable techniques for measuring the visual field in children as well as to give answers to questions about plasticity in response to (early) damage of the visual system.

Summary

The visual field is an assessment or measure of the area that can be seen simultaneously by the eye(s) at any one moment.

Focal damage to the visual system can cause lack of vision in part of the visual field. The pattern of this is closely related to the site and extent of the underlying damage. In cerebral visual impairment, visual field impairment is common. The area of lack of vision is commonly upside down and back to front with respect to the site of the causative brain damage, and is similar for both eyes (or homonymous). Most commonly, damage to one side of the brain can lead to lack of visual field on the other side, whereas damage to the top of the brain at the back on both sides (just above the lateral ventricles in the posterior parietal area) leads to lack of the lower field of vision. Narrowing (or constriction) of the overall visual field is also common.

History-taking, as described in Chapter 8, can provide evidence of visual field impairment.

Confrontation and behavioural methods observe a child's visual responses to a moving target in each quadrant of the visual field. Ideally, the examiner examines from behind while an observer watches for the responses. The target is moved across the visual field in each quadrant until a response is obtained. When a visual field defect is suspected, the repeatability of the observation is tested by moving the target at right angles to the expected boundary of the visual field defect, from the non-sighted to the sighted area.

Visual field impairment and its distribution can be estimated using manual equipment in children from the age of 4–6 years and automated equipment from the age of 7–8 years.

Acknowledgements

It is a pleasure to thank Professor O. van Nieuwenhuizen, child neurologist, and Mrs D. van der Linden, orthoptist, for participation in the study.

This work was made possible by the kind financial support of the ODAS Stichting, Delft, the Netherlands.

Addendum

The term 'visual field *loss*' is used when brain damage is acquired. 'Visual field *impairment*' is a more apposite term for visual field deficits present from birth, as no vision has been lost.

6
ABNORMALITIES OF REFRACTION AND ACCOMMODATION AND THEIR MANAGEMENT

J. Margaret Woodhouse

Long sight, short sight, and astigmatism (collectively called refractive errors) and errors of focusing (defective accommodation) are much more common amongst children with disabilities, including those with brain injury. This chapter will address issues surrounding the high prevalence of these errors, their detection, and their management.

Typically developing children show a wide distribution of refractive errors at birth, and the distribution narrows during the first few years of life. Figure 6.1 shows classic data on

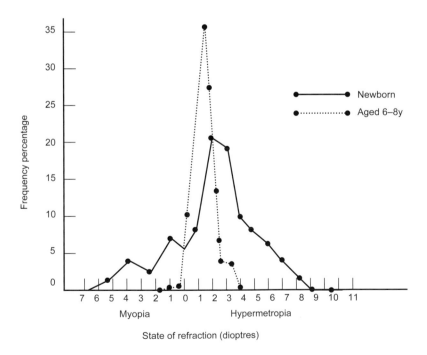

Fig. 6.1 Distribution of refractive errors amongst young children at birth and 6–8 years (Hirsch and Weymouth 1991).

spherical refractive errors (long and short sight) of newborns and children aged 6–8 years that illustrate this marked change.

By primary school age, most children's refractive state clusters around 0 to 1 dioptre (emmetropia or low hypermetropia). Only about 6% of children in Western countries have errors sufficient to warrant spectacle correction at school age. The process by which children grow out of the infantile errors is known as 'emmetropization'. The mechanism is not fully understood, but it is known to be an active process (rather than passive growth) that (in animal studies) requires a reasonable level of vision.

The distribution of refractive errors among newborns is statistically normal, whereas the distribution among older children is far from normal, being highly peaked around emmetropia. The refractive state of an eye is determined by a combination of factors, mainly the curvature of the cornea, the power of the lens, the depth of the anterior chamber, and the axial length of the eye. All of these factors must have the appropriate relative value in order for light to be focused at the retina (i.e. for the eye to be emmetropic). Amongst older children, each of these components has a normal distribution, while the combination of the factors (the overall refractive state) does not. When children have a refractive error, it is usually the axial length of the eye that is out of alignment with the other components. In general, hypermetropic (long-sighted) eyes have a short axial length, whereas myopic (short-sighted) eyes have a long axial length (see Fig. 6.2).

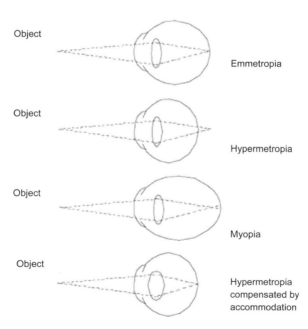

Fig. 6.2 Diagrammatic representation of refractive errors.

Published studies of refractive errors amongst children with brain injury appear to be restricted to children with cerebral palsy and to children with cerebral visual impairment (CVI). The prevalence of 'significant' errors in cerebral palsy has been reported as 76% (Altman 1966), 60.9% (Lo Casio 1977), 40% (Duckman 1979), and 50% (Black 1982). Such figures must be treated with caution because the criteria for a 'significant' refractive error differ amongst studies and none of the studies published comparative data from typically developing children. Some of the studies set the criteria for hypermetropia as low as >+1.00D. It is quite clear from Figure 6.1 that the majority of control children would thus be classified as having a 'significant' refractive error! A 'significant' refractive error would more usefully be defined as one that warrants spectacle correction in the usual case – but even this is not straightforward to determine. Although guidelines exist, such as those published by the American Academy of Ophthalmology in its 'Preferred Practice Series', the values are arrived at by consensus and are not evidence based. The American Academy makes the point that 'there are no scientifically rigorous published data for guidance' (American Academy of Ophthalmology 2002).

The most useful data on refractive errors amongst children with cerebral palsy are those presented alongside values for age-matched comparison children, and the most comprehensive are provided in an unpublished PhD thesis by McClelland and are reproduced in Figure 6.3.

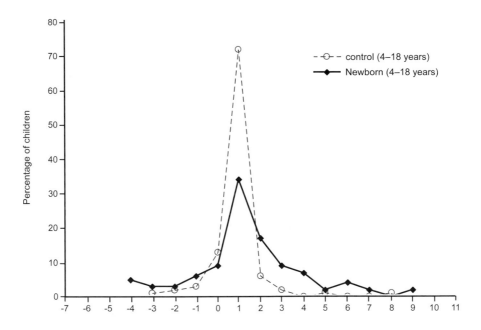

Fig. 6.3 Spherical refraction amongst 128 typically developing children and 95 children with cerebral palsy, both groups aged 4–18 years (McClelland 2004).

As Figure 6.3 shows, mean refractive error is similar in both groups, but the children with cerebral palsy show a much higher prevalence of both myopic and hypermetropic refractive errors. Defining significant hypermetropia as ≥+3.00D and myopia as ≤–0.50D (which might be considered reasonable limits for spectacle prescription in children of school age), McClelland reported a prevalence of 40% amongst children with cerebral palsy and 9.5% amongst comparison children. Astigmatism, too, was more common amongst children with cerebral palsy in McClelland's study. Defining significant astigmatism as ≥1.00D, the prevalence was 36% amongst the cerebral palsy group and 4% amongst the comparison group.

Children with CVI have been studied as part of a larger group of children with visual impairment. Du et al (2005) reported that, amongst 224 children with CVI, 70% had 'significant' refractive errors, defined as ≥1.00D. Remembering that the peak refraction in typical children lies at +1.00D, this is not a useful statistic. However, the authors do quote published normal values from the literature of <20%. In the Du et al (2005) study, other groups of children with visual impairment show similar high prevalence of refractive errors, so it is not clear whether it is the association with poor vision or the brain injury that is the important factor.

Thus, children with brain injury (at least those with cerebral palsy) are at greater risk for refractive errors of all three types (myopia, hypermetropia, and astigmatism) than are typically developing children. The aetiology of the refractive errors has yet to be established but as brain injury happens most commonly at or around the time of birth, it is reasonable to assume that the distribution of refraction at birth is similar in these children to that amongst comparison children. It follows, therefore, that the high prevalence of refractive errors at school age represents a failure of the emmetropization process.

Measuring refractive error
The standard procedures for measurement of refraction in typical adults and older children are static retinoscopy followed by subjective questioning. Neither process is feasible for young children or those with cognitive impairment; instead, the two alternative techniques of cycloplegic and Mohindra retinoscopy are used.

Cycloplegic refraction involves using drops to paralyse the muscles that control accommodation (focusing) and thus make the refractive state stable. It is, of course, an invasive technique that is uncomfortable or even distressing for the child. The Mohindra technique relies on the observation that, in total darkness, the eyes adopt a stable small amount of accommodation (that can be predicted and taken into account; Saunders and Westall 1992). The technique is therefore much more child-friendly, and it is also quick because there is no waiting time for drops to take effect.

Studies show that the cycloplegic and Mohindra techniques give equivalent findings in infants and children (Saunders and Westall 1992, Woodhouse et al 1997). However, the greatest advantage for the Mohindra technique comes from allowing measurement of near functions and accommodation on the same occasion. Cycloplegic refraction, on the other hand, because it sets out to prevent focusing at near, requires a second visit if near functions are to be considered.

Accommodation

Accommodation is the process by which the eye adjusts focus for the different distances of viewing. When the object of interest is at distance (usually defined as 6m or more from the viewer), the lens within the eye is in its thinnest, least powerful, state. When the object of interest comes close, the eye accommodates and the lens thickens and becomes more powerful, by virtue of the action of the ciliary muscle, which surrounds the lens. In this way, objects at all distances can be brought into sharp focus, although there is a limit to the amount by which the lens can change shape, giving rise to the 'near point', the closest distance at which the eye can focus. The lens becomes more rigid throughout life, so that with increasing age the near point recedes. Most people are familiar with the onset of 'presbyopia' (difficulty in focusing at near) that seems to happen suddenly as middle age approaches. In fact, the deterioration in near point is progressive from childhood; the apparent sudden onset happens when the near point coincides with one's usual reading distance.

Accommodation can be used to overcome hypermetropia. By exerting the appropriate amount of accommodation, the image in a hypermetropic eye that would otherwise fall behind the retina (Fig. 6.2) can be brought into sharp focus at the retina.

Most typically developing children will have a very close near point and ample accommodation to carry out sustained near tasks. They can also compensate for low to moderate amounts of hypermetropia and, as Figure 6.1 suggests, most do. Thus, guidelines for prescribing refractive corrections for children tend to set the criterion on the hypermetropic side to quite high amounts. For example, the American Academy of Ophthalmology (2002) sets the hypermetropic criterion to ≥+4.50D for 2- to 3-year-olds. In addition, it is standard practice for hypermetropic prescriptions to be reduced by 1.00–2.00D, leaving the child with a small amount of error that can be overcome by accommodation. (The above criteria apply to children without strabismus. When a strabismus exists, the criterion for prescribing may be set lower and the full hypermetropic prescription given; a comprehensive discussion of prescribing for strabismus is beyond the scope of this chapter.)

When prescribing refractive corrections for children with brain injury, there is no justification for failing to correct errors on the grounds that learning or cognitive impairment limits ability and there is no need for spectacle correction. At the very least, practitioners should use the same criteria for prescribing as they would for typically developing children. However, as accommodation is often defective in children with brain injury, there may be valid grounds for prescribing spectacles more readily in these children than in ordinary children.

As with refractive errors, the literature on accommodation amongst children with brain injury is confined to those with a diagnosis of cerebral palsy. Further, some studies have relied on assessment of the near pupil response to estimate accommodation (e.g. Altmann et al 1966), which may be unreliable. The most recent studies have used direct measures of accommodative accuracy by dynamic retinoscopy. It is an objective technique which does not rely on a child's verbal responses and which can therefore be used with even the youngest or least able child. Because this will be an unfamiliar technique for many practitioners, it warrants a full description.

The child wears his or her distance refractive correction if appropriate and looks at a target designed to stimulate accommodation – this may vary with the age and ability of the child but could incorporate pictures with fine detail. The target is presented at a close distance (most usefully the child's habitual working distance) mounted on a rule. The retinoscope is placed alongside and the practitioner notes the reflex. If the retinoscopy reflex is neutral, the child is accommodating accurately. An 'against' movement indicates over-accommodation, whereas a 'with' movement indicates under-accommodation. Keeping the target still, the practitioner moves the retinoscope (towards the child in a case of over-accommodation and further from the child in under-accommodation) to find the neutral point. This represents the point to which the child is actually accommodating. The distance between the target and the neutral point (converted to dioptres) is the discrepancy in accommodative accuracy. The technique has been shown to be a valid and repeatable technique when compared with autorefraction measures of accommodation (McClelland and Saunders 2003). Leat and Gargon (1996) measured accommodation at three distances in 43 individuals with cerebral palsy (aged 3–35 years) and compared responses with control data reported separately (Leat and Gargon 1996). Accommodative responses were outside the normal range in 42% of participants, all showing under-accommodation. McClelland et al (2006) used the same technique and viewing distances with 85 children with cerebral palsy and 125 normal comparison children (all of school age), with mean results shown in Figure 6.4.

When comparing the data with normal ranges, McClelland et al reported that only 42% of the children with cerebral palsy showed normal accommodation at all three distances. Whilst some children with cerebral palsy appear to have the ability to focus and to sustain focusing on near tasks, the majority do not.

Figure 6.4 shows mean values and demonstrates that, on average, a child with cerebral palsy observing a target (such as school work) at 17cm will be out of focus by 2.00D

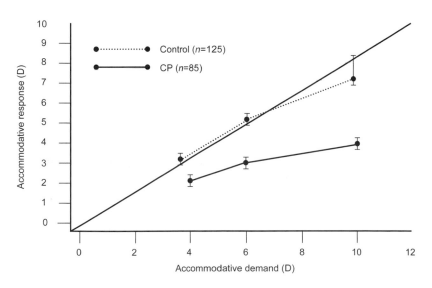

Fig. 6.4 Accommodative responses recorded by dynamic retinoscopy among school-age children with cerebral palsy and control children (McClelland et al 2006).

– a considerable disadvantage for learning. Poor accommodation also has implications for hypermetropia. Although this has not been directly measured, it is a valid assumption that children who cannot accommodate accurately for near tasks may be unable to accommodate to overcome hypermetropia. These children may, therefore, require spectacle correction for small amounts of hypermetropia that would not be needed for a typically developing child.

It is therefore essential that eyecare practitioners, when dealing with children with cerebral palsy (and other forms of brain injury), consider accommodation as a routine part of the eye examination. The decision on prescribing for a refractive error, particularly hypermetropia, must take accommodation into account. Practitioners should not assume that all children can overcome small amounts of hypermetropia, or can focus well on near tasks.

Aetiology of the accommodative deficit

No studies have yet addressed this issue, but sensory or motor defects may be involved. Children with visual impairment are more likely to have an accommodative deficit than children with normal vision (Leat and Mohr 2007). Reduced visual acuity leads to a greater depth of focus, and a greater optical blur can be tolerated. However, the under-accommodation shown in children with visual impairment usually exceeds that predictable on depth of focus alone. Leat (1996) showed that, amongst her participants with cerebral palsy, poor visual acuity was the factor 'most strongly associated with reduced accommodation', so a sensory deficit may contribute in brain injury too. Similarly, McClelland (2004) found a significant association between the accommodation deficit and visual acuity. However, almost 20% of Leat's participants with good acuity also showed poor accommodation, so acuity does not provide the full explanation.

A motor deficit would imply poor control of the accommodative response. Leat (1996) described 'physical ability' (estimated by walking ability from parental reports) as associated with accommodative deficits in her subject group. McClelland (2004) showed that children with more severe motor impairments (as noted from medical records) were more likely to have accommodative deficits. However, in McClelland's study, under-accommodation was also associated with intellectual and communication disabilities. It is likely, therefore, that the aetiology of poor accommodation in children with brain injury is multifactorial.

Managing reduced accommodation

If an accommodation deficit persists when there is no distance refractive error, or when distance errors are corrected, then an additional correction for near tasks should be considered. Separate near glasses, bifocals, or varifocals are all feasible strategies for children. Small-scale studies of children with cerebral palsy show the benefits and success of near corrections (Ross et al 2000, McClelland 2004). Children with Down syndrome are also at risk of accommodative deficits (Cregg et al 2001), although the aetiology of the problems may be quite different. Children with Down syndrome wear bifocals successfully and gain benefit in terms of accommodative accuracy (Stewart et al 2005).

Aetiology of refractive errors

As described above, studies have reported a high prevalence of refractive errors amongst children with cerebral palsy and children with visual impairment (including CVI). Children with Down syndrome are also at risk of refractive errors. All three populations also exhibit accommodative deficits. It is tempting to assume a causal relationship between refractive errors and accommodative deficits. Children with Down syndrome who have accurate accommodation are much more likely to be emmetropic (Stewart et al 2007). McClelland (2004) reported a significant association between accommodative dysfunction, hypermetropia, and astigmatism in cerebral palsy, which, by implication, suggests that children with good accommodative responses are more likely to be emmetropic. Animal studies suggest that successful emmetropization requires a focused retinal image (Nevin et al 1998), so we can imagine that in humans, too, only eyes with a good accommodative response can undergo the emmetropization process. However, the data from children with Down syndrome show that the children with accurate accommodation are emmetropic in early infancy, rather than acquiring emmetropia (Stewart et al 2007) and, to date, no longitudinal studies of refractive error progression exist for cerebral palsy. We are, therefore, some way from understanding the relationship between refractive error and accommodation.

Summary

Children with brain injury are at greater risk than typically developing children of refractive errors (long sight, short sight and astigmatism) and defective accommodation (focusing for near tasks). Refractive errors and accommodation can readily be measured in a routine eye examination, by practitioners experienced in dealing with children. Spectacle correction for defects can, and should, be considered for all children.

7
CLINICAL FEATURES OF PERCEPTUAL AND COGNITIVE VISUAL IMPAIRMENT IN CHILDREN WITH BRAIN DAMAGE OF EARLY ONSET

Gordon N. Dutton, with Elisabeth Macdonald, Suzannah R. Drummond, Shohista Said-kasimova, and Katherine Mitchell

Introduction

The human visual system is served by an input system and a processing system. The input system connects the eyes to the occipital lobes, and its disorders are well understood by the ophthalmic professions (Hoyt and Good 2001). Disorders of the processing system, however, are complex and may be elusive, and thus may not be identified.

Damage to the visual brain can impair visual acuity and contrast sensitivity, and may restrict visual fields (Good 2001, Matsuba and Jan 2006), whereas damage to the higher visual processing centres causes perceptual and cognitive visual impairment. These visual systems can be damaged separately, or together, resulting in poor acuity, visual field impairment, and perceptual visual dysfunction in any combination or degree. Perceptual visual impairment can also occur in the context of normal visual fields and normal or near-normal visual acuities. Such damage may affect white or grey matter or both, and cause visual dysfunction, which varies in nature and degree. In children this can cause multiple problems, including impaired recognition of people and shapes and objects, orientation difficulties, difficulty handling complex visual scenes, and inaccurate visual guidance of limb movement (Dutton et al 1996, 2004, Jacobson et al 1998, Gronqvist et al 2001). The visual system may be the only part affected, or there may be associated damage to other brain structures, resulting in cerebral palsy and/or other developmental problems.

Cerebral visual impairment (CVI), which is now the most common cause of visual impairment in children in developed countries, is increasing in prevalence, probably as a result of improved perinatal care and survival of young children with profound neurological disease. Moreover, the diagnosis is increasingly being recognized.

As described in Chapter 2.1, many causes of brain damage in early childhood can produce CVI. The most common are periventricular leucomalacia (Jacobson et al 2002, Kapellou et al

2006), hypoxia and ischaemia, hydrocephalus (Houliston et al 2000), meningitis, encephalitis, traumatic brain injury, metabolic disease, and the secondary effects of drugs and radiation (Dutton and Jacobson 2001, Edmond and Foroozan 2006, Hoyt 2007).

Visual processing

Higher visual processing primarily takes place in brain areas adjacent to the occipital lobes. As described in Chapter 1, two pathways are central to this process – the dorsal and the ventral stream. The dorsal stream integrates occipital lobe and posterior parietal lobe function. It thus brings about subconscious analysis of the visual scene, integrating this with analysis of data from other sensory inputs. This brain area computes the location of components of the visual scene, and thereby facilitates visual attention and visual guidance of movement by analysing the three-dimensional spatial coordinates of what is being looked at, in order to plan and bring about movement of the body and, via the frontal eye fields, to generate rapid, accurate head and eye movements to chosen targets in the visual scene. When a part of the scene is chosen, for example a pen, the information is passed to the frontal lobes, where the choice is made for the head and eyes to look at it. The pen's coordinates are passed to the motor cortex, which initiates hand movement and accurate reach with pre-adjustment of finger position to grasp the pen (Goodale and Milner 2004). As described in Chapter 1, this process is automatic, 'online', accurate, and rapid, is not afforded conscious awareness, and is not founded in memory, and thereby allows us to move through, and interact with, the surrounding world with immediacy.

The posterior parietal cortex contributes significantly to attentional visual function. Severe bilateral posterior parietal pathology gives rise to simultanagnosia, in which there is profound difficulty registering the presence of any object which is not being attended to. Affected individuals are unable to interpret the totality of the scene despite a preserved ability to see individual portions of the whole picture. It is not possible to move the eyes from one element of a scene to another, probably because the multiple elements are not seen. This inability to move the eyes voluntarily from one element of the scene to another, despite having a normal substrate for bringing about eye movement, is called apraxia of gaze. This is commonly accompanied by impaired visual guidance of movement (optic ataxia). The acquired condition in adults is known as Balint syndrome (Drummond and Dutton 2007). Visual neglect on one side, most commonly on the left, is seen as a sequel to unilateral, particularly right-sided, posterior parietal damage.

The ventral stream connects the occipital lobes to the temporal lobes, which contain the brain's 'visual library'. Information transmitted here allows recognition and visual memory of what is being looked at. Recognition of faces involves visual information passing along the ventral stream into the temporal lobes (commonly the right), where it is compared with data concerning all known faces stored in the fusiform gyrus. If there is a match, the face is recognized. Recognition of shape and form and the ability to recognize and follow routes are likewise temporal lobe functions.

Damage can affect any part of this overall visual system, giving rise to a wide range of patterns of visual dysfunction (Trobe and Bauer 1986, Stasheff and Barton 2001).

The clinical features of visual–perceptual dysfunction in children
Knowledge concerning how the human higher visual system works and is affected by disease is primarily founded in the plethora of literature which describes the specific visual dysfunctions that arise following focal damage to the visual adult brain. This is backed up by the results of experimental work. On the other hand, when pathology affects the developing visual brain, the resultant behavioural manifestations resemble those described in the adult literature, but they are different in nature and degree. The reasons for this include the following.

- Early-onset damage to the brain is commonly diffuse in nature, and thus affects a range of functions.
- Brain growth and development, and brain recovery taking place after the injury, probably modify the manifestations significantly by affording a degree of recovery.
- The behavioural adaptations which the developing child makes to compensate for focal brain dysfunction affecting vision may mask the underlying deficit, unless that specific dysfunction is stressed, by either tiredness or a scenario which isolates the disordered function.
- Habilitational strategies may enhance both functional and behavioural adaptations.
- All young children 'know' that their vision is 'normal' to them, and thus they do not present with visual symptoms. The visual problems are inferred from their behaviour.
- Parents may accept their child's visual performance as 'normal' because he or she grows up with it. This can result in criticism of the child's visual behaviour, which in turn affects the child, who cannot understand what is wrong and cannot 'improve'.

Thus, adult models of interpretation of the features of cognitive visual dysfunction in children have significant limitations, and models of interpretation founded upon observation of children's visual behaviour are needed to provide the foundation for both diagnosis and management of affected children. This subject is in its infancy. Most psychological visual testing strategies tend to be founded upon a presumption of normal visual acuities and visual fields (which is commonly not the case in children with damage to the visual brain). They are also designed to detect aberrance from 'normality'. Apart from specifically designed strategies of investigation (Chapter 8), they are not designed to identify specific dysfunctions, and to characterize and quantify them. Thus, there is a paucity of investigations which can be employed to characterize the wide range of perceptual and cognitive visual problems that parents commonly describe in their children. Detailed history-taking (Chapter 9) can reveal the nature and degree of the visual problems, which can then be corroborated by observation of the child's behaviour in the appropriate contexts.

Performance in tasks requiring visual search, visual attention, and visual guidance of movement can be reduced on account of tiredness, distraction, and stress, presumably on account of diminished functional reserve. This results in considerable day-to-day variation in performance in these areas, which may be incorrectly attributed to lack of concentration.

PERCEPTION OF MOVEMENT

The centres serving perception of movement are found in the middle temporal lobes, in the region of the occipitoparietal–temporal junction. Bilateral damage can cause impaired or absent perception of movement. Only the static visual world is appreciated in this situation. In contrast, individuals in whom this area is intact, despite severe damage to the occipital lobes, may exhibit movement perception as the only visual function because function persists in this area in addition to the areas responsible for reflex visual perception – the superior colliculi and the pulvinar (Goodale and Milner 2004).

Recent research has shown that damage to the periventricular white matter in the parieto-occipital region causes difficulties with perception of the forms of motion required to recognize biological movement (Pavlova et al 2006), and that some aspects of motion perception can be deficient (e.g. the perception of linear motion) while other aspects (such as seeing radial and circular motion) may be intact in children with periventricular white matter pathology on brain imaging (Morrone et al 2008).

DORSAL STREAM DYSFUNCTION

Table 7.1 lists the common visual problems which are seen, often in combination, as a sequel to impaired dorsal stream function. The ability to handle complex visual data improves with age. If this is dysfunctional, the child may demonstrate difficulty in finding an object of interest when the visual scene is too complex, for example a toy in a toy box or on a patterned bedspread (Dutton et al 1996). A similar problem arises with food mixed together or presented on a patterned plate. Seeing objects in the distance is difficult, as the further away things are, the more visual information there is in the scene. For this reason, children with dorsal stream dysfunction like to get very close to the television, presumably so that they can give visual and auditory attention to the individual elements of the moving scene. Busy environments like supermarkets, shopping centres, or swimming pools present complex visual scenes. Children may react to such environments in different ways, becoming either frightened or disruptive.

Reading may be affected, particularly when print size diminishes and print crowding increases with each school year. The progressive crowding of the text increases the complexity of the visual scene. (Spectacles for long-sightedness magnify, which diminishes crowding. Children with mild problems accessing text on account of visual crowding are often helped by wearing a spectacle correction for long-sightedness, which would not normally be prescribed.) Copying information can be very difficult. Impaired visual search means that it is difficult to find the place both in the text to be copied and in the text to be written, while the requirement to employ visual memory, and difficulties splitting attention between these two tasks, can render the overall exercise extremely difficult.

Inaccurate movement through three-dimensional space may occur. Mobility problems result from an inability to differentiate a floor boundary (e.g. between carpet and linoleum) from a step. The child is reluctant to cross it without prior careful exploration. Black-and-white tiled floors can be frightening and large patterns on carpets can be difficult to cross. Stairs and kerbs are problematic as the foot is lifted to the wrong height, too early or too late. Going down stairs can be particularly difficult because of difficulty in judging depth. Inaccurate

TABLE 7.1

Features of dorsal stream dysfunction

Feature	Problems
Impaired ability to handle complex visual scenes	Finding a toy in a toy box
	Finding an object on a patterned background
	Finding an item of clothing in a pile of clothes
	Finding food on a plate
	Seeing a distant object
	Reading, particularly crowded text
	Identifying someone in a group
	Tendency to get lost in crowded locations
Impaired visually guided movement	Negotiating floor boundaries
	Walking over uneven surfaces
	Negotiating steps and kerbs, particularly going down
	Using escalators, with problems getting on and off
	Inaccurate visually guided reach
	Colliding with obstacles
Impaired attention	Performing more than one visual task at a time
	Performing a visual and an auditory task at once
	Marked frustration at being distracted

reach and grasp may also manifest. Such specific impairment of visually guided movement has been ascribed the term 'optic ataxia'.

Attention is often impaired. This becomes evident when the child has to simultaneously perform more than one task, such as talking and walking. This can cause marked frustration at being distracted, to the extent that a child with dorsal stream dysfunction who is trying to work hard and who is disturbed may react violently.

The range of visual dysfunction in children because of impaired dorsal stream function is considerable. Children with profound visual impairment associated with quadriplegic cerebral palsy may appear to be able to attend to only one aspect of a visual scene at a time, and this may explain why they respond well to a single illuminated target in a darkened room. At the other end of the spectrum is the preterm child who is unable to see his mother in a group of people when he is being collected from school, and who relies on his unaffected twin to do this for him, yet has no other visual difficulties.

There appears to be a wide range of expression for dorsal stream dysfunction, in which any or all of the features listed in Table 7.1 may be manifest, in any combination or degree. Dorsal stream dysfunction has been identified as being a significant complication in children born very preterm, both with and without the radiological identification of periventricular white matter pathology (Fazzi et al 2004, Jakobson et al 2006, Atkinson and Braddick 2007). It is also a feature of Williams syndrome (Atkinson et al 2004) and explains the visual behaviours of affected children, who may well benefit from the strategies described in Chapter 15 and the appendix of this book.

It is likely that, as knowledge of this specific form of visual dysfunction develops, a range of other disorders, such as those within the autistic spectrum disorder in which impairment of movement perception has been identified (Milne et al 2005), will be found to show evidence of dorsal stream dysfunction, which may in part explain the behaviours. For example, in our clinical experience, children with dorsal stream dysfunction associated with periventricular pathology find it difficult to look at people's faces while communicating (perhaps because of difficulties splitting their auditory and visual attention) and they commonly line up their possessions as an adaptive strategy to impairment in visual search.

VENTRAL STREAM DYSFUNCTION

Table 7.2 lists the visual difficulties which are seen in children with ventral stream dysfunction. Recognition problems commonly result in difficulty identifying faces (Dutton et al 1996). The child may be unable to recognize even close family members or people seen out of context. This may also lead to identification of strangers as being known. Identification of people in photographs is challenging, as is seeing, interpreting, and understanding the meaning of facial expressions. Similar difficulties include identifying animals, objects, shape, and form.

Orientation problems are common and affect route finding. The child may get lost and require help, even in well-known locations. The difficulties are more marked in new environments, such as shops or hotels, resulting in the child becoming frightened, withdrawn, or disruptive. Children with impaired orientation due to ventral stream problems have great difficulty finding their way around, even in places they have been many times before. (In contrast, children whose dorsal stream dysfunction makes it difficult to find their way around in crowded environments are able to orientate themselves and know where they are and where they are going when there are few distractions.)

Ventral stream dysfunction usually accompanies dorsal stream dysfunction; but, when there is extensive bilateral damage to occipito-temporal pathway damage from an early age, the paradox is created in which an affected person appears not to be able to know what he is looking at, but has remarkably good visuomotor abilities (Lê et al 2002) (Chapter 1).

TABLE 7.2

Features of ventral stream dysfunction

Feature	Problems
Impaired recognition	Recognizing people in person or in photographs
	Interpreting the language of facial expression
	Recognizing animals
	Recognizing shapes and objects
Impaired orientation	Getting lost in both known locations and new environments

Variability of dorsal and ventral stream dysfunction

Unlike visual acuity, which tends to remain stable, disorders of dorsal and ventral stream function in children with damage to the brain tend to be fatiguable, with better visual performance in the morning while the child is wide awake and poorer visual performance towards the end of the day when the child is tired. If the child is distracted and thinking about other things, visual function suffers. Thus, the visual difficulties are typically very variable, which can lead to misinterpretation and misunderstanding.

Case histories

The following set of four anonymous case histories give examples of the typical visual difficulties experienced by children with posterior periventricular white matter pathology on magnetic resonance imaging (MRI) (Saidkasimova et al 2007), and the fifth and sixth case histories describe how early-onset focal hypoxic–ischaemic encephalopathy can cause profound dorsal stream dysfunction similar to that described in adult Balint syndrome (Drummond and Dutton 2007). The sixth case shows evidence of additional ventral stream dysfunction.

PATIENT 1

A male, aged 4 years 6 months, with mild spastic diplegia was born at term with normal delivery despite a threatened labour at 29 weeks' gestational age. His visual acuities were 20/20 in each eye unaided. He presented with a history of tripping over obstacles, frequent falls, and difficulty with steps, stairs, and kerbs greater than expected from his motor disability alone. He was described as not reacting to fast-moving objects such as traffic. He could not identify an item of clothing in a pile of clothes or find a chosen toy either in a toy box or against a patterned background such as a carpet or a bedspread. He was frightened of crowded environments and had difficulty combining tasks such as watching television and talking. It was difficult to break his attention. He had peripheral lower visual field impairment on visual field examination to confrontation. MRI performed at the age of 3 showed limited posterior periventricular white matter injury (Fig. 7.1a and b).

PATIENT 2

This male, aged 4 years 6 months, born at full term, had developmental delay, intellectual disability and partial seizures – controlled on medication when required – and a partially accommodative convergent strabismus. His visual acuities were 20/25 in each eye unaided. His problems included difficulty handling complex visual scenes: he did not tolerate crowds, which precipitated temper tantrums; he had difficulties seeing objects in the distance; finding toys on a patterned background; and identifying his mother (whom he recognizes well) in a group of parents. He also had visuomotor difficulties: he often tripped over obstacles and had difficulty negotiating kerbs and going up and down stairs. He had a short attention span and was easily distracted. Neuroimaging at the age of three demonstrated the presence of moderate periventricular white matter injury (Fig. 7.1c and d).

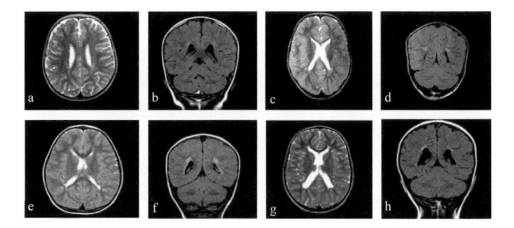

Fig. 7.1 (a–h) These images comprise paired horizontal and vertical transverse (coronal) MRI scans from patients 1 to 4 described in the text. They show very similar patterns of evidence of white matter damage adjacent to the lateral ventricles. (a) Mild periventricular leucomalacia (PVL) (patient 1). T2-weighted axial image of brain at the level of the lateral ventricles demonstrates increased signal in the posterior periventricular white matter of the centrum semiovale bilaterally. The ventricles are of normal size. (b) Mild PVL (patient 1). Fluid-attenuated inversion recovery (FLAIR) coronal image of brain through the posterior lateral ventricles. There is abnormal periventricular white matter signal bilaterally, corresponding to the area identified on the T2-weighted axial sequence (a). (c) Moderate PVL (patient 2). T2-weighted axial sequence of brain at the level of the lateral ventricles. There are features of established PVL, with abnormal increased signal in the peritrigonal white matter. There is white matter volume loss, especially on the right, and this is associated with some irregularity of the ventricular contour. (d) Moderate PVL (patient 2). FLAIR coronal sequence of brain shows abnormal increased signal in the posterior periventricular white matter, adjacent to the trigones. (e) Moderate PVL (patient 3). T2-weighted axial image of brain shows features of moderately severe established PVL, with abnormal periventricular white matter signal, deep white matter loss, and some irregular outline of the ventricular margins. (f) Moderate PVL (patient 3). FLAIR coronal image of brain shows abnormal periventricular white matter signal bilaterally around the trigones of the lateral ventricles. (g) Marked PVL (patient 4). T2-weighted axial image of brain at the level of the lateral ventricles, showing features of severe established PVL. There is abnormal increased signal in the peritrigonal white matter and extending into the centrum semiovale. There is loss of periventricular white matter and ventriculomegaly with irregular outline of the ventricular walls. (h) Marked PVL (patient 4). FLAIR coronal image of brain through the trigone region of the lateral ventricles. This shows the abnormal increased periventricular white matter signal, lateral ventricular dilatation, and central white matter loss.

PATIENT 3

This 9-year-old male with partial seizures (controlled with carbamazepine) was born at 36 weeks' gestational age. He had no recorded neurological deficit. His vision was 20/30 right eye (RE) and 20/17 left eye (LE) with a small hypermetropic correction (+1.50 RE, +0.75 LE). He had difficulty walking over kerbs and going down stairs and frequently tripped over obstacles. He also had difficulty seeing moving objects, and identifying objects in a crowded environment. His behaviour always became difficult in a crowd. He struggled to read crowded text and frequently missed out words. MRI at the age of 4 demonstrated the presence of moderately severe periventricular white matter injury (Fig. 7.1e and f).

PATIENT 4

This female, aged 5 years 6 months, was born at 34 weeks' gestation. Her neonatal period was complicated by jaundice and she required tube feeding in the intensive care unit. Her neurological examination was normal. She had undergone bilateral medial rectus recessions for congenital esotropia. Her visual acuities were 20/32 in each eye with correction of +3.00/+0.50 at 90° for both eyes. By the age of 5 it became apparent that she had difficulties walking over uneven ground or going down stairs or a slope. She occasionally reached incorrectly for things. She appeared to have difficulty seeing moving objects and had problems in crowded visual scenes. She had considerable difficulty identifying her mother in a small group of people (but could do so without difficulty on a one-to-one basis) and locating objects that were pointed out in the distance. She easily lost her way in new locations, but had no problems with orientation in places which she knew. She had difficulty combining tasks and became very frustrated if she was distracted while engaged in another activity. MRI at the age of 5 showed marked periventricular white matter injury (Fig. 7.1g and h).

PATIENT 5

The following case history describes a male with simultanagnostic visual behaviour as a sequel to perinatal hypoxia causing damage both to the optic nerves and to the posterior parietal area of the brain, bilaterally (Drummond and Dutton 2007).

A 7-year-old male was known to have visual impairment as well as intellectual disability and a communication disorder. He had been born at 38 weeks' gestation after an uneventful pregnancy. He was of low birth weight (2.2kg) and developed neonatal hypoglycaemia. At 72 hours, he sustained a respiratory arrest from which he was resuscitated. He subsequently developed poor vision with nystagmus.

On initial ophthalmic assessment, he was accorded a 'diagnosis' of bilateral optic atrophy. At the age of approximately 4 years, a 'normal MRI of the brain' was reported. Two years later, he was referred to the regional paediatric ophthalmology centre for assessment of possible glaucoma. At this time, his binocular visual acuity was measured at 6/30 (logMAR). There was manifest horizontal uniplanar jerk nystagmus and no ocular deviation. There was no objective evidence of congenital glaucoma and the bilateral optic disc pallor was attributed to neonatal hypoglycaemia, autosomal dominant optic atrophy, or an intrauterine event.

When seen in another centre the following year, vision was measured at 6/60 with both eyes open. The patient was unable to identify a 10mm white target in any part of the lower visual field below the horizontal midline. He had slightly reduced contrast sensitivity but normal colour vision, indicating good optic nerve function. He was able to recognize objects and was well orientated, but showed marked difficulty viewing complex scenes: he could not find an object on a patterned background; although he could read, he could not find a word in a page of words; in a crowd, he could go up to the wrong person thinking that she were his mother, although ordinarily he would not have problems recognizing known faces; and he was unable to identify toys in his toy box.

He was unable to judge the edge of the pavement and was unable to tell whether or not a boundary between floor coverings was a step (even when looking directly at it) and had to test it with his foot. Thus, to compound his lower field loss, he appeared to have difficulty using vision to guide lower limb motion. As all these problems could be attributed to a specific dorsal stream disturbance commonly caused by a superior/posterior parietal lobe insult and, because the previous MRI had been reported as normal, review of the MRI at the original hospital was requested (Fig. 7.2).

The following report was issued: 'There is evidence of atrophy and encephalomalacia affecting the posterior parietal and the superior aspects of the occipital lobes bilaterally. There is loss of white matter bulk in this region. There appear to be mature areas of ischaemic damage in the parietal and occipital regions bilaterally.' The child was diagnosed as having additional cerebral visual impairment, and appropriate additional assistance was provided.

PATIENT 6

A female first presented at the age of 5 years with a history of bumping into things just in front of her and treading on objects on the floor. She had difficulty negotiating steps and kerbs. She had been born weighing 2.6kg with an Apgar score of zero, and ultrasound examination showed evidence of cerebral oedema. By the age of 6 it became evident that she could not identify a close friend or relative in a group, and had additional difficulty recognizing faces. Copying words and drawings was difficult, as was naming colours and identifying basic shapes. These difficulties remained evident by the age of 15, when visual acuities, contrast sensitivity perception and stereopsis were all normal, but the Goldmann visual fields were significantly constricted to 30°. Problems using vision to guide movement and to find things in a complex scene had persisted, as did problems recognizing people. These findings are consistent with a pattern of combined dorsal and ventral stream dysfunction. MRI showed evidence of 'cerebromalacic change in the right occipital lobe, superomedial to the occipital pole of the right lateral ventricle'.

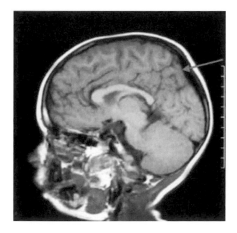

Fig. 7.2 Vertical anteroposterior (sagittal) section of MRI, revealing evidence of damage (atrophy and encephalomalacia) affecting the top of the brain at the back (the posterior parietal and the superior aspects of the occipital territory [arrow]).

115

Conclusion

These case histories show how children with focal dysfunction of perceptual and cognitive visual dysfunction are disabled by their poor vision. Additional problems due to diminished visual acuities, constricted visual fields, cerebral palsy, and intellectual disability lead to further difficulties, which need to be borne in mind when helping such children fulfil their potential.

Classically, visual impairment due to damage to the brain includes reduced visual acuities and causes visual field impairment. Dysfunction of higher visual function in children is being increasingly recognized. The clinical model which describes impairment of both dorsal stream and ventral stream function not only facilitates initial diagnosis through history-taking, but also improves understanding of the wide range of day-to-day difficulties experienced by affected children. This, in turn, provides a structure to allow habilitational strategies to be custom designed for each child.

Addendum

Parental consent has been given to publish these case histories, and consent has been accorded by the *Journal of American Association for Pediatric Ophthalmology and Strabismus* to publish the illustrations.

8
IMPAIRMENT OF COGNITIVE VISION: ITS DETECTION AND MEASUREMENT

8.1 STRUCTURED CLINICAL HISTORY-TAKING FOR COGNITIVE AND PERCEPTUAL VISUAL DYSFUNCTION AND FOR PROFOUND VISUAL DISABILITIES DUE TO DAMAGE TO THE BRAIN IN CHILDREN

Gordon N. Dutton, with Julie Calvert, Hussein Ibrahim, Elisabeth Macdonald, Daphne L. McCulloch, Catriona Macintyre-Beon, and Katherine M. Spowart

A large proportion of the human brain is employed to analyse and understand the visual world, and to visually guide movement of the body. The occipital lobes process visual information serving resolution, colour and contrast perception, visual field analysis, and perception of movement. As described in Chapter 1, higher visual processing primarily takes place in the posterior parietal lobes (which analyse the complexity of the visual scene and guide body movement) and the temporal lobes (which serve visual recognition and route finding). Damage to these areas, or their interconnecting pathways, limits their function, causing characteristic visual behaviours. Children with such damage from early childhood tend to be unaware of visual difficulties, but observation of their behaviour by parents and carers provides information that can help lead to a diagnosis which can be corroborated by further observation, neuropsychological testing, and imaging. The data obtained can be employed to plan habilitative strategies.

The mechanisms within the human brain responsible for vision are complex. However, a simplified working model of the higher visual pathways provides a means of thinking about the questions to ask concerning children whose brain dysfunction causes visual behaviour which may be difficult to understand and manage (Fig. 8.1.1).

Retinal image data are conveyed by the primary visual pathways, via the lateral geniculate bodies and the optic radiations, to the occipital cortex, where primary visual processing takes place. In addition, subconscious visual processing takes place in the superior colliculi and pulvinar of the thalamus, which also receive visual input (Grusser and Landis 1991).

Damage to the primary visual pathways and the occipital lobes results from a range of causes (Chapter 2) and leads to impairment of the basic functions of visual acuity, colour and contrast perception, detection, and analysis of motion and the visual fields (the pattern of visual field defect usually allows identification of the site of damage) (Dutton 2003).

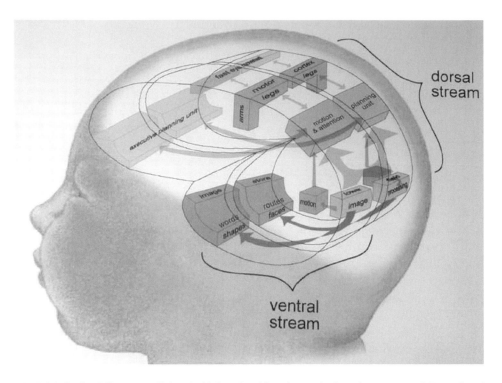

Fig. 8.1.1 Stylized diagram outlining the higher visual functions and where they are served. Reproduced with permission from Dutton (2003).

The posterior parietal lobes serve the functions of overviewing a visual scene; identifying an element within it, giving attention and bringing about gaze towards that element, as well as 'online' subconscious visual guidance of movement of the body through the three-dimensional world. Damage to this area of the brain impairs three visual functions: the ability to identify an element, such as an object or person, within a crowded scene (simultanagnostic visual dysfunction); the ability to accord selective visual attention; and the ability to bring about visually guided movement (optic ataxia) (Milner and Goodale 1995, Gillen and Dutton 2003, Dutton et al 2004, Goodale and Milner 2004). The temporal lobes of the brain serve recognition of what is being looked at and route finding. Damage impairs these functions (Trobe and Bauer 1986). Thus, it is difficult or impossible to recognize people's faces (prosopagnosia), to recognize objects such as the family car (object agnosia), and to distinguish one animal from another. This may be associated with profound impairment of the ability to route find (topographic agnosia).

These visual problems can occur in any degree or combination. During the last 20 years, we have seen a large number of children with damage to the brain leading to visual symptoms consistent with both dorsal stream and ventral stream dysfunction (with dorsal stream dysfunction being more common) (Dutton et al 1996, Houliston et al 1999). The children's

TABLE 8.1.1

Inventory of questions to ask parents/carers of children with cerebral visual impairment and acuities of 6/60 or better

For each of the items listed, the box which best accords with the child's behaviour is ticked.
Question 23 relates to the final category of questions but is located where it fits conceptually with its position in the questioning strategy.

		Never	Rarely	Sometimes	Often	Always	N/A
Questions seeking evidence of visual field impairment or impaired visual attention on one or other side							
Does your child...							
1. trip over toys and obstacles on the floor?							
2. have difficulty walking down stairs?							
3. trip at the edges of pavements going up?							
4. trip at the edges of pavements going down?							
5. appear to 'get stuck' at the top of a slide/hill?							
6. look down when crossing floor boundaries, e.g. where lino meets carpet?							
7. leave food on the near or far side of their plate?	near/far						
If so, on which side?							
8. leave food on the right or left side of their plate?	right/left						
If so, on which side?							
Does your child...							
9. have difficulty finding the beginning of a line when reading?							
10. have difficulty finding the next word when reading?							
11. walk out in front of traffic?							
If so, which side?	right/left/both						
12. bump into doorframes or partly open doors?							
If so, which side?	right/left/both						
13. miss pictures or words on one side of a page?							
If so, which side?	right/left/both						

TABLE 8.1.1 (continued)

Inventory of questions to ask parents/carers of children with cerebral visual impairment and acuities of 6/60 or better

	Never	Rarely	Sometimes	Often	Always	N/A
Questions seeking evidence of impaired perception of movement						
Does your child...						
14. have difficulty seeing passing vehicles when he or she is in a moving car?						
15. have difficulty seeing things which are moving quickly, such as small animals?						
16. avoid watching fast-moving TV?						
17. choose to watch slow-moving TV?						
18. have difficulty catching a ball?						
Questions seeking evidence of difficulty handling the complexity of a visual scene						
Does your child...						
19. have difficulty seeing something which is pointed out in the distance?						
20. have difficulty finding a close friend or relative who is standing in a group?						
21. have difficulty finding an item in a supermarket, e.g. finding the breakfast cereal he or she wants?						
22. get lost in places where there is a lot to see, e.g. a crowded shop?						
23. get lost in places which are well known to him or her?						
24. have difficulty locating an item of clothing in a pile of clothes?						
25. have difficulty selecting a chosen toy in a toy box?						
26. sit closer to the television than about 30cm?						
27. find copying words or drawings time-consuming and difficult?						

Questions seeking evidence impairment of visually guided movement of the body and further evidence of visual field impairment						
28. When walking, does your child hold on to your clothes, tugging down?						
29. Does your child find uneven ground difficult to walk over?						
30. Does your child bump into low furniture, such as a coffee table?						
31. Is low furniture bumped in to if it is moved?						
32. Does your child get angry if furniture is moved?						
33. Does your child explore floor boundaries (e.g. linoleum/carpet) with his or her foot before crossing the boundary?						
34. Does your child find inside floor boundaries difficult to cross?						
34a. If so... boundaries that are new to him or her?						
34b. ... boundaries that are well known to him or her?						
Questions seeking evidence of impairment of visually guided movement of the upper limbs						
35. Does your child reach incorrectly for objects, i.e. does he or she reach beyond or around the object?						
36. When picking up an object, does your child grasp incorrectly, i.e. does he or she miss or knock the object over?						
Questions seeking evidence of impaired visual attention						
37. Does your child find it difficult to keep to task for more than 5 minutes?						
38. After being distracted does your child find it difficult to get back to what he or she was doing?						
39. Does your child bump into things when walking and having a conversation?						
40. Does your child miss objects which are obvious to you because they are different from their background and seem to 'pop out' (e.g. a bright ball on the grass)?						

121

TABLE 8.1.1 (continued)

Inventory of questions to ask parents/carers of children with cerebral visual impairment and acuities of 6/60 or better

	Never	Rarely	Sometimes	Often	Always	N/A
Questions seeking evidence of behavioural difficulties associated with crowded environments						
41. Do rooms with a lot of clutter cause difficult behaviour?						
42. Do quiet places/open countryside cause difficult behaviour?						
43. Is behaviour in a busy supermarket or shopping centre difficult?						
44. Does your child react angrily when other restless children cause distraction?						
Questions evaluating the ability to recognize what is being looked at and to navigate						
Does your child....						
45. have difficulty recognizing close relatives in real life?						
46. have difficulty recognizing close relatives from photographs?						
47. mistakenly identify strangers as people known to them?						
48. have difficulty understanding the meaning of facial expressions?						
49. have difficulty naming common colours?						
50. have difficulty naming basic shapes such as squares, triangles, and circles?						
51. have difficulty recognizing familiar objects, such as the family car?						

visual behaviours, as described by parents, vary considerably, but they are consistent, and it has become apparent that history-taking can often lead not only to an appreciation of the location of the damage, but also to an understanding of the underlying visual dysfunction and approaches to compensate for the visual problems.

This section of the chapter describes approaches to structured history-taking from parents of children with cerebral visual impairment (CVI) and measurable visual acuities, and from parents of those with profound visual impairment. These models have been assembled as a sequel to our team having seen large numbers of affected children. The information accrued not only facilitates identification, further investigation, and diagnosis, but also contributes to management plans. The question sets are designed for use with children who show evidence of CVI, for example otherwise unexplained reduced visual acuities, or peripheral lower visual field impairment, and positive responses must be clarified and properly interpreted.

Structured clinical history-taking inventories

Structured history-taking is a foundation of medical practice. While the questioning strategies for many medical diagnoses are internationally recognized and applied, there are no standardized question sets for CVI.

Assessment of a child's visual behaviour is limited by time and the child's behaviour at the time. Parents and carers have a long-term perspective and experience of their child's behaviour, which they commonly volunteer. However, they can be unaware that their child's behaviour could be related to visual dysfunction, or they may not even recognize the problem, having grown up with it.

We have found structured history-taking for visual difficulties to be indispensable both in identifying perceptual and cognitive visual dysfunction and in delineating the pattern of visual disability. The information obtained can help guide the design of appropriate educational and habilitative strategies.

We have developed two question inventories which we use routinely.

1   Seven sets of questions, which have been assembled and validated for reliability. These help to characterize the visual problems and complement the results of measurement of visual function and assessment of the child (Table 8.1.1). They can be employed for those with visual acuities of 6/36 to 6/60 or better. They seek evidence of:

- visual field impairment, or impaired visual attention on one side;
- impaired perception of movement;
- difficulty handling the complexity of a visual scene (dorsal stream dysfunction);
- impairment of visually guided movement of the body (dorsal stream dysfunction) and further evidence of visual field impairment;
- impaired visual attention (dorsal stream dysfunction);
- behavioural difficulties or distress associated with crowded environments; and
- the ability to recognize what is being looked at and to navigate by means of visual recognition (ventral stream dysfunction).

The responses which are sought comprise 'Never', 'Rarely', 'Sometimes', 'Often', 'Always', and 'Not applicable'. The questions are designed in such a way that the answer 'Always' indicates the greatest dysfunction. Ongoing investigation is showing reliability and consistency.

When using this inventory it is common to find a set of difficulties highlighted by one or two groups of questions. Features of dorsal stream dysfunction without ventral stream dysfunction are commonly elicited. Such children have considerable difficulty entering a crowded environment such as a supermarket or a children's party and may react adversely. Combined dorsal and ventral stream dysfunction is the next most common, while isolated ventral stream dysfunction related to bilateral temporal lobe dysfunction is, in our experience, rare.

There are a number of potential confounders to the interpretation of the results. For example, children with poor hearing may get close to the television in order to hear better, and children with intellectual disability may have disabilities which are identified by this form of history-taking, while children with lower limb motor problems also have difficulty with steps and pavements. We have also elicited positive responses in children with autistic spectrum disorder. This is a topic which warrants future study. Thus, expertise is required to interpret the responses in the context of the child as a whole and to avoid incorrect diagnosis. Nonetheless, although the underlying causation of unusual visual behaviour may not be strictly 'visual' in origin, consistent identification of specific visual disabilities can guide management.

In our experience, a small group of questions which probe the range of visual difficulties that are described most frequently provides a rapid clinical method of identifying children who warrant more detailed evaluation. The answers to the following five questions provided no false positives and no false negatives. Positive responses (of 'Often' or 'Always') were obtained for three or more of these questions in all cases in a series of 40 children with cognitive and perceptual visual impairment, whereas no more than one such positive response was obtained from an unaffected control population of over 150 children.

Q2. Does your child have difficulty walking down stairs?

Q18. Does your child have difficulty seeing things which are moving quickly, such as small animals?

Q19. Does your child have difficulty seeing something which is pointed out in the distance?

Q24. Does your child have difficulty locating an item of clothing in a pile of clothes?

Q27. Does your child find copying words or drawings time-consuming and difficult?

Further research is required to develop and define optimal clinical questioning strategies which both assist diagnosis and provide useful information to guide management.

VISUAL SKILLS INVENTORY

Name:

Please help us by answering the questions relevant to your child and bring this to your next visit.

SPECTACLES (please tick)

		Yes	No
1	Should your child wear spectacles?		
2	Does he or she wear them?		

PATCHING

		Yes	No
3	Does your child wear an eye patch?		
4	Is it difficult to patch the eye?		
5	Do you understand why your child's eye is patched?		

VISION

		Yes	No
6	Does your child follow your movements around a room when you give him or her no sound clues?		
7	Does he or she react to you approaching him (without sound clues)?		
8	Does he or she react to a light being switched on? (Making sure there is no sound of the switch.)		
9	Does he or she screw up his eyes when taken into bright sunlight?		
10	Does he or she return your smile when you smile without any sound?		
11	Does your child reach for a drink bottle when you hold it in front of him or her?		
	Does he or she become excited but does not reach for the drink bottle?		
12	Is he or she aware of a spoonful of food coming towards his or her mouth?		
	If yes, do you think he or she sees it?		
	... smells it?		
	... or both?		

Figure 8.1.2 Inventory of questions asked for children with profound cerebral visual impairment

		Yes	No

13	Is he or she aware of himself in a mirror?
	If yes, at what distance:
	   6 feet?
	   4 feet?
	   3 feet?
	   2 feet?
	   1 foot?
	   less?		

Please tick

		Yes	No
14	Does your child reach for a small bright noisy object (e.g. rattle, slinky)?		
15	Does your child reach for a large bright noisy object?		
16	Does your child reach for a small bright silent object?		
17	Does your child reach for a large bright silent object?		

18	Does he or she see a large silent bright object (e.g. ball)?
	If yes, at what distance:
	   more?
	   4 feet?
	   3 feet?
	   2 feet?
	   1 foot?		

19	Does he or she see a small silent bright object (e.g. toy)?
	If yes, at what distance:
	   12 inches?
	   6 inches?
	   3 inches?
	   nearer?		

20	Does your child's vision seem better in bright light? Or in dim light?		
21	Do you think your child knows and recognizes your face?		
22	Does he or she recognize other faces of familiar people?		

Figure 8.1.2 (continued) Inventory of questions asked for children with profound cerebral visual impairment

2   A separate set of questions to help characterize profound visual impairment (Fig 8.1.2). These children can manifest variable visual function or may not be able to oblige. The responses to the questions closely relate to behavioural and electrophysiological measures of visual function, and provide a means of corroborating or even substituting for measurement (McCulloch et al 2007). They can also assist management planning.

THE USE OF QUESTION INVENTORIES

Structured history-taking is standard practice in many branches of medicine. The lists of questions are not questionnaires because the concepts being explored are complex and often require additional discussion with the parents/carers to clarify what is meant by both the questions and the responses.

An efficient way to use these question inventories is to supply one in advance of the clinic visit, or in the waiting room. Positive responses can then be identified, clarified, and acted upon.

Parents may not have thought about their adaptations to their child's behaviour because they have evolved slowly. Structured questioning can help parents become aware of how they have adapted to their child's behaviour. This can help them understand their child's problems. Providing the questions in advance allows parents and carers to consider the salient issues and to discuss the responses with teachers and carers. They often volunteer additional unique information about their child's visual behaviour and adaptations.

The patterns of visual dysfunction elicited by structured history-taking are unique for each individual. This information guides subsequent observation of the child's visual behaviour, and the choice of tests of perceptual visual function, as required, to validate the clinical diagnosis (Steirs et al 1999, 2002, Fazzi et al 2004, Atkinson and Braddick 2007). The combined information can then be used to design the management plan, which takes into account all the visual and behavioural difficulties (Dutton 2003). The question sets are not fully comprehensive and other visual difficulties may need to be considered.

A major benefit of interpretation and explanation of the responses to structured history-taking is that a child's behaviours, which were ill understood or even criticized (e.g. 'Look where you're going!', 'Pay attention, your shoes are right in front of you!') are now understood, and it is often like a light bulb being switched on. The resultant change in parents' behaviour can much improve a child's self-confidence and self-esteem.

The reader is welcome to use these question inventories (and to modify them as required), with the recommendation that they are used by trained personnel only because interpretation and use of the information in the correct context is essential.

Examples of common 'symptom complexes' elicited by this strategy

The 6-year-old male has dorsal stream dysfunction due to posterior parietal pathology occurring as a sequel to a respiratory arrest during the first week of life, giving rise to focal hypoxic–ischaemic encephalopathy. He is able to recognize friends and relatives, but cannot find a toy in a toy box (compensating by tipping out the toy box to find the one he wants, or calling a parent to do this for him) nor can he see something pointed out in the distance (the farther away things are, the more there is to see). He is unable to identify his mother in a small group of people but is able to recognize her on a one-to-one basis and in photographs. The child has a full visual field yet has to probe the ground ahead with his foot at floor boundaries outside the home, in order to elicit whether a step is present or not. The floor boundaries at home are well known and cause no problems. If furniture at home is moved it is bumped into. The parents do not take their child to the supermarket because they know that he will not be able to cope with excessive auditory and visual stimulation, yet he is happy sitting quietly in the countryside fishing with his father. The visual problems are worse in the evening when the child is tired, and the parents describe a more marked visual problem than the teacher does. Recognition that dorsal stream dysfunction clinically impairs overall information processing of both auditory and visual information means that simplification of presentation of all forms of information may reap dividends.

A 10-year-old female was born at 26 weeks' gestation and developed intraventricular haemorrhage, causing hydrocephalus and requiring a shunt. This child cannot recognize close relatives, such as her mother, and has great difficulty understanding the meaning of facial expressions. For this reason, she does not look people in the eye when they are talking to her, and she is getting into trouble for this. The underlying reason is damage to the right temporal lobe.

8.2 OBJECTIVE BEHAVIOURAL AND ELECTROPHYSIOLOGICAL MEASURES FOR ASSESSING VISUAL BRAIN FUNCTION IN INFANTS AND YOUNG CHILDREN

Janette Atkinson and Oliver Braddick

Introduction

Cerebral visual impairment should not be considered an all-or-nothing phenomenon. The brain basis of visual processing is complex, and perinatal brain injury can lead to a range of deficits from profound impairment to more subtle deficits of specific visual functions. Evaluation of impairment cannot be restricted to the basic sensory processes of vision; the boundaries between these and wider perceptual, cognitive, spatial, and motor function are not well defined and, in any case, what is important for the child is the way that visual impairment may impact on integrated cognitive and sensory motor function.

The rationale behind our research is to develop safe, reliable measures of assessment over the entire range of visual abilities. Some tests are for specific visual deficits, related to the development of particular eye–brain mechanisms. A broader goal is to gauge brain plasticity in recovering from early brain damage, and to assess the value of visual measures as 'early infant surrogate outcome measures' in predicting later cognitive outcome and assessing the effectiveness of early treatment and intervention. These approaches have been reviewed by Atkinson (1989, 2000) and Atkinson and van Hof-van Duin (1993). They have been applied to infants who have undergone hemispherectomy to relieve intractable epilepsy (Braddick et al 1992, Morrone et al 1999), to infants born very preterm (Atkinson 2003, Atkinson and Braddick 2007), and to infants with perinatal focal infarcts (Hood and Atkinson 1990, Mercuri et al 1996b, 1997b, 1998, 2003) and hypoxic–ischaemic encephalopathy (HIE) (Mercuri et al 1997b, 2004) and their prognostic value examined (Mercuri et al 1998, 1999, Atkinson and Braddick 2007).

The tests of cerebral visual impairment described here fall into several different categories.

- **Functional visual cortex (behavioural and electrophysiological) tests**. These gauge local cortical processing of visual attributes such as orientation and direction of movement. These are intended for use in normally developing infants, older children in this mental age range, and children with very limited communication skills.
- **Global cortical visual processing tests for infants and children**. These tests are designed to target specific visual processes beyond the level of primary visual cortex.

- **Functional vision tests**. The Atkinson Battery of Child Development for Examining Functional Vision (ABCDEFV) is designed to assess a wide range of age-appropriate visual behaviour in children whose developmental age is between birth and 5 years.
- **Attention and executive function tests**. These assess key areas of visual behaviour, and ones that are especially sensitive to neurological damage, such as maintaining and switching visual attention.
- **Spatial cognition (specifically, location memory) tests**. These assess how young children obtain, from vision, an understanding of spaces and objects around them.

Model of normal visual development

Visual defects and developmental problems can be gauged only if the normal course of development is understood. From our work on typically developing children, we have established and refined neurobiological models of early normal visual development (Atkinson 1984, 1998, 2000, Atkinson and Braddick 2003) which provide visual milestones against which to estimate the degree of delay or deficit in individual infants. Figure 8.2.1 presents a schematic of our current model. The stages, marked by numbers on the diagram, are as follows.

1. Newborn Orienting to a Peripheral Target

The newborn's subcortical visual system (in particular the superior colliculus in the posterior upper midbrain) underpins orientating to salient stimuli in the near periphery (provided there is no competition from stimuli in the central field), and tracking salient stimuli with saccadic eye movements. Another aspect of subcortical function is seen in newborns' visual optokinetic responses when viewing a large field of movement. In binocular viewing, the response can be seen in both directions, but with monocular viewing the newborn shows an asymmetry in optokinetic response, with each eye giving responses only to nasalward pattern movement. This is what would be expected if it is controlled purely by a crossed subcortical pathway via the nucleus of the optic tract. The monocular response to motion in the opposite temporalward direction (away from the nose) is not seen until 3–4 months post-term age. The idea that this depends on development of a cortical pathway is supported by studies of infants with early hemispherectomy (Braddick et al 1992, Morrone et al 1999), who show a persisting asymmetry because cortical control fails to develop for the damaged hemisphere.

2. Cortical Processing: Local and Global

Processing in visual cortex can be divided into 'local' and 'global'. The input from the retina arrives first in the primary visual cortex, or area V1, where visual information is processed locally over separate small regions of space. Areas of extrastriate cortex, such as area V5, carry out global processing, integrating information over extended regions. Within extrastriate cortex, there is a major division between the dorsal and ventral streams of processing, as described in Chapter 1. The developmental model of Figure 8.2.1 indicates processes developing separately in the two streams, although we should not lose sight of the importance of coordination between the two streams in development and in everyday perception (see reviews by Atkinson 2000, Atkinson and Braddick 2003, Braddick et al 2003).

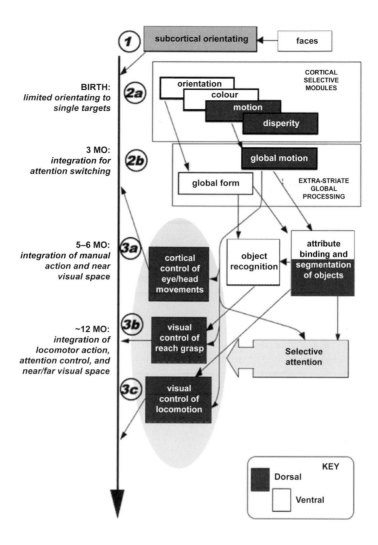

Fig. 8.2.1 Schematic of the Atkinson and Braddick model of early visual development. Functions of the dorsal and ventral streams are coded with distinctive shading. Circled numbers refer to explanatory material in the text.

2a. Local processing in V1

Detection and discrimination of colour, orientation, direction of movement, and binocular disparity depends on sensitivity in specific populations of neurons in the primary visual cortex (V1) and in extrastriate areas (e.g. V2, V3, V3A, V4, V5). Each of these cortical processes has its own functional time course in normal development within the first few months of life. Orientation and colour processing can be demonstrated in newborns in the first few weeks of life. Cortical responses that discriminate directions of movement emerge in infants over 2 months post-term age (Wattam-Bell 1991, 1992, Braddick et al 2003). Binocular correlation and disparity discrimination (three-dimensional stereo vision) can be demonstrated from 4 months post-term age, with sensitivity increasing with age (Braddick et al 1980, Birch 1993, Braddick 1996).

2b. Global processing
Global processing of different forms of information (pattern and motion) takes place in specific extrastriate cortical areas. We describe below tests we have developed, which vary the coherence of global form and motion patterns, to study the emergence of global processes in infants in the first year of life and their development during childhood.

3. ATTENTION AND ACTION MODULES
This model of human development allows not only for differential timing of functional development between the two major cortical streams, but also for differential development between different modules within each stream. In infants, the multiple 'action' modules within the dorsal stream – controlling head, eyes, arm, hand, legs, and body movements – each shows their own developmental time course (as shown schematically in Fig. 8.2.1).

3a
The first visuomotor action module to become functional controls exploratory eye movements, shifting attention through head and eye movements from one object to another seemingly 'at will'. To assess selective attention we developed the fixation shift paradigm (FS, described below).

3b and 3c
This is followed in development by the action modules controlling exploratory reaching and grasping, and then the action module controlling independent walking starts to function. Each of these action systems takes months or years to develop to adult levels. All these systems involve spatial analysis of the visual layout, but the different systems require quite different scales of spatial representation. For reaching and grasping, the infant needs only a spatial representation of space which is relatively near to the body. However, this space may need to be extended if the child starts to use tools to extend the spatial area of control of the hands in order to manipulate objects at a distance. For independent walking, both peripheral vision and spatial layout some distance from the child must be represented to enable the child to find objects in spatial locations further away than arm's length. Vestibular and peripheral optic flow information must be integrated with complex coordinated leg and trunk movements, together with mechanisms for analysing depth and distance seen in central field, for successful walking to a target location.

As well as these overt action systems, there are internal covert systems of attention and memory. While some draw an imaginary line between 'perception' and 'cognition', processes for decoding incoming sensory information rather than those for categorizing and storing this information in visual memory buffers, in this neurobiological approach it becomes a continuum, with feed-forward and feedback loops particularly involving the mechanisms of visual attention.

Within the framework of this model, the methods available to assess the different components of visual development during infancy and early childhood can be described.

Specific tests of cortical function

ELECTROPHYSIOLOGICAL MEASURES (VEP/VERP)

Visual evoked potentials (VEPs) or visual event-related potentials (VERPs) are electrical responses, picked up from electrodes on the scalp, which reflect the brain's response to visual stimuli. They do not require a controlled motor response from the child, although they do depend on the child being able to maintain gaze on the visual display. Repetitive stimulus events, of various kinds, can be presented to elicit an electrical response which can be detected

TABLE 8.2.1

Different forms of visual evoked potential/visual event-related potential recording, designed to elicit responses related to specific forms of visual processing

Stimulus	Process indicated	Age at onset	Reference
Flash	Response to light – does not depend on cortical processing	Preterm	
Pattern reversal	Response to spatial contrast – input to cortex, does not necessarily reflect cortical processing	Late preterm/term	
Orientation reversal	Local cortical pattern processing	~1–3mo (frequency dependent)	Braddick et al (1986), Braddick (1993)
Direction reversal	Local cortical motion processing	~2–3mo	Wattam-Bell (1991), Braddick et al (2005)
Onset of coherent form or motion	Global integration by extrastriate cortical mechanisms	Later than 2mo (4–6mo), global motion response before global form	Atkinson et al (2005), Braddick et al (2006), Braddick and Atkinson (2007)

as time-locked to the visual event. Flash and pattern-appearance VEPs are standard techniques in clinical electroencephalography departments. However, the use of stimulus sequences designed to pick out specific aspects of cortical processing can provide more detailed information about the development of visual mechanisms and capacities. Table 8.2.1 presents a series of different stimuli, a number of which have been developed in our own work, as indicated by the references, which elicit responses from different subcortical and cortical processes.

The conventional flash VEP usually gives a large signal–noise ratio. The response demonstrates that this child's visual system is responding to light, but cannot be interpreted as a measure of cortical function. A child with severe cortical damage may still give a strong VEP to a flash stroboscopic stimulus so long as the signal from the retina to the brain is reasonably intact. A pattern of stripes or chequerboard, reversing in contrast, indicates the presence of pattern vision. However, the simple response to contrast is characteristic of levels of processing below the visual cortex (retinal ganglion cells or thalamus), and so even though it is picked up at the input to the cortex it does not indicate that specifically cortical processes are functional. However, cortical neurons, unlike those earlier in the visual pathway, are tuned to different orientations and so a VEP response that is time-locked to changes in orientation, rather than simple contrast changes, indicates basic cortical processing and functioning (Braddick et al 1986, Braddick 1993). This is the orientation reversal stimulus (OR-VEP) in Table 8.2.1. A response to the direction reversal stimulus (DR-VEP) indicates the later-developing cortical selectivity for the direction of visual motion, which we have found to be specifically delayed in infants born preterm (Birtles et al 2007). Recently, we have developed stimulus sequences that isolate the response of higher level cortical processes to the onset of globally coherent structure, in either pattern (form) or motion displays (Braddick et al 2006); these have yet to be used in a clinical context, but we anticipate that they will enable the assessment of deficits in these higher level functions, which may be present even if local processing is intact.

Behavioural Measures of Cortical Function

Forced-choice preferential looking (FPL) and habituation methods have shown infants' ability to discriminate orientation at a few weeks of age (Atkinson et al 1988) and discrimination of directional motion from 8 weeks of age upwards (Wattam-Bell 1992, 1994). However, these methods are not well suited to individual clinical assessment. A different test of cortical function, which proves to be revealing for developmental deficits, is the fixation shift (FS) test. This measures the response time of infants to make saccadic shifts of attention, from a foveated target to one appearing in the left or right peripheral field, either when the initially foveated target disappears (non-competition) or when it remains visible (competition), and so the infant has to disengage attention from one target to attend to the other (Atkinson et al 1992). Studies with hemispherectomized infants have shown non-competition responses on both sides but specific impairment of the competition response on the side corresponding to the removed cerebral hemisphere, supporting the theory that the non-competition response can be subcortically mediated, but that cortical involvement is necessary to cope efficiently with competing targets. The FS test, therefore, provides an indicator of the maturation and asymmetries both of the subcortical mechanism, which directs attention to a salient stimulus when there is no competition, and of the cortical mechanism necessary for controlling shifts of attention under competition. Typically developing infants under the age of 3–4 months show difficulties disengaging from the central target under conditions in which the central and peripheral targets simultaneously compete for attention.

USE OF THESE CORTICAL MEASURES
We have used the OR-VEP and fixation shift under competition, in a number of clinical populations, to gauge the plasticity of recovery from early brain damage, and to predict later visual and cognitive outcome.

In very preterm infants (under 32 weeks' gestation) we found a delayed onset time for the OR-VEP response in those who showed abnormalities on cerebral ultrasound (Atkinson et al 1994), but a normal onset time in those with normal ultrasound results (Atkinson et al 2002a).

In a series of longitudinal studies on term infants with focal cerebral lesions or hypoxic–ischaemic encephalopathy (HIE), identified on neonatal serial brain MRI and neurological examination, infants with HIE more frequently manifested abnormal measures of cortical visual function (Mercuri et al 1995b, 1996b). However, poor visual outcome is not necessarily most strongly associated with specific damage to classically 'visual' areas of the brain, and certain focal lesions in early visual areas can, to some extent, be compensated for by the immature brain. Isolated lesions in specific parts of basal ganglia, as seen on MRI, were generally associated with a more severe visual outcome than isolated cortical lesions. This supports the idea that certain circuits between subcortical and cortical areas are essential for normal visual development, and that there is little plasticity of recovery in the circuits involving the basal ganglia (Mercuri et al 1997b).

In 46 term infants with brain lesions visible on MRI, we found that one-half of our cohort did not show a significant cortical OR-VEP at 5 months of age (Mercuri et al 1998). This response would normally be expected by 3 months of age (Braddick et al 1986, 2005). A total of 14% of the cohort showed continuing delayed onset of cortical function using this indicator between 6 and 12 months of age, and in 34% the VEP responses were always abnormal. Infants with focal infarction or haemorrhage on MRI tended to show normal or only mildly delayed cortical responses, while grade 2 or 3 HIE tended to be associated with persistent abnormalities of VEP responses. Ninety-six per cent of those who had shown 8Hz OR-VEP by 5 months were neurologically normal at 3 years, compared with 57% of those who attained the response by 12 months and none of those in whom it was still absent at 18 months (Mercuri et al 1998).

OR-VEP and fixation shift testing of 29 infants with HIE gave consistent prediction of Griffiths developmental quotient <80 at 2 years (OR-VEP sensitivity=100, specificity=79, positive predictive valve [PPV]=63, negative predictive valve [NPV]=100; FS sensitivity=100, specificity=59, PPV=47, NPV=100).

We have used these cortical indicators in cohorts of children born very preterm (before 32 weeks) who had undergone neonatal and term MRI. Diffuse excessive high signal intensity (DEHSI) is a common feature of the white matter in very preterm infants who are scanned around term, although it cannot be readily identified earlier or after about 3 months post term. The presence of white matter damage (either periventricular leucomalacia [PVL] or DEHSI) was noted and the degree was classified as mild, moderate, or severe depending on the extent and intensity of areas visualized with DEHSI alongside identification of focal lesions and intraventricular haemorrhage and dilatation. Some children with a diagnosis of cystic PVL were included in the group classified as severe on their MRI results. OR-VEP testing of this group of 24 such infants gave a sensitivity of 86% and specificity of 65% in predicting Griffiths developmental quotient <80 at 2 years. Fixation shift results gave similar values, showing that both tests can be useful in predicting later developmental outcomes (Atkinson and Braddick 2007, Atkinson et al 2008).

TESTS FOR GLOBAL CORTICAL PROCESSING – FORM AND MOTION COHERENCE
Integrative processing beyond primary visual cortex can be studied through the ability to detect global coherence. In a pattern like that shown in Figure 8.2.2, local processes can detect the orientation of individual line segments, but the overall circular structure can be detected only by a process that combines information across an extended area. The sensitivity of this process can be measured by testing a participant's ability to detect the structure when a percentage of the line segments are randomly orientated (60% in the example of Figure 8.2.2). In an analogous test for global motion sensitivity, the task is to detect the common pattern of movement in a display of dots, where the 'coherence' is the percentage of dots moving according to the pattern while the remaining percentage move randomly.

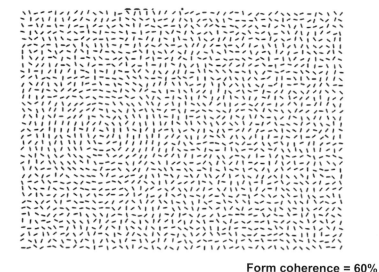

Form coherence = 60%

Fig. 8.2.2 Stimulus of the type used to test form coherence sensitivity. Within one region of the display, a percentage of the line segments are arranged tangentially to concentric circles. This percentage is the measure of 'coherence'; coherence threshold is the minimal percentage required for a participant to identify the concentrically organized region.

Neurophysiological studies of the monkey brain suggest that global processing of form and global processing of motion are functions of extrastriate areas in the ventral and dorsal streams, respectively. We have used patterns of this kind in fMRI studies on adults to locate the brain areas which respond differently to coherent versus incoherent form and motion (Braddick et al 2000, 2001). These studies show that primary visual cortex (V1) does not differentiate coherent from incoherent because its neurons respond only to the local orientation or directional motion. Independent, extrastriate brain systems are activated by global form and global motion; the motion system includes extrastriate areas V3A and V5 in the dorsal stream, and the areas activated by global form include anatomically ventral areas in the lingual and fusiform gyri. These results suggest that behavioural or VERP responses to form and motion coherence in children will be revealing about the development of the two streams.

GLOBAL PROCESSING IN INFANTS

Global motion thresholds have been measured in normal infants using preferential looking for a display of oppositely moving strips of dots with varying coherence (Wattam-Bell 1994, Mason et al 2003), showing marked improvement over 9–20 weeks of age, following the age at which direction discrimination first emerges (Wattam-Bell 1992, 1994). These results suggest that very soon after local motion signals are first processed in the developing brain, the processes which integrate them into global representations are operating quite efficiently. It may be that the connectivity between V1 and extrastriate areas on which this integration is based exists early, at least in a crude form, awaiting the organization of local directional selectivity in V1 – perhaps because the latter requires some minimum level of temporal performance in the developing visual pathway before it can function. We have also used behavioural and VERP methods in infants to show early processing of global form information (Braddick et al 2002, Atkinson et al 2005, Braddick and Atkinson 2007); at this first stage, ventral stream integration of form appears to develop more slowly than dorsal stream integration of motion. This differential development may reflect the importance of global motion for segmentation and depth organization of the visual world. Current research is recording infants' VERPs to the onset of global motion or global form, using a high-density geodesic array of 128 electrodes. This method should enable us to separate topographically the motion and form responses in the infant brain, and hopefully identify anomalies in development when specific brain areas have suffered perinatal damage.

RELATIVE DEVELOPMENT OF GLOBAL FORM AND MOTION DURING CHILDHOOD

We have created versions of coherence sensitivity tests as computer games which can be successfully used with children as young as 4 years. For motion coherence, in the 'road in the snowstorm' test, the child has to find the 'road' on the left- or right-hand side of the computer screen, a segmented strip with dots moving coherently in the opposite direction to the rest of the screen. In the 'ball in the grass' task, the 'ball' is the static or rotating concentric area on the left or right of the screen surrounded by either randomly oriented small line segments for form coherence, as in Figure 8.2.2, or randomly appearing dots (for motion coherence). We have compared development of normal children between 4 and 11 years using these tests and have found that, using either computer display ('the road' or 'the ball') for measuring motion coherence thresholds, these show a slower maturation to adult levels than form coherence measures (Gunn et al 2002, Atkinson and Braddick 2005).

These tests have been used to compare motion and form coherence thresholds in a number of clinical populations, relative to typically developing children of the same chronological or developmental age. The first group we studied was children with Williams syndrome. This developmental disorder, related to a specific deletion on chromosome 7, shows a very characteristic cognitive profile, with relatively strong expressive language abilities combined with unusual semantic knowledge and social sensitivity, good face recognition, but very poor spatial cognition (see, for example, Bellugi et al 1999, Klein and Mervis 1999, Atkinson et al 2001). This profile suggests the possibility of a deficit in dorsal compared with ventral stream function, supported by our findings that many children with Williams syndrome show a relative deficit in global motion compared with form coherence processing. The motion coherence deficit persists into adult life in Williams syndrome (Atkinson et al 2006). Further support for a dorsal stream deficit is found in children with Williams syndrome in the 'mail-box' task, which tests the use of orientation information to control an action (posting a letter through an oriented slot – dorsal task) compared with a perceptual judgement (to match the letter's orientation to that of the slot – ventral task). Children with Williams syndrome are relatively poorer on the posting task than on the perceptual matching task (Atkinson et al 1997).

However, further studies showed that deficits specific to global motion processing are not unique to Williams syndrome. Children with hemiplegia, despite normal IQ levels, showed significantly poorer global motion performance for age than typically developing children, while global form sensitivity was normal (Gunn et al 2002). A similar impairment of motion relative to form sensitivity has also been found in a group of children with autism (Spencer et al 2000), in children with developmental dyslexia (Cornelissen et al 1995, Stein et al 2000, Ridder et al 2001), and in children with fragile X syndrome (Kogan et al 2004). As this motion coherence deficit appears to be a common feature across a wide variety of paediatric disorders with very different aetiologies and neurodevelopmental profiles, we have suggested that it represents a general early vulnerability in the motion processing stream (Braddick et al 2003). This suggests that measures related to motion and to dorsal stream function more generally are likely to offer the most sensitive measures of early neurological problems, a view supported by our findings on the delays in directional responses in preterm infants (Birtles et al 2007).

A functional vision battery
To evaluate the degree and impact of children's visual impairment, whether from cerebral damage or other causes, it is necessary to have a battery of tests which not only assesses the basic parameters of vision such as acuity and visual fields, but also examines the behavioural abilities appropriate to the child's age which reflect his or her use of vision for cognitive, spatial, and visuomotor function. We have developed such a battery – the ABCDEFV (Atkinson et al 2002b) – for assessments of functional vision, for children with either normal or abnormal general development. The battery spans the mental age range from birth to 5 years. Of course, for clinical populations, the chronological age range of children for whom the tests are useful may be much wider.

TABLE 8.2.2

Component tests in the ABCDEFV battery

Core vision tests

Test	Function assessed
1. Pupil responses	Responsiveness of pupils to light assessed as a basic indicator of neurological integrity
2. Diffuse light reaction	Orientation to light as an indicator of minimal visual function in very young infants and cases of suspected total blindness
3. Lateral tracking	Visual attention and eye movements (either saccadic or smooth pursuit accepted)
4. Peripheral refixation – lateral fields	Visual attention and extent of lateral visual fields
5. Symmetrical corneal reflexes	Binocular alignment. Manifest strabismus may be associated with ocular and/or neurological problems
6. Convergence to approaching object	Binocular function; failure may indicate neurological or ophthalmic problems
7. Attention at distance	Sustained visual attention possible at moderate distance; failure may be related to distance acuity or to neurological attentional problems
8. Defensive blink to approaching object	Development of visuomotor response related to distance perception
9. Visually follows falling toy	Visual cognition: early stage in development of object permanence

Core vision tests (optional)

Test	Function assessed
10. Optokinetic nystagmus	Reflex eye movements associated with subcortical mechanisms
11. Acuity cards	Measurement of visual acuity
12. Videorefraction	Accommodation, attentional shifts, and refractive error

TABLE 8.2.2 (continued)
Component tests in the ABCDEFV battery

Additional tests

Test	Minimum age	Function assessed
13. Lang test	2y	Stereoscopic vision
14. Batting/reaching	4mo	Visuomotor development
15. Pick up black and white cotton	12mo	Visual control of fine hand and finger movement (including pincer grasp); crude test of contrast sensitivity
16. Retrieval of partially covered object	6mo	Visual cognition: intermediate stage in development of object permanence
17. Retrieval of totally covered object	6mo	Visual cognition: intermediate stage in development of object permanence
18. Shape matching with form board	2y	Shape recognition, recognition of spatial relations, visual planning, and control of manual actions
19. Embedded figures	2y	Figure–ground segmentation and shape recognition
20. Placing letter in envelope	2y	Recognition of spatial relations, visual planning, control of manual actions
21. Block construction – free play	12mo	Requires recognition of spatial relations, visual planning, control of manual actions
22. Copying block designs	18mo	Graded test of recognition of spatial relations, visual planning, and control of manual actions. Identifies developmental problems of 'constructional apraxia'

The rationale of these tests is that different parts of the battery tap different aspects of sensory, perceptual, motor, and cognitive vision. The battery is transportable, so that it can be used in different settings. We intend it as a diagnostic starting point for pinpointing areas of concern in visual development in individual children. The tests are divided into core vision tests and additional tests. All children are assessed on the core vision tests while the additional tests are more restricted in use because the functions they assess require the child to be capable of reaching and grasping (at least with one hand with the other as support) and to have a mental age of beyond 6 months. Table 8.2.2 lists both the core and additional tests included in the battery. Full descriptions of the tests are available (Atkinson 2000, Atkinson et al 2002b) along with the normalization over the developmental age range. Experience of using the battery with a number of different clinical groups is outlined below.

ABCDEFV in Follow-up of Vision Screening Tests

We have used the ABCDEFV in follow-up of normally developing children with marked refractive errors including hypermetropia at 9 months of age, identified in the Cambridge Infant Vision Screening Programmes (Atkinson et al 1984, 2007, Anker et al 2003). In the second programme, we screened a population of around 5000 healthy infants, representing 80% of infants born in a geographically defined district over a 2-year period. Around 5% of these children showed significant hypermetropia and were followed up at 6-monthly intervals to 7 years of age alongside a control group of normally developing infants without refractive errors recruited from the same population. We found that children who had been significantly hyperopic in infancy performed significantly worse than comparison children on a number of the visuoperceptual, visuocognitive, and visuospatial tests in the ABCDEFV at 14 months and 3 years 6 months, although there were no significant overall differences between the groups on the Griffiths Child Development Scales, MacArthur Communicative Development Inventory, and British Picture Vocabulary Scales (Atkinson et al 2002c), in which both groups performed in the normal range. Although infant hypermetropia was associated with the development of amblyopia and strabismus, excluding children with these conditions from the analysis did not substantially alter these results, suggesting that the differences between groups were not a direct causal consequence of these early visual disorders, but that the failures had an underlying common cause across visual, visuomotor, visuocognitive, and visuospatial domains. These results indicate that early hypermetropia is associated with a range of developmental deficits that persist at least to age 5 years 6 months, the effects being concentrated in visuocognitive and visuomotor domain rather than in the linguistic domain.

ABCDEFV in Clinical Populations

We have used the ABCDEFV across various clinical groups and for children referred to us with suspected visual problems in the appropriate mental age range. We have been able to complete the core vision tests with nearly all children. We have found some of the optional core vision tests to be particularly useful for many clinical populations. For example, one pervasive deficit found across many clinical populations with suspected cerebral damage (whether it be severe or mild) is an inability to change focus (accommodate) on targets at different distances, in the absence of any marked refractive error measured using videorefraction (Chapter 6). It seems likely that networks involving accommodative mechanisms in conjunction with cortical systems have never developed normally in infancy. Whether this is a result of deficits in the accommodative control system per se, or whether it reflects more central damage to cortical attentional systems, cannot be determined from these measurements alone.

CHILDREN WITH SUSPECTED SEVERE CEREBRAL VISUAL IMPAIRMENT

We have used the ABCDEFV battery core vision tests to assess children referred to our unit with suspected CVI, alongside the OR-VEP and FS measures of cortical functioning described above. Many of these children do not show any consistent shifts of attention in the FS paradigm even under non-competition, nor do they show a significant OR-VEP response. Table 8.2.3 summarizes three case histories to illustrate the kind of information that can be gained from the combination of these tests.

CHILDREN BORN PRETERM BEFORE 32 WEEKS' GESTATION

We have also used the ABCDEFV to follow longitudinally a cohort of children born very preterm (<32 weeks' gestation) who have also undergone neonatal and term cerebral MRI. Generally, the more severe the identified damage, particularly to white matter (including DEHSI on T2-weighted images) on MRI, the poorer the capabilities indicated by the ABCDEFV tests. We find that many of the children with indications of only mild brain abnormality fail on the spatial tests of copying constructions of block designs and other visuocognitive tests, for example where the child has to identify embedded figures or match shapes in a puzzle (Atkinson et al 2003, Atkinson and Braddick 2007), indicating the sensitivity of these parts of the battery to damage which is not apparent on assessing more elementary visual functions.

Tests of attention and executive control

Visual function is not a passive reception of stimuli; normal functional vision depends critically on the individual's ability to deploy his or her visual processing resources efficiently to meet the demands of the task in hand. Components of this capability are known as visual attention and executive function.

The most basic form of visual attention is assessed in the fixation shift test – the infant's controlled orienting towards a salient target, including the ability to disengage fixation from a prior target. We have mentioned the limitations shown by this test in hemispherectomized infants, reflecting the role of cortical control. The failure to disengage and to make eye and head movements to a salient peripheral target when a central target is still visible is a common finding in many children with perinatal brain damage involving parietal and frontal areas. When damage extends to subcortical networks, then, even without competition, shifts of gaze (and presumably attention) can be absent and/or slow. This means that the fixation shift test can be used across the whole range of severity of cerebral visual impairment as the most basic test of attention.

TABLE 8.2.3

Example case histories of tests with children with cerebral visual impairment

Case 1 – background: born at term, umbilical cord round neck, hypoxic and resuscitated, neonatal seizures, classified severe hypoxic–ischaemic encephalopathy

Age at test	Eye movements	Fields	Blink	Accommodation	PL acuity	VEP	Fixation shifts	Additional tests
8mo	Nystagmus, alternating divergent strabismus, diffuse light reaction only			Fixed hyperopic focus	No response	Pattern –ve	Non-competition –ve, competition –ve both R and L	Not possible, no reaching or grasping
12mo	Nystagmus, alternating divergent strabismus, diffuse light reaction only			Fixed hyperopic focus	No response	Pattern –ve, OR –ve	Non-competition –ve, competition –ve both R and L	Not possible, no reaching or grasping
19mo	Nystagmus, alternating divergent strabismus, diffuse light reaction only	Narrow, R<L	Absent	Fixed hyperopic focus	No response		Non-competition –ve, competition –ve both R and L	Not possible, no reaching or grasping
31mo					1 c/deg	pattern –ve, OR –ve		
43mo					1 c/deg		Non-competition –ve, competition –ve both R and L	
55mo		Narrow, R<L			2.5 c/deg			Not possible, no reaching or grasping
Conclusions	Severe CVI, subcortical visual responses at best, but some improvement from 19mo when seizures improved

143

TABLE 8.2.3 (continued)

Example case histories of tests with children with cerebral visual impairment

Case 2 – background: born at term, emergency Caesarean, reduced amniotic fluid in pregnancy, intrauterine growth retardation. Neurologically normal at birth, poor feeding and glycaemic control at 2 days. MRI microcephalic, EEG normal

Age at test	Eye movements	Fields	Blink	Accommodation	PL acuity	VEP	Fixation shifts	Additional tests
10mo	Left convergent strabismus	R absent, L narrow		Fixed myopic focus	<1 c/deg	OR +ve	Non-competition +ve Competition –ve	Not possible; no reaching or grasping
13mo	Left convergent strabismus	R and L narrow	Absent	Fixed myopic focus		OR +ve	Non-competition +ve Competition –ve	
Conclusions	Primary cortical responses, but very poor control of attention (likely parietal deficit)							

TABLE 8.2.3 (continued)

Example case histories of tests with children with cerebral visual impairment

Age at test	Eye movements	Fields	Blink	Accommodation	PL acuity	VEP	Fixation shifts	Additional tests
Case 3 – background: born at term, large left intraventricular haemorrhage. Seizures in first week. Developing hydrocephalus but no shunt required								
9mo	Alternating convergent strabismus, no tracking to R	Both narrow, L<R	Present	Fixed hyperopic focus	Not possible	Pattern +ve, OR +ve	Non-competition –ve, competition –ve	
15mo	ACS, full eye movements	Both narrow, R<L		Fixed hyperopic focus	Not possible		Non-competition –ve, competition –ve	
21mo	ACS, full eye movements	Both narrow, R<L	On camera		4 c/deg		Non-competition –ve, competition –ve	Retrieved totally covered object, no pincer grasp
30mo	ACS, full eye movements	Full	On camera		5 c/deg		Refused	
42mo	ACS, full eye movements	R<L	Hyperopic focus		21 c/deg		Refused	Shape sorter +ve, Griffiths boxes +ve, block construction 18mo level
Conclusions	Progress from 1yr; continuing field loss, acuity normal, but about 18mo visuocognitive delay							

L, left; R, right; OR, orientation reversal; ACS, alternating convergent strabismus; c/deg, cycles per degree (acuity measure; 30 cycles per degree is equivalent to 6/6).

Three different components of attention have been identified from neuropsychological, cognitive, and imaging studies, each with rather different neural underpinnings. The first component is selective attention as deployed in visual search tasks. The second is 'sustained attention', which can be measured in vigilance tasks. The third involves inhibition of a pre-potent response to switch or maintain attention to a new strategy, an essential element of what is called executive control. Many of these inhibitory tasks are believed to have their underpinnings in frontal lobe circuitry. Developmental trajectories for different components have been found to differ (e.g. McKay et al 1994, Kelly 2000, Rueda et al 2004). The Test of Everyday Attention for Children (TEA-Ch; Manly et al 2001), for normal children between the age of 6 and 16 years, supports the notion that distinct attentional components exist in childhood with differential impairment of these components in clinical samples including attention-deficit–hyperactivity disorder (ADHD) (Heaton et al 2001, Manly et al 2001) and traumatic brain injury (Anderson et al 1998).

A number of tasks have been developed to examine executive function in young children, requiring the child to inhibit a prepotent response, for example a direct reaching response in the Detour Box (Hughes and Russell 1993, Biro and Russell 2001); a familiar verbal label in the Day/Night test (Gerstadt et al 1994); and a response to falling objects in the Gravity Tubes (Hood 1995). We have also devised a new spatial inhibitory task, called 'counterpointing', in which the child first points as rapidly as possible to a target which appears to either the left or right of a fixation target. The rule is then changed and the child is asked to point as rapidly as possible to the opposite side to where the target appears. On this test inhibitory control is achieved on average by 4 years of age in typically developing children.

We have used these tests to analyse visuospatial components of executive function in children with Williams syndrome (Atkinson et al 2003) and ex-preterm children (Atkinson and Braddick 2007). The children with Williams syndrome generally showed much poorer performance on counter-pointing and the Detour Box than on the verbal inhibition task (Day/Night), suggesting that they have a particular deficit in the visuospatial aspects of executive function. In a cohort of very preterm infants and children tested between 2 and 5 years, less than 50% performed in the normal range for their chronological age on these preschool executive function tests. It may prove possible to relate performance on these tests to subsequent attentional deficits (e.g. ADHD).

To provide a wider assessment of the abilities of preschool children on the different components of attention, we have devised and normalized a new battery for the 3- to 6-year-old range of developmental age (Breckenridge et al 2007). Work applying this battery to children with Williams and Down syndrome is in progress; initial results suggest that we can success-fully characterize different developmental profiles across the component processes of attention for these neurodevelopmental disorders.

Tests of visuospatial representation in memory
Children with a range of risk factors and neurodevelopmental disorders show deficits which are often most marked in the visuospatial and visuomotor domains. The origin of these may lie in basic visual mechanisms, in executive control processes, or in the various modules in

between these levels that translate visual information into spatial representations used for action and for cognitive operations. One of the latter is the representations, stored in memory, of the spatial layout of the environment. These representations require translation between different 'frames of reference': a location may be encoded relative to the child's viewpoint (egocentric), or relative to local landmarks or the room layout (allocentric), and the child may be able to update egocentric information by 'path integration' based on his or her own movement through the environment.

Work in our group has developed the 'town square' task, measuring location memory to tap these different levels of spatial representation for children in the developmental age range of 3–6 years. The child sees a small toy hidden under a cup in a random array of 10 identical cups on a square board with colourful toys around two sides of the board which can serve as 'landmarks' for the hiding location. The child then has to find the hiding place from the starting location (allowing egocentric coding to be used), or, by moving, from a different viewpoint (requiring allocentric coding or path integration), or also from a different location and with the board rotated (requiring use of a landmark-based frame of reference). Age norms have been established for these progressively more difficult conditions (Nardini et al 2006a). Relative to these norms, a group of 6-year-olds who had been born at 25–30 weeks' gestation had an average delay of more than 1 year across conditions (Nardini et al 2006b). Their average deficit was as large for external frames of reference (landmarks) as for egocentric recall. However, correlations with other cognitive and motor tests indicate the existence of subgroups with differential patterns of impairment. Impairments to spatial updating for changes of viewpoint produced by walking may be predicted by poor detection of coherent motion (related to visual processing of optic flow), whereas performance on the 'perspective problem' (when changes of viewpoint are produced by movement of the array) is correlated with 'executive control' tests of inhibition and response selection, suggesting that this task requires a 'frontal' inhibition of a more dominant frame of reference.

We have also compared the development of 'egocentric' and landmark-based recall in children and adults with Williams syndrome. We found that these frames of reference were combined anomalously in development, and that adults with Williams syndrome showed only marginal ability to use local landmarks to solve the 'perspective problem', solved by typical children at 5 years (Nardini et al 2008). Visuomotor, localization, and constructional deficits in Williams syndrome (e.g. Atkinson et al 1997, 2001, Vicari et al 2006) may thus be related in part to the unusual integration of different frames of reference in development, and the poor ability to select local landmarks even in adulthood.

Conclusions

In summary, cerebral damage, or atypical brain development, may affect visual and visuospatial capabilities at many levels, and both the normal and atypical development of visually controlled behaviour must be considered as the product of integrated brain systems running from the input to primary visual cortex, to spatial cognition and memory, motor control, attention, and frontal executive function, and extensive feedback from one processing level in the brain to another. Deficits in one area can have cascading effects in both feedforward processing and feedback. In this chapter we have described a number of tests, both behavioural and electrophysiological, which aim to assess and distinguish functions at all these levels. In our experience, these have proved valuable in diagnosing specific deficits and assessing the impact on everyday function of varying degrees and types of cerebral visual impairment. We have also established that methods of cortical visual function which can be applied in the first months of infancy can help to predict broader cognitive and neurological outcome at a later age, and thus will be of potential value in measuring the effective outcome of early interventions and therapies in at-risk infants.

Summary

The complexity of visual function and its disorders means that a structured approach to the clinical assessment of vision is required to ensure that each aspect of visual dysfunction is recognized and measured for the purposes of diagnosis, determination of morbidity, and planning rehabilitation.

Acknowledgements

Work described here was supported by programme grants from the Medical Research Council. We thank Dr John Wattam-Bell and other colleagues both within and beyond the Visual Development Unit, in particular Shirley Anker, Dee Birtles, and Marko Nardini; clinical colleagues from the Neonatal Unit in the Hammersmith Hospital – Lily Dubowitz, Eugenio Mercuri, David Edwards, Francis Cowan, Mary Rutherford, Leigh Dyet; and Giovanni Cioni and Andrea Guzzetta (Stella Maris Institute and University of Pisa), whose work has contributed to these studies; and the families whose cooperation makes our work possible.

8.3 PSYCHOMETRIC EVALUATION OF HIGHER VISUAL DISORDERS: STRATEGIES FOR CLINICAL SETTINGS

Peter Stiers and Elisa Fazzi

It is well established through studies of adult patients that focal brain damage can result in selective impairment of isolated aspects of visual processing (Farah 1990). However, it has only been since the early 1990s that it has become more widely accepted that selective visual–perceptual dysfunction can result from congenital brain disorders, such as brain malformation, cortical damage due to birth asphyxia, white matter damage in preterm infants, and even genetic disorders. These disorders affect the visual brain before it is fully differentiated and operational. Initial studies have focused on lower aspects of visual functioning, and visual acuity in particular, mostly in children following birth complications (Dobson et al 1980, Scher et al 1989, Birch and Bane 1991, Schenk-Rootlieb et al 1992, Pike et al 1994, Lanzi et al 1998). Soon after, reports of general visual–perceptual dysfunctioning appeared (Menken et al 1987, Koeda and Takeshita 1992, Goto et al 1994, Ito et al 1996) and, later, impairment in specific subfunctions of visual processing, such as object categorization (Stiers et al 1998, Van den Hout et al 2000, Stiers et al 2005), motion perception (Atkinson et al 1997, Gunn et al 2002, Pavlova et al 2003), saccadic control (Fedrizzi et al 1998, Fazzi et al 2007a), and visuomotor integration (Fazzi et al 2004, 2007a), were described. Although the nature and range of dysfunctions have yet to be well established, they have increased the need for practitioners to evaluate visual abilities beyond the lower aspects of vision that are typically assessed by the ophthalmologist. Higher visual abilities have long been the domain of neuropsychology, but the field of congenital brain disorders has attracted the attention of neuropsychologists only in recent years, and many practitioners working with these children have no neuropsychological background. The need exists, therefore, for information on how to assess visual–perceptual disorders in the clinical evaluation and diagnosis of the individual patient. The information in this chapter stems from long practical experience in clinics and research on cerebral visual impairment in children.

The major problem in the psychometric evaluation of higher visual functions in children with congenital brain disorder is that the disorder does not affect the brain focally. For many children, there is extensive and diffuse damage to the developing brain. As a result, they suffer from multiple neuropsychological disabilities. This makes it difficult to establish whether a reduced score on a particular visual perception test is due to a visual processing disorder or to other disabilities that the child may have. In this chapter, we address this general neuropsychological problem, and present a way to circumvent it. After this, we discuss some additional aspects of visual–perceptual evaluation that need to be taken into consideration in the diagnosis of higher visual disorders.

Evaluating visual abilities in children with multiple disabilities
How well a person performs on a visual perception task is dependent not just on the part of the brain that is involved in visual processing, but on many parts of the nervous system, ranging from the retina to the prefrontal lobes, with many cortical and subcortical structures in between. Damage to any component of this complex neural system may result in reduced performance on visual–perceptual tasks. In more clinical terms, this means that a child with an ocular disorder as well as a child with a cognitive disorder (among others) may obtain scores on a visual–perceptual task that are below those for age, without there being (primary) dysfunction of brain areas directly involved in the processing of visual information. Thus, with some oversimplification, the core problem in evaluating visual–perceptual dysfunction is that the processes of interest are intermediate between basic visual functions (fields, acuity, contrast, etc.) and higher integrative and cognitive abilities, with a high frequency of comorbidity on both sides (see, for example, Fazzi et al 2007a). In what follows we will mainly focus on distinguishing between visual–perceptual and 'higher' disabilities. The interference of basic visual functions in the assessment will briefly be touched upon later because much less is known about it.

Visual and Non-Visual Contributions to Reduced Perception Scores
In this section, we illustrate the assessment problem and introduce a solution by means of presenting data from two children with cerebral palsy. Cerebral palsy is a developmental motor disorder associated with an increased risk for visual processing disorders – estimates of prevalence range between 33% and 66% (Marozas and May 1986, Koeda and Takeshita 1992, Ito et al 1996, Stiers et al 2002). Some clinical characteristics of the two children are presented in Table 8.3.1. Both were born preterm and developed periventricular leucomalacia. One of them, MD, was referred to the multidisciplinary clinic for children with cerebral visual impairment, at the University Hospital, Leuven, Belgium. Visual problems were suspected because she gave unusual interpretations of line drawings and had problems in school doing simple exercises when several were printed on a single sheet. She was verbally orientated, with little interest in puzzles or television. The other child, FE, was selected from a study on visual abilities in children with cerebral palsy (Stiers et al 2002), to match the clinical characteristics of MD. There were no complaints about FE's visual abilities. Both children had some ocular problems, as is common in children with cerebral palsy. These were not sufficient to account for MD's visual problems. Both children also had a non-verbal to verbal intelligence quotient (IQ) discrepancy, which is not unusual for children with cerebral palsy. The two children are presented here by way of an external criterion to evaluate the validity of the psychometric procedure: a psychometric assessment aiming to diagnose visual processing deficits should be able to differentiate between these two children.

Both children were assessed with the visual–perceptual battery L94 (Stiers et al 2001), which comprises eight tasks assessing object categorization (VISM), object recognition under

TABLE 8.3.1

Clinical characteristics of two children with cerebral palsy

	MD (female)	FE (male)
Age at testing	7yr 0mo	6yr 1mo
Neonatal		
Gestational age	30 weeks	29 weeks
Birth weight	1550g	1140g
Apgar score	9 after 1 min	8 and 9 after 1 and 5 min
Neurological		
Ultrasound echography	Increased echo bilateral periventricular	Not available
MRI (age 2y)	Cystic periventricular leucomalacia, with dilated occipital ventricle horns	Bilateral periventricular leucomalacia, frontal and parietal Spastic quadriplegia, right side more affected
Motor development	Discrete spastic diplegia, right side more affected Gross motor dyspraxia	
Cognitive development		
WPPSI-R Verbal IQ	76	87
WPPSI-R Non-verbal IQ	51	60
Language	Language delay of 1y	Delayed language development
School	Special education programme physical disability	Special education programme physical disability
Other	Poor attention and concentration	
Ophthalmology		
Visual acuity (gratings)	10 cycles per degree	16 cycles per degree
Visual fields	Assessment unsuccessful	Not available
Refraction	Normal	Mild myopia
Strabismus	Right convergent + hypotropia	Right convergent
Nystagmus	Latent rotary	No

WPPSI-R, Wechsler Preschool and Primary Scale of Intelligence – Revised.

151

suboptimal circumstances (DEVOS, VIEW, OVERL, NOISE), visuomotor construction (VMI, BLOCKC), and visual discrimination (BLOCKM) (see Fig. 8.3.1). The centile scores obtained by MD and FE on these tasks are presented in the upper panel of Figure 8.3.2. It is clear that both children had impaired performances on several L94 tasks. This illustrates that observing impaired scores on a so-called 'visual perception' test is not enough to validly diagnose visual–perceptual disorders.

As a solution to this problem, we introduce the notion of a 'specific impairment'. This simply means that when a diagnostic evaluation of a patient leads to the conclusion of a functional impairment (e.g. a visual–perceptual impairment), there must be some evidence of specificity in the impairment. That is, the performance impairment should be more severe on tests measuring visual perception, whereas there should be less impairment on tests with less load in that particular function. Or, in other words, there should be covariance between the patient's performance level on the tests and the load of the tests on that function (e.g. visual perception). If no such covariance can be demonstrated, and consequently the patient's performance is equally impaired in a wide range of tests regardless of his or her load in visual perception, then it would be difficult to maintain that the person had a 'visual–perceptual' impairment. An important implication of this approach for clinical assessment is that it cannot be judged from a single test whether someone has a specific dysfunction – more measurements are needed to come to the right conclusions. This is not a minor drawback, for more tests mean longer (or more) test sessions, and more collaboration from the person assessed. This requires a great deal of commitment from all parties involved, particularly in preschool children.

In practice, the evaluation of a particular function is based on comparing the performance on a test with a high load on this function with the performance on a set of baseline tests with a low to intermediate load on that function. The baseline tests serve to establish a reference performance level against which a possible reduction in performance on the high loading test can be judged. To avoid administering too many extra tests, the baseline tests are chosen from the set of tests that are commonly administered in the evaluation of children with multiple disabilities. There are two important criteria in the selection of baseline tasks. First, they must have at least some load on the function of interest. It makes no sense, for instance, to use verbal memory tasks as a reference for evaluating visual perception because any performance discrepancy between these tasks could easily arise as a result of factors other than visual–perceptual dysfunction, such as memory problems. Second, the performance baseline should be based not on just a single task, but on several tasks with some heterogeneity. This is required to rule out the possibility that a single deficit, captured by the one and only baseline task, might compromise the baseline measurement. Given these requirements, our choice fell on non-verbal intelligence subtests. Non-verbal subtests are obviously visual. Nonetheless, they were designed to maximize load not on visual–perceptual processing, but on cognitive abilities. Therefore, they can be assumed to require low to medium visual–perceptual skills. In addition, intelligence subscales comprise several subtests, usually five or six, intended to assess non-verbal cognition from different angles. This lends them sufficient heterogeneity. As an additional advantage, they are generally of high psychometric quality. And, lastly, there is the important practical advantage that they are included in almost every standard clinical assessment protocol. It is important to stress at this point that it does not matter for the above

Visual matching (VISM)

In each of 10 items a target drawing depicting an everyday object is presented for 1s and replaced by four alternatives. One of these, a different exemplar of the target object, must be pointed out.

Overlapping figures (OVERL)

Two, three, or four drawings on top of one another must be found among four, five, or six subsequent alternatives. Each of six items starts with total overlap, but can be shown as partial overlap, touching, or separate (=control drawing).

Unconventional viewpoints (VIEW)

Twenty objects that are depicted from unconventional viewpoints in decreasing levels of unconventionality have to be named. The control drawing is a prototypical representation.

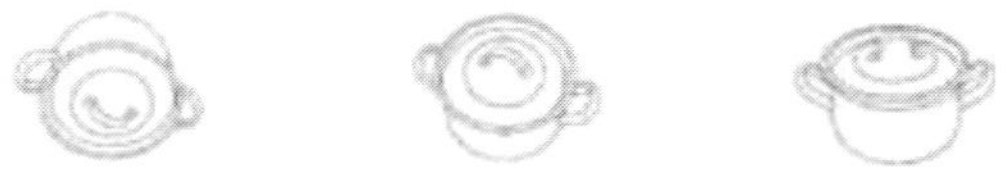

Figure occluded by noise (NOISE)

Objects in drawings partially occluded by noise of small squares have to be named. Each of six items starts at 60% occlusion. This is reducible in seven steps to 0%, which is the control drawing.

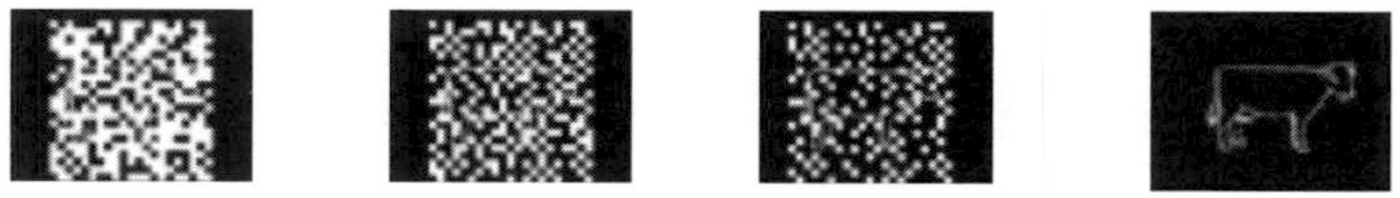

De Vos (DEVOS)

Naming objects that are either embedded in context, partly deleted, drawn in contour-line, missing a typical part, or seen from unusual viewpoint. Each of 43 items contains a prototypical control drawing.

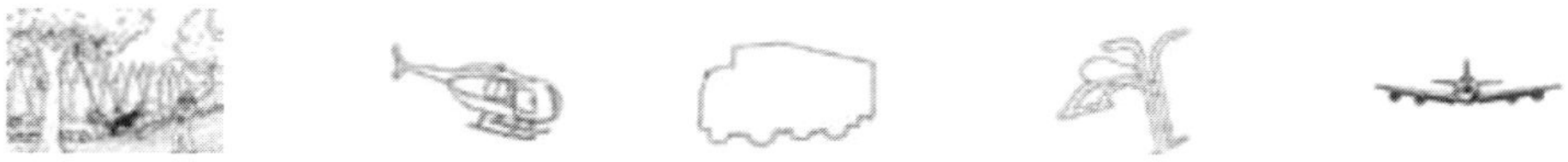

Matching block designs (BLOCKM)

A complex form matching task in which black and white geometric forms (block design patterns) have to be matched to four simultaneously presented similar patterns.

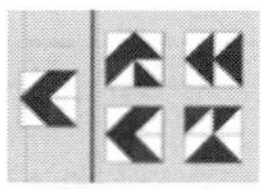

Beery's VMI

Developmental Test of Visual Motor Integration (VMI; Beery 1997). Geometric figures have to be copied with a pencil in a predefined space below each example.

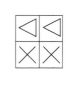

Fig. 8.3.1 Illustration of seven tasks in the visual–perceptual battery L94 (Stiers et al 2001; http://med.kuleuven.be/neupsy/cvi/). The eighth task is 'constructing block designs' (BLOCKC), in which children have to construct block design patterns from examples using two-dimensional blocks. The battery was standardized on a sample of 263 children aged between 2.5 and 6.0 years, in 6-month age groups (see Stiers et al 2001).

153

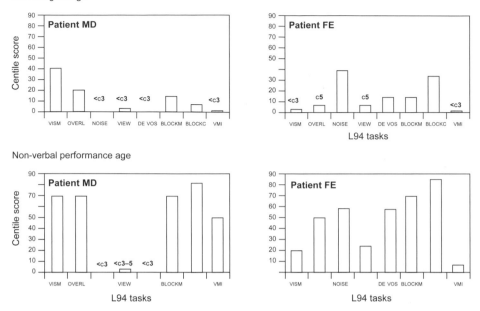

Fig. 8.3.2 Centile scores obtained by patients MD and FE on each of the eight tasks in the L94 visual–perceptual battery (Stiers et al 2001; http://med.kuleuven.be/neupsy/cvi). Upper graphs: raw scores were transformed to centile scores based on the chronological age of the patient. Both patients obtained impaired scores (i.e. at or below the fifth centile) on four of the eight tasks. Lower graphs: raw scores were transformed to centile scores based on the non-verbal performance age, which is the median of the Wechsler Preschool and Primary Scale of Inteligence – Revised (WPPSI-R) non-verbal subtest ages. With this procedure, only patient MD obtained impaired scores on L94 tasks, while all patient FE's scores were above the criterion for impairment (at or below fifth centile). c, centile; VISM, visual matching; OVERL, overlapping figures; NOISE, figures occluded by noise; VIEW, unconventional viewpoints; DE VOS, De Vos; BLOCKM, matching block designs; BLOCKC, constructing block designs; VMI, visual motor integration.

procedure that these tasks were originally designed to assess non-verbal intelligence – a set of other tasks that have nothing to do with intelligence can be used for the same purpose. The crucial point is that the baseline tasks require at least some visual processing, but to a lesser extent than the visual–perceptual tasks. This discrepancy in load will ensure that a discrepancy in performance will emerge between the baseline tasks (as a whole) and a visual perception task, in the case of a visual perception problem.

We can now return to our case study, where the above-described strategy was applied as follows. Each child's raw non-verbal intelligence subtest scores were transformed to an age equivalent, by replacing the raw score with the age of the age group in the normative sample in which the child's raw score equalled the mean score. For each child, the median of these six subtest age scores was determined. We refer to this median age equivalent as the non-verbal performance age of the child. This performance age was used instead of the child's chronological age to determine the entry into the normative tables of the visual–perceptual tasks. Thus, if the child was 6 years old and obtained a performance age of 4 years, he or she was compared with the 4-year-old children in the normative sample. The result of this shift in reference line is shown in the lower part of Figure 8.3.2. It is clear that now we are able to differentiate between MD, the child with visual complaints, and FE, the child without such complaints. Although FE did not obtain a score below the 10th centile on any of the tasks, MD's evaluation yielded significant impairment (at or below the fifth centile) on three of the eight tasks. Note that the impairment that she shows on these tasks is substantial: her scores are below the fifth centile of her already reduced non-verbal performance level. It is therefore justified to call this a specific impairment, amidst several other disabilities of this child.

VALIDATION OF THE PROPOSED SOLUTION

We will now leave the single case description and investigate the validity of the above strategy more systematically, by looking at the visual–perceptual performance in different groups of children. The data presented here were obtained with the L94 battery introduced in the previous section (see Fig. 8.3.1). The procedures evaluated, however, can be generalized to any visual–perceptual test or battery, such as the Test of Visual Perceptual Skills (Martin 2006), the Frostig Developmental Test of Visual Perception (Hammill et al 1993), the Motor-Free Visual Perception Test (Colarusso and Hammill 2003), or the visual–perceptual battery proposed by Bova et al (2007).

We start with a group of children with multiple disabilities due to disorders not commonly associated with visual processing deficits. The group comprises mostly children who have mild to moderate intellectual disability and no substantial loss of vision (Stiers et al 2001). Their clinical histories show no evidence of any visual processing problem. The clinical characteristics of the children in this group are summarized in the left column of Table 8.3.2. Their scores on the L94 tasks, transferred to centile scores based on chronological age, are presented in Figure 8.3.3 (upper left graph). It is immediately clear that, as a group, these children are severely impaired in their performance on these tasks. Given the fifth centile cut-off criterion for establishing impairment, we would expect 5% of typically developing children to obtain a score at or below the fifth centile. The graph in Figure 8.3.3 shows, however, that the frequency of impairment is significantly higher than 5% for each of the tasks. Given the clinical background, it is highly unlikely that these reduced scores truly reflect visual dysfunction. This expectation is confirmed when the specific impairment strategy, as described above, is applied to the raw scores, the result of which is presented in the lower left graph of Figure 8.3.3. Now, the visual–perceptual performance in this group is within the 'normal' range – that is, the range that can be expected given the general non-verbal performance level of each child. This dramatic change in the picture illustrates the magnitude of the diagnostic problem created by multiple disabilities.

While the above result demonstrates that we can control the number of false positives, it still has to be shown that we can detect visual–perceptual problems. Direct proof of this requires an objective way of establishing who has and who does not have visual problems, against which the performance of the new technique can be evaluated. Since no objective criterion exists for visual processing problems, we must use an indirect criterion to establish validity. This is provided by children with birth complications. It is well known that these children are at increased risk for visual problems (Goto et al 1994, Lanzi et al 1998). A psychometric procedure for diagnosing visual processing deficits should at least be able to confirm

155

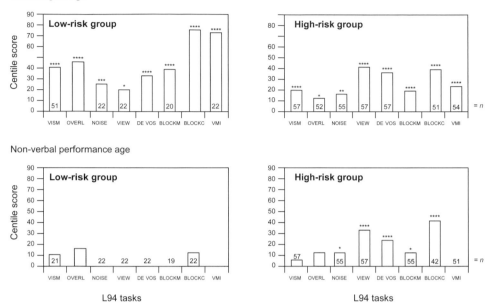

Non-verbal performance age

L94 tasks

L94 tasks

Fig. 8.3.3 Relative frequency of impaired performance for each of the L94 tasks in a group of children with low risk (*n*=22) and a group with high risk (*n*=57) for visual–perceptual impairment. Upper graphs: raw scores were transformed to centile scores based on the chronological age of the children. For each task the frequency of impairment (score at or below the fifth centile) is significantly higher than 5%, in the low-risk as well as in the high-risk group. Lower graphs: raw scores were transformed to centile scores based on the non-verbal performance age. Only the high-risk group shows a significantly increased incidence of impairment on some visual–perceptual tasks. In contrast, the frequency of impairment is not different from the normal criterion (5%) in the low-risk group. Numbers at the bottom of the bars represent number of cases in each bar, i.e. the number of children whose (performance) age was within the normative age range of the task. Asterisks indicate significance of cumulative binomial probability of observed frequency relative to the expected frequency of 5%. *$p \leq 0.05$; **$p \leq 0.01$; ***$p \leq 0.005$; ****$p \leq 0.0001$. VISM, visual matching; OVERL, overlapping figures; NOISE, figures occluded by noise; VIEW, unconventional viewpoints; DE VOS, De Vos; BLOCKM, matching block designs; BLOCKC, constructing block designs; VMI, visual motor integration.

this increased risk. An ideal opportunity to investigate this hypothesis was presented by a follow-up study on visual development at the University Hospital in Utrecht, the Netherlands. This study followed a group of children representing the three major types of birth complication: periventricular leucomalacia and intraventricular haemorrhage in preterm infants, and birth asphyxia (hypoxic–ischaemic encephalopathy) in term infants. The children had been extensively studied during their first 18 months (Eken et al 1994, 1995). A re-examination at the age of 5 included the administration of the L94 visual perception tasks (van den Hout et al 2000, Stiers et al 2001). The clinical characteristics of the group are summarized in the right-hand column of Table 8.3.2, and the L94 results are presented in Figure 8.3.3. Given their clinical characteristics, the results based on chronological age (upper right graph) can be expected to over-rate the occurrence of visual perception problems. However, as the lower

TABLE 8.3.2

Clinical characteristics of two groups of children assessed with the L94 visual–perceptual battery

	Low-risk group	High-risk group
N	22	57
Gender	15 male, 7 female	35 male, 22 female
Chronological age mean (SD)	8.46 (3.54)	5.29 (0.13)
Intelligence		
Impaired (IQ <85)	90.9%	35.1%
Moderate intellectual disability (IQ <55)	63.6%	10.5%
Performance age		
Range	2.33–7.50y	2.59–7.61y
Mean (SD)	4.23y (1.31)	5.37y (1.26)
Pathology	Attention-deficit–hyperactivity disorder: 3	Periventricular leucomalacia: 12
	Down syndrome: 7	Intraventricular haemorrhage: 17
	Other genetic: 3	Hypoxic–ischaemic encephalopathy: 11
	Unknown cause: 9	
Visual acuity		
Impaired (n <25 cycles per degree)	27.3%	10.5%
Low vision (n <10 cycles per degree)	0	0

right graph shows, not all impaired scores disappear when the children are evaluated based on their non-verbal performance age. For six of the eight tasks the frequency of impaired scores is still significantly higher than expected in a normal population. Thus, the proposed procedure does allow us to detect visual–perceptual deficits in at-risk children.

Further considerations for evaluating congenital visual–perceptual disorders
Despite its merits, some considerations have to be made when using this procedure for evaluating visual processing deficits. First, it is not 'the' final solution to the problem of assessing specific deficits. It is merely a coarse clinical implementation of a general principle in neuropsychological research with children with multiple disabilities: inferring particular dysfunctions requires a careful examination of similarities and differences in performance profiles on several tests. Second, our choice for non-verbal subtest as the baseline for visual–perceptual impairment is practically motivated. It does not imply a theoretical statement about the nature of perception or non-verbal intelligence. We claim only that the procedure works well in many cases. In fact, it also turns out to be a fruitful approach in domains other than visual perception. For instance, we have also used verbal and non-verbal intelligence age equivalents as reference performance levels for the evaluation of memory and attention in children with genetic disorders (Stiers et al 2005, Wouters et al 2006) and epilepsy (Wouters et al 2006, Stiers et al 2010). In these cases, the procedure allowed fine distinctions to be drawn between deficits that were not discernible when the children were evaluated in the traditional way relative to chronological age. However, intelligence subtests are not the solution for all evaluations, and the choice of tasks to be used as baseline strongly depends on the function of interest. The more specific the question to be answered, the more carefully the baseline has to be chosen.

A frequent objection is that the baseline tasks (i.e. the non-verbal intelligence subtests) are sensitive to visual–perceptual ability. As explained above, this is not a problem as long as the baseline tasks rely less upon visual processes than the perception tasks do. A bigger problem is that often non-verbal intelligence subtests or subscales are used as a substitute for visual–perceptual tests (e.g. Fedrizzi et al 1993, 1996, Goto et al 1994, Ito et al 1996, Jacobson et al 1996). Given that these subtests use the visual modality to assess cognition, it seems plausible that reduced scores may in some cases come about as a result of visual processing deficits. Nonetheless, we have, up to now, not been able to demonstrate a negative effect of specific visual–perceptual impairment as defined above on non-verbal intelligence scores, not for individual subtests, not for non-verbal or verbal subscales, and not for discrepancies between these subscales. This was investigated with the L94 tasks for the WPPSI, WPPSI-R, WISC-R, SON-R, and MOS (Stiers et al 1999, Stiers and Vandenbussche 2004). So, there is considerable evidence that high or low performance on non-verbal intelligence subtests is not related to deficiency in visual processing ability. Of course, other aspects of visual processing not assessed in the L94 tasks may interfere with non-verbal intelligence subtest performance, but it seems wise to first establish this association empirically, before replacing visual tests with non-verbal intelligence subtests.

Most visual perception tests available today comprise several subtests and provide the opportunity to compute composite perception scores – a perception quotient similar to the IQ. Such a composite score is warranted only to the extent that the contributing subtests assess a common ability. The composite score is intended to capture this common factor. Although more research is needed, it seems that in many cases this assumption is not valid for visual processing. Studies with the L94 show that, for many children, the visual processing deficit is manifest only in some tasks and not in others. Within the group of children with visual–perceptual impairment, those with more pervasive impairment form a small subgroup: 30% are impaired on three or more and 11% on four or more L94 tasks (Stiers et al 2000, 2002). Our clinical experience indicates that this is also true for other batteries, such as the Test of Visual Perceptual Skills (Martin 2006) or the Frostig Developmental Test of Visual Perception (Hammill et al 1993). In the case of selective impairment, the composite perception score will underestimate the existing perceptual problems because the few impaired scores will be averaged with the unimpaired scores on the other subtests. Consequently, it is important to look at the subtest profiles rather than the composite perception score. In addition to the selectivity, there is also large intersubject variability in impairment. As was already evident from Figure 8.3.3, impairment profiles over the eight tasks are highly variable. This should not be a surprise given the large extent and level of segregation of the cerebral visual system. Since lesion position is variable, the visual–perceptual deficits that arise because of them will be variable. The implication for assessment, however, is that administering one or two visual–perceptual tasks will not suffice for an adequate evaluation.

Inferences about the nature of the dysfunction underlying the observed visual–perceptual impairment constitute an area warranting special attention in clinical diagnoses. As discussed above, the making of such inferences always requires contrasting the scores on several tasks. Of course, what can be inferred is highly dependent upon the choice of tasks. An object identification task using video fragments, for instance, may be attractive to children, ensuring good compliance. But, the stimuli provide the child with many parallel routes to object identification (shapes, textures, colours, surroundings, motion, depth, etc.). Consequently, such stimuli may not be very sensitive to visual dysfunction because of the use of compensatory mechanisms, and in the case of impairment it is unclear what aspect of the stimulus is responsible. The response paradigm also has to be taken into consideration. Discrimination paradigms are often used (e.g. the Beery–Buktenica Developmental Test of Visual–Motor Integration, the Motor-Free Visual Perception Test, and Gardner's Test of Visual Perceptual Skills, among others), in which a target stimulus is presented together with several possible solutions. Finding the correct answer requires systematically comparing the visual shapes. This places a load on several additional visual functions such as visual attention orienting, visual search, crowding suppression, space representation, and the perception of visuospatial relations. In some tasks the solutions are presented after the target stimulus has disappeared. This adds working memory load to the paradigm. This is, for instance, the case in the L94 task 'overlapping figures', in which overlapping target drawings are presented for 6 seconds, after which they are replaced by a number of separate drawings among which the child must find the target drawings. In such a paradigm, a child may achieve reduced scores because of memory problems without having visual processing problems (Stiers and Vandenbussche 2004). Given these potential interpretation problems, it is important to carefully consider the choice of tasks and, if possible, to choose tasks with perceptually simple paradigms that target specific visual–perceptual functions. For preschool children, some L94 tasks meet that requirement. And recently, for school-aged children, a new battery of visual–perception tasks has been published that meets this requirement (Bova et al 2007).

Cerebral visual impairment is a major cause of low vision. In Western countries it is the main cause of visual dysfunction in 30.6–45.0% of children with low vision (Rogers 1996, Rosenberg et al 1996, Mervis et al 2000). Because reduced visual acuity may interfere with adequate perception of visual material, the question arises of how well we are able to distinguish between the contribution of visual acuity loss and visual processing problems to reduced performance on visual perception tasks. It is clear that visual–perceptual dysfunction can occur without low vision (van den Hout et al 2000, Fazzi et al 2007a). There is also evidence that low vision and visual–perceptual dysfunction are associated disorders. For instance, in the study of Stiers et al (2002), 39.1% of the children with physical disability who were assessed had a reduced single Landolt-C optotype acuity (>10 and ≤24 cycles per degree), and another 7.6% had low vision (≤10 cycles per degree). The prevalence of impairment on one or more L94 tasks in the children with normal visual acuity was 24%, and these children were, on average, impaired in 1.58 of the eight tasks. In the reduced acuity group, the proportion of children impaired on one or more L94 tasks increased to 50%, and the average number of impaired tasks was 2.0. In the low vision group, 59% of the children were impaired on average on 3.0 of the eight tasks. The reason for this association is as yet not clear, but at least for this subgroup of children with low vision it seems that there is no causal link between low vision and performance in the visual perception tasks. As Table 8.3.3 shows, there is a

TABLE 8.3.3

Incidence of normal visual–perceptual performance on the L94 task in eight children with low vision (binocular single optotype acuity at near distance [57cm])

Subject	Acuity (cycles per degree)	Centile				
		DEVOS	VIEW	VISM	NOISE	OVERL
L1	10					
L2	10					
L3	6					
L4	6	≤5	≤5		≤5	
L5	5	≤5	≤5	≤5	≤5	≤5
L6	4	≤5	≤5		≤5	
L7	3					
L8	2	≤5				
Unimpaired	n	4	5	7	5	7
	%	50.0	62.5	87.5	62.5	87.5

DEVOS, De Vos; VIEW, unconventional viewpoints; VISM, visual matching; NOISE, figures occluded by noise; OVERL, overlapping figures.

sufficient number of children with low vision who are not impaired on each particular task to conclude that low vision itself is not the cause of reduced perception scores in this group, at least for grating acuities of 2.0–3.0 cycles per degree and higher. Rather, it is more likely that low vision and perceptual problems co-occur as two separate dysfunctions. This is a topic of great importance for understanding the nature of visual problems in children with congenital brain disorders and for the clinical assessment of these children. Unfortunately, it has not yet received much research attention.

Summary
Disorders of visual perception due to disorders of the brain in children are being increasingly recognized. However, when interpreting the results of neuropsychological testing, it can be difficult to know the relative contributions of generalized brain dysfunction, impairment of acuity, and impairment of specific higher visual functions. All elements of each test performed must be visible to the child. With this proviso, baseline measurement of non-verbal intelligence is needed to find out whether low scores obtained when using tests designed to investigate higher visual function are specifically related to visual dysfunction or whether low scores relate to an overall cognitive impairment.

9
THE EFFECT OF IMPAIRED VISION ON DEVELOPMENT

Elisa Fazzi, Sabrina G. Signorini, and Josée Lanners

Introduction

The role of vision in human development and human relationships has long been recognized. The Ancient Greeks thought of vision as a vital spirit, which entered and exited the human body through the channel of the pupil and optic nerve, and exercised its function: to explore and analyse the external world. In more recent times, research has supported the importance of visual function and its crucial role in early neuromotor, cognitive, and emotional development: Fraiberg (1977) defines vision as the central agency of sensorimotor adaptation, the 'synthesiser of experience', because of the visual system's capacity to coordinate all the other perceptual–sensory systems.

The visual system allows us to extract information from the environment. It rapidly becomes more efficient in the first weeks of life: the view that newborn infants are functionally blind has long been superseded. On the basis of experimental research, beginning with the early studies of Fantz (1964, 1965), newborn infants are now considered to have a significant level of perceptual competence; they are considered able to respond selectively to different environmental inputs, and to be actively engaged in the acquisition of information through exploration that, while still rudimentary, nevertheless appears to be orientated and controlled. Thus, newborns are no longer thought to be immersed in a chaotic and disorganized world of elementary and fragmentary sensations; instead, they are regarded as a being equipped for relational life and for propositive intersubjectivity, thanks to behavioural systems that, according to the model of infant research (Threvarten and Aitken 2001), are able to evoke, in the caregiver, actions designed to promote interaction in daily life.

Visual function, which is linked to the child's perceptual, motor, and emotional development, is highly influenced by the environment and external experience, as shown by recent research which stresses the role of early experience in the maturation of the visual system. Thus, the visual system, with its plasticity, soon asserts itself as a preferential channel for analysing reality, and the first mental representations are based, largely, on visual experience. Moreover, it is through vision that an object is perceived in a holistic fashion, as a *gestalt*, that information about its shape, size, colour, and contrast is perceived simultaneously.

Vision is characterized by 'tonic' functioning, which allows continuous monitoring of the external world. Other sensory channels, with the exception of proprioception, are activated only in response to appropriate stimulation, and are thus characterized by 'phasic' functioning (in which reality is perceived as a series of partially or totally disconnected perceptions and sensations). The consequence of this dual mode of functioning of sensory systems is that vision becomes the integrator of the various perceptual experiences into a mental representation. It is through vision, above all, that the child becomes conscious of the external world, as being separate from self, and comes to know and recognize his mother's face, with awareness of her movements, and, through observation of her 'comings and goings', attaches meaning to absence–presence experiences. Clearly, difficulties in this process are manifest in the visually impaired child.

The development of visually impaired children has been the focus of many studies, and we cite, in particular, the pivotal work of Fraiberg (1977). From these studies it emerges that congenital or early-onset visual impairment interferes with a series of functions and abilities: organization of sleep–wake patterns, gross and fine motor functions, spatial concepts, cognitive abilities, attention and memory, communicative skills, learning processes, behaviour, and bonding. Moreover, visual impairment can fundamentally impair the development of social responsiveness and communication (Sonksen and Dale 2002).

Beyond the clinical value of these studies and the therapeutic indications they provide, it is also important to appreciate the research value of investigating situations in which the child is deprived, from the earliest stages of life, of one of the main instruments for interacting with the world, particularly in view of the fact that, in the developed world, visual impairment is usually secondary to brain damage, which in turn can involve other functions (motor and cognitive). In fact, one of the biggest questions is that of the extent to which the developmental peculiarities of visually impaired children are a result of possible associated neurological damage. Clinical pictures characterized by the presence of multiple disabilities are extremely complex both diagnostically and from a rehabilitation perspective, not least because affected individuals are little able, or are completely unable, to collaborate with clinical/instrumental investigations and treatments.

The following sections consider the role of visual function in relation to the neuromotor, cognitive, and emotional development of visually impaired children.

Visual impairment and neuromotor development

The problems of early blindness are not limited to the lack of vision. Blind children provide experimental evidence on the essential role of visual information in early motor development and on how and when the absence of vision may be compensated for (Prechtl 2001). It has long been known that the development of blind infants is delayed in various domains, especially self-initiated mobility, posture, and locomotion (Fraiberg 1977, Troster and Brambring 1992, Sonksen 1993b, Fazzi et al 2002). Fraiberg first hypothesized that the peculiar trend of motor development found in the blind child can be attributed to the absence of the incentive which sight represents for all voluntary skills. She suggested that the early motor development of the visually impaired child can be divided into two stages. In the first 6 months of life, achievement of the gross motor milestones is only slightly delayed. However, the delay becomes more marked in the second 6 months of life, a period during which voluntary motor skills are acquired and motor function emerges as a key aspect of sensorimotor experience (exploration, searching, etc.). It is from this moment that the visually impaired child begins to present a delay in the acquisition of crawling, standing, and walking unaided, and to display peculiar motor behaviours (e.g. bottom shuffling), which represent compromise solutions between the desire to explore and maintenance of the postural advantages offered by the sitting position.

In a previous study (Fazzi et al 2002), we assessed early neuromotor development in 20 congenitally blind or severely visually impaired children (nine blind only and 11 blind with multiple disabilities, i.e. cerebral palsy or intellectual disability) in order to work out a strategy for early intervention in these individuals. Their mean age at first observation was 11.4 months (range 4–30mo). The mean follow-up duration was 16.9 months (range 3–36mo). Assessment included developmental history, neurological examination, video-recording of spontaneous activity, administration of the Reynell–Zinkin scales for visually impaired children, and neuroradiological and neurophysiological investigations. Our results confirmed Fraiberg's earlier findings: in the blind-only children, all the milestones were reached with a delay, which increased with age, in comparison with the motor development of the sighted children; these delays were slight for head control and independent sitting, but more marked in the subsequent stages involving the use of functions connected with spatial orientation and standing upright. The blind-only children all learned to walk independently, although later than normal children, at an age ranging from 13 to 32 months (mean 19.8mo). The qualitative aspects of walking were also distinctive: walking around the walls with feet apart on tiptoe, with little fluidity or variability of movement.

Four of the nine (45.4%) blind-only children did not crawl. Of the five who did crawl, two did so at the normal age; one crawled and walked at the same age; and another crawled at 24 months, having learned to walk independently at the earlier age of 23 months; finally, one crawled but was not walking at 26 months.

The profile was very different in the blind children with multiple disabilities. Almost all the neuromotor functions were absent in these children, except in one child with hemiplegic cerebral palsy who succeeded in walking with support at the age of 25 months and a child with septo-optic dysplasia who walked independently at 20 months.

The children with multiple disabilities, compared with the blind-only children, showed a marked postural delay in motor items and a more marked delay in dynamic and locomotor items. In children with visual impairment accompanied by other types of central nervous system damage it is not methodologically possible to distinguish between the pathogenetic role of the sensory impairment and that of the other pathologies. The clinical picture of these children is extremely severe: they present marked postural motor delays, and find it difficult to relinquish reference points in their environment – their contact with the floor or the bed, for example – in order to move towards the outside world.

Motor development in blind children improves only once they become able to reach out for and grasp an object presented to them through sound. The capacity to reach an object presented by sound clue seems to serve as the organizer of motor experience: all the blind children learned to walk independently only after gaining the ability to get their bearings guided by a sound. As regards the development of fine motor skills, Fraiberg (1977) emphasizes that vision and grasping evolve synchronously. Indeed, in the first months of life, the hands of the blind child remain for long periods at shoulder height, as though they were persistently divorced from their exploratory tactile function. They converge on the median line only sporadically because this convergence (or 'fingering game') is strongly reinforced by sight. In our study (Fazzi et al 2002), the use of the hands and 'reach on sound' were achieved by all the blind-only participants at between 8 and 10 months of age, providing proof of their having achieved the union of touching with hearing experience. This ability did not appear to be achieved by the majority of individuals whose visual deficit was associated with other neurological disorders.

However, there is a risk that, as well as the eyes, the hands, too, will become 'blind'. The child, in the early months of life, must manage to overcome a true 'conceptual problem'; in other words, he or she must acquire the ability to attribute an external object with identity and substance, even when this object manifests its presence through only one of its attributes: sound.

From Fraiberg's descriptions it can be deduced that this skill (the ability to grasp an object that has been presented exclusively through the medium of sound) is a real breakthrough in the blind child's development and is at once a condition of, and a catalyst to, all subsequent achievements.

Since, for the blind child, objects do not possess the sensory and perceptual qualities that make them recognizable to sighted children, in order to conceive of grasping a sonorous object, the blind child must do without the visual information relating to that object and form a mental image of it, derived from prior tactile experience.

Visual impairment and cognitive development

According to Piaget (1955), vision is the primary sense used in the construction of sensorimotor intelligence. A visual impairment can interfere with sensorimotor understanding, causal processes, spatial relations, and object permanence. Without vision, which serves specifically to organize and integrate information originating from various sensory channels, development of the first learning processes becomes complex and fraught with difficulty.

In the first years of life, the blind child is obliged to understand the external world, and to interact with it, through alternative channels (Brambring 2001). Furthermore, learning by imitation, a very important process for cognitive development, is impaired. Various authors (Fraiberg et al 1966, Bigelow 1986, 1992) have highlighted a slower acquisition of the object concept in blind as opposed to sighted children. According to Piaget, the child acquires understanding of the object concept through six distinct stages, which cover the period from birth to the age of 18–20 months, and which correspond to the six stages in his theory of the development of sensorimotor intelligence.

By object, Piaget means a multisensory whole, that is as something that can, for example, be seen, heard, or touched, and that continues to exist, for the subject, even outside any perceptual contact with it.

The spatial universe of the infant is qualitatively different from that of the older child or adult, in whom the concepts of space and time have been acquired. In the earliest stages of life, the way a child perceives objects is significant. The mother and objects, in the form of visual representations, begin to populate the mind of the sighted child. The perceptual stability offered by vision becomes linked to a progressive assimilation of cognitive and affective experiences. In the sighted child, vision is able to confer identity on people and objects and to act as a synthesizer of experiences and of the attributes of objects. In the case of the blind child, it is the formation not of a visual image, but of a mental image, that constitutes the first fundamental step in giving meaning to his world.

The visually impaired child has to skip the visual–perceptual stage and accomplish a difficult adaptive adjustment: he or she must acquire the ability, with the help of other compensatory sensory modalities (e.g. hearing and touch), to interiorize his or her experience directly, i.e. in the absence of the visual–perceptual component.

However, not all objects are sonorous; furthermore, sounds cannot always supply us with information on the intrinsic characteristics of the objects that produced them. If we think, for example, of the noise made by an object that falls to the floor, it is easy to appreciate how noise runs the risk of remaining a purely sensory input. The same applies to touch: visually impaired children can grasp an object that is brought into contact with their hands, but if they let it go, it falls into space, it disappears completely – it becomes a datum that cannot be used for the purpose of building up experience. Furthermore, ear–hand coordination is more complex than eye–hand coordination, and is established later. Fraiberg et al (1966) describe how, at 5 months, a blind child, although aware of an object located easily within his or her reach, will often remain indifferent to it. Sighted children, on the other hand, from the age of 5–6 months, will stretch out their arms towards a visually perceived object. Because of this delay, the non-sighted child runs the risk of being, for a time, incapable of acting – of remaining stuck in a sensory void (Willis 1979).

By the age of 7–8 months, visually impaired children will become aware of a sonorous object, their facial expression showing that they recognize it. Yet still their hands are not drawn to the object. Subsequently, such children will begin to unite touching with hearing experience: if you put a musical toy close to a visually impaired child and get him or her to touch it and then take it away for a moment, the child will open his or her hand and move it slightly in an attempt to get it back. When the child is around 11 months old, merely shaking the sonorous object nearby will cause the child to open his or her hand and move it towards the source of the sound: at this point the child is able to attribute substance to the object, even in the presence of only one of its properties. This means that visually impaired children, unlike sighted children, must achieve a certain level of conceptual development before being able to reach out their hand and grasp a sonorous object. To be able to resolve the problem visually impaired children must be equipped with memory and with an emerging concept of the permanence of objects.

It is thus easy to appreciate the risk that visually impaired children will never find the adaptive solution, and will remain 'frozen' at the level at which they focus on their own bodies. When such children acquire the ability to sit unsupported, one should then furnish the space around them with objects that will arouse their curiosity, arranging them in such a way as to encourage the exploratory activity of the hands. This is the phase of the 'reach and touch on sound' milestone, which is crucial for not only fine motor, but also cognitive, development.

Visual impairment and emotional development

Children with congenital visual impairment have an inherent difficulty relating to others and to reality (Fraiberg 1977). Numerous authors (Burlingham 1975, Willis 1979, Brambring and Troster 1992) have stressed that this difficulty persists throughout development, assuming specific significance at different ages, but there is no doubt that the most delicate phase is that of the first years of life. Indeed, vision plays a crucial role in the mother–child relationship: after just a few weeks of life, infants begin to observe their mother's face and to smile when they see it, in this way pleasing their mother and encouraging her attachment to them. The fact that the infant can see his or her mother helps the infant to feel in touch with her, even when she is not tending to him or her; it helps the infant to understand her emotions, and to interact with her in a meaningful way, thereby favouring the development of their relationship.

It is through sight that the first bonding and attachment experiences are established in the child, becoming permanent and natural behaviours. A sighted child is generally able to establish emotionally significant relationships with specific key individuals during his or her first 18 months of life. The development of permanent human bonds in this period is signalled by a series of increasingly discriminatory behaviours towards preferred individuals: social smiling, discrimination between the mother and the stranger, separation and reunion behaviours. All these, without exception, are visually mediated behaviours.

But in a world that is devoid of images, how do visually impaired children learn to tell their mother apart from other people? How do they express their preference for her and the particular value that they attach to her? There is thus a danger that non-sighted children will find themselves in a void, unable to forge the bonds essential for emotional development.

Observing the sequential development of selective and preferential behaviours in a group of non-sighted children, Fraiberg found the following. The familiar voice is the primary activator of smiling: as early as 4 weeks of age, children display a selective, but irregular, smile in response to the voices of their parents, of their mother in particular; the same smile is not evoked by unfamiliar voices. There is no circumstance that can regularly evoke their smile. From 2.5 months to 6 months of age, visually impaired children continue to smile selectively in response to their mother's voice; but smiling, evoked by voice, remains inconstant. From 6 to 11 months of age, the smile of the visually impaired child does not alter substantially compared with the previous phase.

In the course of the first year of life, 'tactile language' is crucial in the construction of object relations. In the first weeks of life, non-sighted children's quest for contact is very similar to that of sighted children (with the exception that, for the latter, tactile experience is just one of a range of possible ways of establishing contact). Non-sighted children, for many months, are able to establish contact with their mother only when she manifests her presence to them, through touch and voice. By the fifth month of life, the child's quest for tactile contact is becoming increasingly discriminatory and intentional.

Between 5 and 8 months of age, non-sighted children begin to use their hands to explore the faces of their parents and of other familiar individuals, and only rarely will they explore the face of a stranger: this is thus a first form of recognition.

Between 7 and 15 months of age, visually impaired children, like their sighted peers, reject strangers, refuse their embraces and care, cry in protest, and will be consoled only by their mother's voice or by physical contact with her.

In the second year of life, sighted children already display some signs of growing independence from their mother, and can tolerate a brief separation from her; in contrast, visually impaired children tend to present episodes of intense attachment to their mother and to develop genuine panic attacks when they are separated from her.

The negative reaction to strangers is regarded as a criterion for evaluating the positive bonds established with the mother and with other preferred individuals, and the age at which separation anxiety manifests itself seems to correspond to the emergence of a concept of the mother's permanence. In blind children, the first manifestations of protest and anxiety appear at the end of the 21st month of life, almost 6 months later than in sighted children. This delay corresponds exactly to the delay with which the blind child reaches the fourth stage of object permanence, according to the theory of Piaget. Indeed, until the mother has been established as an object, clearly there cannot be any concept of 'loss' or of 'absence'.

The direct consequence of this delay is a prolonging of mechanisms of dependence and an entrenchment of feelings of insecurity and inadequacy. The way parents react to their child's visual disability also plays a fundamental role in the development of object relations. It is possible to observe reactions of denial, overprotection, or even profound depression in the mother that prevent effective emotional interaction with the child.

The risk is that visually impaired children, who need to receive extra inputs to compensate for their lack of vision, may receive far less than normal children, and this has important effects on their emotional development.

But sometimes mothers do prove able, from the outset, to read the needs and behaviour of their children, and to adapt to them, keeping interaction going. These mothers' sensitivity to the needs of their children, and the capacity to predict their behaviour, are essential elements for secure attachment.

Some parents, on the other hand, tend to institute a relationship of dependence, hindering the achievement of personal autonomy in daily life.

Visually impaired children, who are slow to interiorize the concept of their mother as an object, may demand that their recently acquired sense of security and protection is constantly reinforced by her physical presence. In this situation, the anaclitic (strongly dependence-based) relationship will last much longer than is normal, veering towards a symbiotic evolution, in which every attempt at separation becomes traumatic because of the fragile framework of the child's personality. The presence of anxieties as strong as these is, in itself, an obstacle to further development and to the correct building of relationships, and this danger looms even larger in situations in which the visual deficit is associated with a picture of multiple disabilities.

Although visually impaired children do not present a typical personality profile, it is possible to recognize certain rather frequent traits, particularly high anxiety levels, a refusal to engage in competition, absence of aggressiveness, and a tendency to isolation and passivity; furthermore, the behavioural traits more often associated with deafness, namely aggressive or angry reactions, are not typical in these children.

There is a danger that the personality of the visually impaired child can remain closed and focused on bodily sensations and that the bridge with the external world may be unstable or, worse, never even built. In a world devoid of substance and permanence, bodily sensations become the only certainty, the only aspect that possesses continuity (Willis 1979).

On the basis of what has been said, it is clear that severe, early damage to the visual system can impair the development of the early mental and emotional processes, which are the ones that allow children to organize their experiences and develop different areas of learning.

Visual impairment and developmental setback

Children with profound visual impairment are at risk of developmental setback. In one group of children with visual impairment of mixed aetiology, setback occurred between 15 and 27 months and was frequently accompanied by impaired social communication, an increase in stereotypies, and behavioural difficulties (Cass 1994). A fifth of children with profound visual impairment due to 'peripheral visual impairment' suffer a deceleration in developmental quotient, mainly in the domains of verbal comprehension, expressive language, and sensorimotor function. Setback is more strongly associated with more profound visual impairment, while the presence of perception of form and motion appears to exert a protective effect on early cognitive and language development (Dale and Sonksen 2002).

In addition to developmental delay, children with profound visual impairment are at risk of developing features similar to those seen in children with autism spectrum disorders (Fazzi et al 2007).

Developmental risk signs in the visually impaired child

Tustin (1972) suggests that the situations in infancy that really predispose a child to psychosis are those in which 'bonding' experiences are either not established or very precariously established. And it is in this context that we must consider the risks facing the visually impaired child. We know that, in reality, many children with a severe visual impairment nevertheless show healthy and substantially harmonious development. In this regard, authors emphasize the positive role that is played by an intuitive mother, who, overcoming her own anxieties and depression, manages to create a valid and gratifying emotional atmosphere, in which other equally effective modes of interaction compensate for the child's visual impairment. However, it has been found that very early-onset severe visual impairment may affect a child's development and lead to the onset of autistic-like pictures. Hence, early developmental abnormalities in visually impaired children, such as the delayed acquisition of symbolic play and social and communicative skills, might reflect the influence of the visual deficit on early interactive experiences, rather than the coexistence of a primary impairment of social interaction and communication.

A greater understanding of this issue may allow the development of specific strategies of intervention in children with visual impairment, strategies designed to reduce these children's withdrawal behaviours, to encourage alternative channels of communication, and to promote environmental exploration (Fazzi et al 2007b).

In view of this, it is clearly crucial that the professionals who come into contact with these children are able to recognize the signs of developmental risk. The main ones are the presence, persistence, and entrenchment of a whole series of behaviours, which are expressions of considerable social isolation.

These behaviours include the maintenance of floor postures, lack of attention to environmental stimuli, and absence of smiling (or difficulty eliciting smiling).

Other risk signs include poor adaptive use of the hands to explore and recognize objects, absent or poor 'reach on sound', and persistence of excessive and non-functional use of the mouth as the main interface with the environment.

The tendency to create an exclusive bond with the mother, and the presence of fits of anxiety related to the experience of separation, are also to be interpreted as signs of difficulty progressing beyond the symbiotic stage of affective development.

In older children, an excessive production of speech (with declarative rather than communicative intent), serving to fill an emotional void, must also be considered one of the risk signs.

The most typical risk signs in visually impaired children are stereotyped behaviours whose frequency is such that they deserve specific consideration in a separate section.

Stereotyped behaviours in the visually impaired child

The presence of stereotypies in blind or severely visually impaired children has been observed and reported in numerous studies, and we might recall, in particular, those of Fraiberg (1977), Willis (1979), and Fazzi et al (1999). The terms 'stereotypy' and 'mannerism', which emphasize the characteristic repetitiveness of these traits, have now replaced the term 'blindism', since these behaviours are not observed exclusively in non-sighted children.

The stereotyped behaviours typically observed in visually impaired children are usually divided into motor stereotypies (e.g. repetitive hand/finger movements [fluttering], head/body rocking, thumb sucking, jumping, and twirling) and oculo-digital signs. The latter, almost exclusively encountered in blind or severely visually impaired children, include eye poking (pressing the eye with the fingers), eye pressing (pressing the eye with the palm of the hand), and eye rubbing. These gestures, which target the visual system, can have a series of consequences, including infections, keratoconus, and corneal scarring.

The literature contains several interpretations of stereotyped behaviours. In particular, with regard to oculo-digital signs, Jan et al (1994a) suggest that these behaviours are particularly marked and frequent in children with a peripheral visual deficit, as in cases of retinopathy of prematurity or Leber's congenital amaurosis. Oculo-digital signs can be interpreted in the light of their capacity to stimulate the production of light sensations, or 'phosphenes' (pressing on the eyeball stimulates the optic nerve and activates the still intact visual cortex). These authors have suggested that these behaviours have more to do with a desire on the part of the child to increase his or her pain threshold ('stress-induced analgesia'), through an increased secretion of endogenous opioids, than with the condition of visual impairment specifically.

Zentall and Zentall (1983), on the other hand, suggest that stereotyped behaviours can act as modulators of the state of arousal, increasing or reducing the level of stimulation to which the individual is submitted, thereby allowing him or her to maintain an optimal level of vigilance.

A correlation has, indeed, been observed between the type of stereotyped behaviour and the situation in which it manifests itself. Troster et al (1991), for example, observed that eye pressing and thumb sucking occurred prevalently in situations in which the child was left alone, or was bored, whereas other stereotypies, such as repetitive hand movements and jumping, were more likely to occur when the child was excited or having fun. In the light of Zentall and Zentall's above-mentioned theory, it has thus been hypothesized that behaviours such as eye pressing and thumb sucking, typically observed in situations of reduced stimulation, may be interpreted as ways of increasing the level of stimulation, and other behaviours, for example jumping and repetitive hand movements, as ways of reducing it, allowing the individual to maintain an optimal level of vigilance.

Stereotyped behaviours are generally more reversible in children with isolated visual deficits than in those with multiple disabilities (Fazzi et al 1999) or in individuals affected by intellectual disability and/or psychosis. In the latter, indeed, stereotyped behaviours seem to be more rigid, tending towards irreversibility, and to be less responsive to stimuli and environmental changes. Furthermore, even the type of stereotypy appears to be different, conditioned by the presence and severity of the associated disabilities.

In a study of visually impaired children with additional associated disabilities (Fazzi et al 1999), the stereotyped behaviours observed were characterized by a poor motor repertoire (archaic motor patterns and a lack of fluidity of movement). Furthermore, unlike the blind-only children, these individuals did not present the so-called oculo-digital signs: on the whole, their stereotyped behaviours, which did not target the eye, took the form of grimacing and thumb sucking.

In children with isolated visual impairment, on the other hand, more complex repetitive motor behaviours have been reported, probably correlated with a cognitive level that allows them to evaluate the relationship between cause and effect, and thus to anticipate the consequences of a given behaviour.

Summary

Vision plays a central role in early development and is pivotal in (1) the development of object location and permanence, (2) differentiation between self and surroundings, (3) interaction with, bonding with, and understanding of others, (4) according meaning to what is observed, (5) guidance of body movement, (6) providing incentive for exploration and learning, (7) understanding causal process, (8) learning through imitation, (9) synthesizing experience into meaningful representations for learning and memory, and (10) cognitive development.

The visually impaired child is at risk of impaired development of sleep–wake patterns, gross and fine motor functions, posture, self-initiation of mobility and loco-motion, spatial concepts, cognitive abilities, attention and memory, communicative skills, learning processes, behaviour, and bonding, and requires alternative channels to gain the requisite experiences. There is, effectively, a risk of the blind child becoming 'stuck in a sensory void'.

For the blind child, lack of, or alternative forms of, motor development and locomo-tion, such as bottom shuffling, become progressively evident in the second 6 months of life. Walking is delayed, lacks fluidity, and tends to be with feet apart, on tiptoes.

In potentially mobile visually impaired children with central nervous system dam-age, the impairment of motor development can be profound, but it is not possible to determine the contribution of each causative element. For security, such children need to be in tactile contact with known reference points, and sound can provide the bearings needed to bring about locomotion through exploration. For such children, objects, too, need the catalyst of being provided with localization through sound as a substitute for vision, in order to initiate 'reach on sound' which unites, integrates, and accords mean-ing to the experiences of touch and hearing. Lack of discovery of such cross-referencing for meaningful experience, during the early months of life, leads to the risk of the hands becoming 'blind' on account of not having had the opportunity to accord a structured mental image through tactile exploration.

Vision plays a crucial role in the mother–child relationship, in the differentiation between familiar and unfamiliar people, and in the development of emotional language through the progressive recognition of the language in facial expression and gesture. For the blind child, voice is the principal substitute, with the child selectively smiling at known voices from an early age, later exploring the parents' faces through touch. The concept of the mother's object permanence, however, tends to take 6 months longer to develop, and the relationship can become highly dependent.

The risks facing visually impaired children concern their early interactive experi-ences, which may be affected by impaired ability to connect with others (or the ability to establish only insecure bonds). It is crucial to detect signs of developmental risk in these children and, if necessary, to adopt specific preventative and therapeutic strategies of intervention, to minimize isolation, to encourage the creation of alternative chan-nels of communication, and to promote exploration of, and familiarity with, the world around them (Sonsken 1993b, Sonksen et al 1991, 1999). Another possible preventa-tive approach could revolve around the potentially pivotal role of the development of a meaningful auditory linguistic framework (akin to 'radio language' – for which closing the eyes does not impair understanding), from the start of the child's life. Clinical and empirical experience suggests that families who adopt 'non-visual' referencing of lan-guage, commencing at the earliest opportunity, have considerable success in negating the adverse effects of blindness.

Acknowledgements

I wish to thank the team at the Centre of Child Neuro-ophthalmology, Department of Child Neurology and Psychiatry, 'C. Mondino Institute of Neurology' Foundation, University of Pavia, for its continuing collaboration and support, and my friend, Catherine Wrenn, for her help with my English.

10
PSYCHIATRIC CONSIDERATIONS IN CORTICAL VISUAL IMPAIRMENT

Roger D. Freeman

Background

It was only in the mid-1980s that publications began to emerge which described the complexity of cortical visual impairment (CVI) as distinct from ocular impairment. Prior to that time, it was thought that this referred only to a small group of children with profound intellectual disability. We now know that many children with CVI have near-normal eyes, with acuity ranging from light perception to almost normal. Their CVI typically arises from hypoxic–ischaemic injury associated with preterm birth, but also from brain maldevelopment, hydrocephalus, infections, or sometimes battering (Edmond and Foroozan 2006, Ricci et al 2006).

This chapter will consider adaptations of children with CVI, especially those that may be easily misunderstood, and an approach to psychiatric symptomatology, diagnosis, and its consequences. At the outset, one needs to know that there is very little about CVI – if indeed anything – in the psychiatric literature.

The conventional psychiatric focus is on *abnormality* of adjustment or behaviour, specifically interpreting symptoms and using pattern recognition to make diagnoses. This immediately poses a problem because it presumes a reference point of normality, arguably unavailable in this group of children whose behaviour might be unpredictable and confusing. Because of great variability and complexity, a routine psychiatric evaluation by a clinician unfamiliar with CVI may be worse than useless; the delineation of biological, psychological, or social factors that constitute the basis for meaningful psychiatric formulations of problems may be severely limited or distorted.

The psychiatric study of a person with CVI may be attempted by a psychiatrist, or by another clinician who is available and whose training, experience, or job description overlaps that of a psychiatrist. A person may be known to have CVI and have been assessed by a qualified team, CVI may be suspected but incompletely delineated, or may be unknown at the time. There may have been conflicting assessments. The parents may consider themselves to be expert either in general, or about their child's behaviour, or with varying levels of ignorance. Clearly, then, it is difficult to generalize about the initial situation that brings the child to attention. The terminology of CVI is itself still subject to confusion and debate (Hoyt and Fredrick 1998, Jan and Freeman 1998).

There are, nevertheless, several focal points.

A child who has a disability from birth or early life, has initially to accommodate to life as he or she finds it (until it is possible for the child to actively modify his or her own environment). The parents and family, however, will have an unusual and often confusing child to whom to adjust.

Although the understanding of CVI may be a special case of multiple disabilities, there are special features, detailed below.

- Visual function may evolve over time (usually improving) (Salati et al 2002, Hoyt 2003, Matsuba and Jan 2006). However, certain symptoms and problems can interfere with the optimal development of visual function that can be accomplished through early stimulation and intervention (Jan 2001).
- The child's behaviour will not generally be like that of a child with ocular visual impairment, even if ocular impairment is also present.
- The child's behaviour in accommodating to his or her unusual way of visual functioning is highly likely to be misunderstood by all concerned, and wrongly attributed to another comorbid diagnosis, to a psychiatric disorder, to inappropriate parental care, or to late diagnosis and intervention.

The child is highly likely to have impairments other than visual, that is comorbidity (mainly neurological). The results are likely to be interactive, not only additive.

Case studies

Case Study 1

A male patient was followed in neuropsychiatry from the age of 8 to 17. He was born preterm, weighing 4 pounds 12 ounces, and at birth had respiratory distress and pneumothorax. Spastic quadriplegia was diagnosed in his first year. It was noted that he tended to be in his own world much of the time. At age 3 he was diagnosed with CVI and demonstrated visual crowding, problems with depth perception, and eye rolling, with an abnormal electroencephalogram (EEG). He also had anxiety and difficulty both falling and staying asleep. A hyperactive gag reflex, bruxism, and episodic rages, aggressive acts, and self-biting in response to frustrations or changes in routines were noted. His pervasive developmental disorder was diagnosed only at age 8, as was obsessive–compulsive disorder (OCD). Psychological testing showed average intelligence but areas of specific intellectual disability and very repetitive questioning (later categorized as a non-verbal intellectual disability). At age 13 he was reassessed and no longer met formal criteria for CVI (eye movements and acuity had improved). After orthopaedic surgical interventions, he developed complications and chronic pain, aggravating his sleep disorder and anxiety; avoidance of movement aggravated the orthopaedic problems. After 2 years at the same school, he continued to make wrong choices at a junction with his wheelchair (a line in the concrete could mislead him into getting lost). A combination of more successful surgery and a new school, which allowed more flexibility, eventually led to significant improvement.

Comments

Here, one can see the pattern of improvement in visual functioning, but additional and continuing problems in many complex areas of neurodisability, as well as some residual cognitive visual impairment, all over-ridden by severe chronic pain and anxiety. Also apparent is the powerful effect of the change in one or more negative factors, despite the presence of so many others.

CASE STUDY 2

An 11-year-old male was referred for anxiety. He was a preterm infant who had a streptococcal infection in the post-natal period and required ventilation. He developed spastic diplegia followed later by orthopaedic surgery, abnormal EEG without seizures, and strabismus surgery on three occasions; however, these factors were overshadowed by severe OCD and sleep disorder. Any stress provoked phobic and general anxiety and horrific negative thoughts. He had average general intelligence on standardized testing, but significant specific intellectual disability (difficulty with categorization and social cues, weak visual memory and visual–perceptual functioning less than one centile). In addition, he had tactile and auditory hypersensitivities as well as motion sickness. He had great difficulty finding his way around despite adequate visual acuity, and had weakness in making mental maps, easily becoming lost. He was diagnosed with CVI with visual crowding effects. Hand-flapping and finger-flicking patterns were also noted and mild autistic disorder was also diagnosed. On follow-up 7 years later, he continues to have severe anxiety, easily becomes lost, and is receiving both medication and cognitive behavioural therapy for OCD.

Comments

Again, there is severe anxiety, easily aggravated by any stress or change, and specific intellectual disability in addition to cognitive visual impairment. This renders his current cognitive behavioural therapy of limited benefit.

Parental and family adjustment

As can be seen in the two case studies, the overall burden on families can be enormous. It is common for additional diagnoses to be made – and to require parental understanding and emotional adaptation – as the child develops. The visual problems are only one part of this, but are highly likely to be misunderstood, especially by schools. However, it is the parents who are likely to know and understand their child's confusing behaviour and the strategies used to cope with it effectively, usually better than anyone.

SPECIAL FEATURES

Many of the adaptations of children with CVI could be interpreted as something else, such as blind mannerisms, autistic stereotypies, compulsions, or avoidances. These are confusing and may lead to wrong diagnoses, but there are also differences in behaviour between those with primarily ocular impairment and those with primarily CVI (Jan and Groenveld 1993). Such compensatory adaptations can be a rich source of information for habilitation and advice from experts in this field (Jan 1991, Hoyt and Fredrick 1998). The most important difference is that the children do not appear blind: they show *highly variable visual function*, *short visual attention span*, *compulsive light-gazing* and *light sensitivity* (Jan et al 1993), no eye-pressing, *preserved colour perception* (and therefore seek coloured objects to view), and, more commonly, *peripheral field losses*. They may have problems with route-finding in unfamiliar places, forgetting where objects were located, and difficulty recognizing faces or shapes (Edmond and Foroozan 2006). A position with the head hanging down may further restrict visual input. Unusual head postures may be compensatory and should not be interfered with unless their function is understood (Jan and Groenveld 1993). Children with CVI may *turn their heads to the side while reaching* for an object, as if using their peripheral fields (Jan et al 1987). Close looking occurs in both ocular visual impairment and CVI, but in CVI eliminates the *'crowding effect' of too much visual input* to process (Groenveld et al 1990, Dutton 1994). *Stereotyped behaviour* may be a consequence of the need for visual or other input to facilitate neurological maturation (Jan and Groenveld 1993). Compensatory mechanisms may be invoked to deal with several visual and neurological problems simultaneously (Jan 1991). *Prolonged light-gazing* occurs in about 60% of children with CVI with significant impairment in visual acuity (Jan et al 1990a). Some children may even gaze into the sun. Finger movements in front of the eyes against a light source may be an indication of CVI. *Body-rocking* was reported to be more common in CVI than in ocular visual impairment (Jan and Groenveld 1993). About one-third of CVI children show bright light sensitivity (Jan et al 1987). *Attraction to colours* is common and is thought to be due to bilateral hemispheric representation, requiring fewer functioning neurons than form perception. These, and other important but variable features, are tabulated in Table 10.1. In addition, lesions affecting various circuits can influence sensory responsiveness and alter children's responses in other ways (Baranek et al 2007).

COMORBIDITY

Almost all – if not all – individuals considered in the CVI category will have multiple factors in the aetiology of their cortical damage, and very likely multiple neurodevelopmental diagnoses (e.g. cerebral palsy, seizure disorder, and intellectual disability or specific intellectual disability) will have been applied. Some have hearing impairment.

DIAGNOSTIC CONSIDERATIONS

Because there is, as yet, no generally accepted and simple way to assess CVI, especially in children with neurological impairments, CVI may be missed and its consequences attributed to some other factor or diagnosis. One must consider whether the symptom pattern represents a primary psychiatric illness, or a phenocopy (in this case a pattern of reaction to overwhelming stress). Some criteria for psychiatric disorder may be uninterpretable for purposes of diagnosis in children with CVI. Behavioural descriptions or conclusions abstracted from context may not be helpful. Here, a good history of symptoms in relation to the timing of changes in the patient's life may provide some guidance. As visual function is very easily affected by unfamiliarity of place and situation, assessment in a more natural environment, such as at home, is ideally more helpful (Freeman 1967). At home, a child is more likely to demonstrate his or her capacities than in an unfamiliar, and perhaps frightening, office.

TABLE 10.1

Special features and adaptations common in cerebral visual impairment in children with low visual acuities

Area	Frequency	Mechanism	Misunderstanding	References
Other disabilities	Almost universal	Damage to central nervous system	Interplay between pathologies may not be appreciated	Jan et al (1987), Huo et al (1999), Matsuba and Jan (2006)
Ocular and visual pathway lesions	Common, in up to two-thirds	Multiple factors	Cerebral visual impairment (CVI) and ocular impairment are a complex combination	Groenveld et al (1987, 1990), Jan et al (1987), Good et al (2001)
Variable visual function	Common	Complexity of visual information, unfamiliarity; medication, seizures, fatigue	Motivation may be suspected; attention may be involved	Jan et al (1987), Good and Hoyt (1989), Jan and Wong (1991), Good et al (1994)
Impaired head control	Common in cerebral palsy	Changes gaze and visual functions	May seem depressed or uninterested	Jan et al (1987)
Visual input	Commonly view things (e.g. television) from close up	Reduces crowding, copes better with fewer items	Reason not ocular; may not be known	Groenveld et al (1990), Jan and Wong (1991), Dutton (1994)
Direction of gaze	May be averted	Looking away to see better; ?use of peripheral vision	Lack of interest or sociability	Jan et al (1987), Jan and Wong (1991)
Visual attention	Often brief or seemingly absent	Complex	Lack of interest	Jan and Wong (1991)
Light-gazing	14–60%; may stare at sun	Unknown	Important behavioural sign of CVI	Jan et al (1987, 1990), Jan and Wong (1991), Good et al (1994)
Light sensitivity/ photophobia	In about one-third; prolonged dazzle possible	Unknown	Can paradoxically occur with light-gazing	Cummings and Gittinger (1981), Jan et al (1987, 1993), Jan and Wong (1991)
Spatial sense and motion perception	Often impaired	Visual processing, of what is seen, impaired	Capacity may be underestimated	Jan and Wong (1991)
Contrast and colour preference	May be strong	?Bilateral representation	Another way to pay visual attention that may be confusing	Jan and Wong (1991), Dutton and Jacobson (2001), Good et al (2001, 2004)
Stereotyped behaviour	Common	Different theories	May be assumed autistic or tics	Jan et al (1977, 1983, 1990b)

Autistic spectrum disorders (ASDs), depression, lack of motivation and visual attention, anxiety, impulsivity, and angry outbursts with frustration are frequent causes for concern.

- **Anxiety**. The high anxiety level that is so common in children with multiple neurodevelopmental disabilities can become a source of conflict between parents or between parents and schools, especially when theories of causation differ. Family history of psychiatric disorder may be of interest, but may be irrelevant to the child's diagnosis. It may be important, however, in considering the burden of care carried by family members. The difficulty the child has in making sense of his or her environment and of the expectations of others, and the much longer time these may require, can easily be underappreciated. Cognitive limitations and lack of incidental learning during development may make explanations that would otherwise reduce the child's anxiety less effective or impossible.
- **Autistic spectrum disorders**. With the broadening of the criteria for autistic disorder, there has been a large increase in diagnosis that has led to speculation of a recent 'epidemic' of autism. One needs to be aware, therefore, that the suspicion of ASD is highly likely, sometimes raised by parents and teachers. Its likelihood is increased when eye gaze peculiarities and self-stimulating behaviours are present. However, the instruments used to diagnose ASD were never based on a CVI or even ocular visual impairment population, so diagnosis is inherently difficult. Furthermore, blind 'mannerisms' or stereotypies are very common in children with early ocular impairment (Jan et al 1977, Freeman et al 1991), but stereotyped behaviour is also part of one of the criteria for autism, and its presence often increases the suspicion of autism.
- **Depression**. We depend, to a large extent, on mutual visual contact in judging mood. When that is lacking, delayed, or inconsistent, depression may be suspected. Children with CVI may look at people with their peripheral vision, with their head tilted or in a position suggestive of lack of engagement or interest (Jan 1991, Jan and Groenveld 1993). Periods of marked mood change (somnolence, apathy, or agitation with sleeplessness, combined with a family history of bipolar disorder) may arouse a suspicion of masked bipolar disorder (Jan et al 1994b, Freeman and Jan 1996).
- **Tics and Tourette syndrome**. Stereotyped or repetitive behaviour may be wrongly assumed to be tics. On the other hand, tics may take the form of not only the well-known eye-blinking, -winking, and -rolling, but also conjugate eye movements (Binyon and Prendergast 1991). Tics are common in children with neurodevelopmental disorders, and may be mistaken for stereotypies, leading back to a suspicion of autism.

TREATMENT
What are treatment targets? Medication for anxiety, OCD, sleep disorders, and possibly irritability may be helpful, although probably less often than in a non-disabled population, and always with consideration of other medications and with close monitoring (Stores and Ramchandani 1999). When medication is tried it should be at the lowest dosage initially and the physician has an obligation to be available to deal with adverse or unusual reactions and

side-effects. It is not sufficient to prescribe a new medication and immediately go on holiday or delegate management to a family physician. Greater vulnerability of the child's nervous system increases the risk of unusual reactions and of impairing already marginal functioning. The presence of pain that cannot be described or located by some children must also be kept in mind. Advocacy for services to lessen family burden and to minimize misunderstandings is very important and should never be neglected.

Conclusions

Treatment or management is mostly non-specific and could be applicable to many children with multiple disabilities, except that CVI alters behaviour in confusing ways and adds another level of uncertainty. Multiple theories can usually be generated to account for problematic behaviour. Many taken-for-granted meanings and interpretations must be avoided or used only with great care. One should not forget that a useful role for the psychiatrist can be to *remove* a previous diagnosis for sufficient reason and after careful study, not only to make a new one. Assessment of a child with CVI is not the role of a solo clinician or one with limited time.

Approaches that are recommended include the following:

1 Ensuring that the patient's profile of symptoms, disabilities, and details of visual function have been competently assessed by a coordinated team effort, including input from teachers, as many children with CVI remain undetected or inadequately diagnosed.
2 Awareness of the medical–surgical history and issues that might maintain anxiety and stress in a patient, or in his or her family or school.
3 Never assume that identified factors are the complete or necessary ones.
4 Awareness of the child's delayed or impaired coping skills.
5 Identify patterns of behaviour in relation to triggers in the life history.
6 Consider environmental modification of identified sources of stress.
7 Medication is usually a last resort, and requires unusually careful monitoring and consideration of both adverse effects and interactions with other medications.

Having outlined the many challenges and obstacles, it is also appropriate to point out that, under the right circumstances, the assessment and treatment of children with CVI can be rewarding and lead to refinement of the clinician's skills.

11

CHILDREN WITH SEVERE BRAIN DAMAGE: FUNCTIONAL ASSESSMENT FOR DIAGNOSIS AND INTERVENTION

Jenefer Sargent, Alison Salt, and Naomi Dale

Introduction

Severe brain damage may cause cerebral (or cognitive) visual dysfunction arising from the cortex, subcortical structures, and posterior visual pathways, which may be severe or profound. Visual disorders of the peripheral visual system (globe, retina, and anterior optic nerve) are also commonly accompanied by intellectual disability. Over three-quarters of children with severe visual impairment have additional non-ophthalmic disorders or impairments which may give rise to other functional deficits (Rahi and Cable 2003).

A major challenge for clinicians concerned about brain damage and visual difficulties is identifying visual disorders when a child has more generalized brain damage and intellectual disability, and intellectual disability when a child has severe visual impairment. Particularly in cases of severe damage, it can be difficult to distinguish whether functional deficits arise from visual or intellectual disability or both. This has implications for clinical assessment, diagnosis, and intervention to help the child.

Drawing on the clinical experience and research of the developmental vision team of Great Ormond Street Hospital in London, UK, this chapter describes a systematic approach to assessing and diagnosing visual difficulties in the context of severe brain damage and intellectual disability. This includes the assessment of functional visual skills using a developmental framework, whether or not in the presence of additional motor and communication disorders. Three case examples illustrate the main arguments and show how intervention can be tailored to the assessment and its findings.

Severe brain damage: what are the consequences?

Traditionally, diagnostic classification and definitions of paediatric disorders have focused on unitary or 'pure' deficits, and have thereby potentially minimized recognition of co-occurring conditions. This is now being redressed in certain classifications; for example, the recent update in the definition of cerebral palsy acknowledges the increased risk of other deficits (Bax et al 2005).

From a clinical viewpoint, severe brain – or cerebral – damage is a non-specific term. Severity may refer to the form and extent of structural damage, the range of different cognitive functions affected, and/or the degree to which each is impaired. Functionally, cerebral damage may affect motor skills, sensory–perceptual ability (e.g. vision, hearing), higher cognitive skills including language, memory, attention, perception, social cognition, and other skills. The specific consequences of cerebral damage will depend on the areas of the brain involved. However, the relationship between structural damage and function is far from clearcut. In addition to medical investigations of brain structure and function, a child will require systematic and detailed clinical assessment of functional ability, including both vision and general learning. The evidence provided directly informs decisions on habilitation and education.

The specific consequences of brain damage on visual function may include reduced acuity (arising from damage to any structure within the posterior visual pathway), refractive errors, strabismus, oculomotor impairment, impairments of accommodation, visual field defects, difficulties with maintenance or shift of visual attention, and difficulties with recognition or interpretation of visual images (Mackie et al 1998, Houliston et al 1999, Sobrado et al 1999, Jacobson and Dutton 2000, Pennefather and Tin 2000, Jan et al 2001, Salati et al 2002, Andersson et al 2006). The functional consequences may be variable according to the presence or absence of other difficulties, and assessment and intervention approaches will therefore need to be tailored according to individual need.

Severe visual impairment and intellectual disability
Vision is viewed as the major integrative sense for all sensory experience in infancy, and the acquisition of many developmental skills in infancy and the early years appears to be strongly 'driven' by, or dependent on, vision. These include fine motor skills, gross motor skills and mobility, social, communication and language skills, play, and concepts of the material world. Our developmental vision team and others have recorded cumulative impacts of functional deficits in all areas of development in infants and young children with congenital severe visual impairment (Reynell 1975, 1978, Sonksen et al 1984, McConachie and Moore 1994, Brown et al 1997, Sonksen and Dale 2002). These deficits have been recorded in children whose visual impairment derived from congenital disorders of the peripheral visual system ('potentially simple' CDPVS), as well as in those of cerebral origin. Although some eventually achieve normal or superior development in line with their fully sighted peers, a significant proportion show continuing delay or deviance across their early years (Dale and Sonksen 2002). At least one-third of those with profound visual impairment show a significant developmental setback with prolonged plateauing and/or regression of early developmental skills, followed by long-term intellectual disability and autistic features (Cass et al 1994, Dale and Sonksen 2002, Sonksen and Dale 2002, Dale 2005).

The relationships between vision, visual impairment, and brain development are far from understood, but a number of studies have shown positive correlations suggesting a link between brain substrate, peripheral visual impairment, and developmental outcome in children with optic nerve hypoplasia (Brodsky and Glasier 1993) and in heterogeneous children with 'potentially simple' CDPVS (Waugh et al 1998).

Multidisability and visual impairment: consequences for function
Children with multidisability, arising from brain damage affecting multiple systems of the brain, are at greater risk of deficits in vision and other impairments, including oromotor, fine,

and gross motor skills, because of the extent of brain damage. Although the capacity and plasticity of the brain to compensate when severely damaged is debated (Lebeer and Rijke 2003), a cumulative impact of damage to different brain systems is conceivable. For instance, infants may rely on visual, auditory, and manipulative skills for interacting with and learning about their world. Reduced motor skills would limit such natural learning opportunities and the impact of this may be even more devastating if the child cannot see (Schenk-Rootlieb et al 1993).

Children and adults with motor impairments benefit from assistance in developing communication skills using alternative or 'augmentative' methods, which supplement or replace speech and writing. Techniques include unaided methods (e.g. gesture/facial expression, formal sign language, 'yes'/'no' responses, and eye-pointing) and aided methods (e.g. vocabulary presented as objects, photos, symbols or text, ranging from simple single message systems to complex electronic voice output communication aids) (Sclosser 2003). Aided methods of communication depend on the use of multiple visual functions and behaviours. These include sufficient *acuity* to resolve images presented, maintaining *accommodation* for near targets, *recognizing and interpreting* visual images, maintaining visual attention and controlled shift of *gaze* for eye-pointing, executing controlled *eye movements* to inspect and search across visual arrays, and the *social use of gaze* for joint attention with the other communicator.

Functional visual impairment can therefore constrain vital opportunities for communication and learning in children with motor impairment, and identification of such problems is vital for guiding habilitation. In the authors' experience, functional visual difficulties of varying degrees are often unidentified or misinterpreted in children with multidisability. The reasons for this are several, and will be discussed below.

Current challenges for assessing vision in brain-damaged children

Children with multidisability will often be seen by multiple professionals, and whilst integrated multidisciplinary assessment is seen as the ideal, this is often difficult to achieve in practice. Where this is not possible, paediatricians are well placed to take on the role of attempting to draw together the findings from multiple specialists to form a cohesive and functional picture of a child's strengths and weaknesses. However, many school-aged children may not be in current contact with any medical services (Msall et al 2003). There are a number of potential challenges and pitfalls when assessing vision in children with brain damage.

First, information derived from unidisciplinary professional assessments may be designed to answer a specific question, such as documentation of organic pathology. A pathology-orientated examination will not necessarily predict functional skills. Ophthalmological assessment is required before a diagnosis of cerebral visual impairment can be considered. In children with multidisability, it is not uncommon for a normal eye examination to be mistakenly taken by others as proof of normal visual function. Such beliefs are then difficult to dislodge and visual behaviour is not appropriately interpreted.

Second, professionals may attribute a functional problem on the basis of apparent difficulties in one area of functioning, without considering the whole child. It is not uncommon to hear that children with multidisability, including cerebral palsy, are diagnosed as having 'visual–perceptual problems', 'visuospatial problems', 'poor spatial vision', or 'visual processing problems'. Scrutiny of the basis for these diagnoses often shows that there has been very little systematic measurement, that the observations of the child's performance could be interpreted in alternative ways, and that, even if standard psychometric tests have been used, they have not always been considered within the child's overall development.

Third, there is a paucity of scientifically robust tools and methods for assessing functional vision and general development in children with visual impairment (and, even more so, multidisability). Those standardized tests that do exist, for example semi-standardized Reynell–Zinkin scales for young children (Reynell 1978), may be outdated in content and norms (Dale and Sonksen 2002, Sonksen and Dale 2002, Salt et al 2006). This potentially limits their usefulness for planning habilitative and educational programmes. The lack of adequate testing tools makes the diagnosis of visual and intellectual disability much more challenging and reliant on skilled clinical judgement.

Fourth, ascertaining what a child can or cannot do depends on what functional behaviours can be performed physically. Direction of gaze (or eye-pointing) in a forced-choice task can be used to measure the cognitive or linguistic understanding of a child with severe motor impairment who is unable to talk. However, this avenue of communication (and assessment) is reduced or removed entirely if the child has severe visual impairment and cannot view the visual material. The issue of potential skill interdependence for assessment is also of great challenge, as the level of one skill is often demonstrated through the use of another type of skill. For example, the level of a child's language understanding may be usually demonstrated by the child's use of manipulative skills to carry out a specific instruction or to select a target object, or through the use of speech to respond. If a child cannot manipulate or talk, it may lead to premature assumptions on developmental or visual level.

A framework for clinical assessment

The neurodisability service at Great Ormond Street Hospital for Children, involving a multidisciplinary team (neurodisability paediatrics, psychology, speech and language therapy, and occupational therapy), has gained considerable experience of children with isolated visual impairment, and those with visual impairment and other disabilities. The developmental vision team is an integrated clinical and research service and has developed and published on several systematic, scientific methods for assessing vision and development. These methods have permitted the systematic research of developmental and visual trajectories especially in the early years (Sonksen and Dale 2002). More recently, the team has published the new developmental framework and intervention programme (*Developmental Journal for Babies and Children with Visual Impairment*) for the 0- to 3.5-year-old population of children with severe visual impairment in England and Wales as part of the UK governmental Early Support programme (Salt et al 2006). Our augmentative communication service, which is another specialist team, has extended the understanding of the challenges faced by motor-impaired children in acquiring functional skills for learning, communication, and play (McConachie and Ciccognani 1995, Cass et al 1999, Pennington and McConachie 2001).

The cumulative experience of the developmental vision team has led to development of a framework of multidisciplinary assessment which aims to answer the clinical questions listed in Table 11.1. This framework can be applied to any child with visual impairment and also with multidisability.

The route to answering these questions is a thorough functional assessment of vision, cognition, and, where appropriate, motor development. A joint team of a paediatrician, clinical neuropsychologist, and occupational therapist or speech and language therapist work collectively to integrate the paediatric and psychological perspective and assessment methods.

The assessment focuses on function or behavioural use; thus, *functional vision* is defined as the *behavioural use of vision*. The functional assessment of vision has two aspects: (1) the collecting of information on, and observation of, how the child uses his or her vision in everyday situations and (2) standard measurement of the child's use of vision. The latter permits comparisons in an individual child over time, comparison with other children, and, where available, comparison with developmental norms. In the last 20 years, preferential looking techniques have provided a methodology for use in infants and children who are intellectually too young to match optotypes (Teller 1979). The clinical experience of our team suggests that, for infants and preschool children with severe visual impairment, a functional scale that allows measurement of vision lower than the lower limits of other scales (e.g. grating acuity 0.18 cycles/degree at 38cm – less than 6/1000 Snellen equivalent) is essential if the developmental needs of this population are to be met (Sonksen and Dale 2002). A 10-point functional scale (the scale of near-detection vision) has been developed, which permits formal grading of these lower levels of vision (Sonksen 1983, 1993a).

The initial part of the assessment involves collecting information from the parent or caregiver and local professionals involved with the child, such as the specialist teacher for the visually impaired, about the child's use of vision and general development. The *Developmental Journal* for infants and children with severe visual impairment (Salt et al 2006) provides a developmental framework and record for parents to fill in at home and to chart their infant or young child's development across the first 3–4 years of life (www.earlysupport.org.uk – select 'Early Support materials and resources') The framework can also be used with children with multidisability who are still within this developmental age range.

TABLE 11.1

Key questions for clinical assessment of functional vision and development

---

Does the child have cognitive impairment?

Does the child have motor or hearing impairment?

What are the implications of the child's impairments for choice of assessment tools and interpretation of assessment?

Does the child have visual impairment and, if so, what aspects of vision are impaired, and to what extent?

Is the child's visual development in line with his or her general development?

How do the child's combined impairments impact on function?

What are the implications of the child's impairments for habilitation methods, and what intervention will promote development and/or vision?

The second part of the assessment involves a structured assessment using a particular set of measures and observations which are carried out in a playful approach so that it is fun for the child. It is important that the interaction with the child is relaxed, playful, and encouraging, to enable the child to participate and engage positively. The order of assessment is necessarily flexible.

Functional vision assessment begins with observations of the child's ability to sustain visual fixation or interest, and whether this is influenced by task content or visual surroundings. An assessment room in which background decoration and foreground clutter are kept to a minimum is recommended. Standard measures of detection vision and acuity (preferential looking or optotype methods), at near and distance, are used. Eye movements, both smooth pursuit and saccades, are elicited using a motivating visual lure; visual fields are assessed using confrontational techniques for more able children and a modified distraction technique for younger children. Vision for objects is tested with a selection of real, everyday objects at a standard distance, and vision for pictures with the standardized Sonksen Picture Guide to Visual Function. Attention to the developmental skill level required for particular visual tasks is essential (Table 11.2). For further reading about these methods, see Sonksen (1983), McDonald et al (1985), Teller DY et al (1986), Sonksen and Macrae (1987), Sonksen and Silver (1988), Hodes et al (1994), and Sonksen et al (2005).

In addition to, and complementing, the functional visual assessment, we carry out an assessment of cognition, social development, and communication/language. The purpose of this assessment is to identify the child's current level of developmental functioning and to use this information to aid interpretation of the child's functional use of vision. Since functional vision is a neurodevelopmental process in which advances in acuity, visual interest, and visual attention occur during the early years, it is important to separate out delays and deficits in functional vision from general developmental aspects of the child. In addition, cognitive assessment identifies the child's current developmental needs and how his or her visual or learning environment may need to be adapted to promote and support his or her developmental progress (taking into account the child's current level of vision and visual impairment).

The cognitive assessment begins with play-based observations and then moves on to semi-standardized and standardized forms of assessment, including the Reynell–Zinkin scales for young children with a visual handicap (Reynell 1978) and, for older children, the Intelligence Test for Visually Impaired Children (Dekker 1989). Other standardized cognitive tests which have been designed for sighted children are used partially or in full, depending on the child's

TABLE 11.2
Cognitive skills/developmental age required for visual tasks

Naming objects	From 18mo
Naming pictures	From 21mo
Matching symbols	From 30mo
Naming symbols	Pictograms from 33mo
	Letters from 42mo

level of vision, developmental level, and motor impairment, with cautious interpretation because such tests do not have norms for children with severe visual impairment. Verbal test items may be used with children with very limited vision; non-verbal pictorial reasoning items may be used with children who can see the material but cannot manipulate it physically. The decision on what test material to use is discussed jointly by the psychologist and paediatrician to ensure that the test material best meets the child's needs and the ceiling of performance reflects cognitive and not other constraints.

By linking the functional vision assessment with cognitive assessment, and by extending it beyond measures of acuity alone, we aim also to document the level and quality of vision available for development and learning. The functional vision assessment identifies what kind of visual promotion is needed to help the child achieve maximum visual development. The evidence-based intervention programme for visual promotion (Sonksen et al 1991) is incorporated in the work of our clinic. The cognitive assessment provides the framework for establishing appropriate developmental and educational goals, and guidance on how these can be achieved. Assessment findings can also be linked to the parent–professional *Developmental Journal* (Salt et al 2006), which provides detailed activity suggestions for promoting vision and development.

ADAPTING THE ASSESSMENT FOR THE CHILD WITH MULTIDISABILITY

This functional assessment approach may have to be adapted when assessing a child with a potential multidisability. A main clinical risk is that the child's current capacity and potential for learning is either underestimated or overestimated by parents, caregivers, and professionals because the child is very individual and complex and difficult to compare with other children. Test materials can be adapted for the individual child; however, this may mean that the original standardization conditions of the test construction are no longer met and the test has reduced validity.

To increase reliability and validity, we use a number of different tests (or subtests of different tests) and supplement these by systematic and careful observations of the child's behaviour in different task situations. Careful observations or reporting of the child's visual and cognitive behaviour in different settings help build up a picture of the child's current functioning. Charting the child's progress over time also increases reliability and confidence in the assessment findings and the child's rate of learning.

The most challenging child to assess is one with very limited behavioural output (Porro et al 1998a). A starting point is to systematically observe and record the child's responses to everyday familiar situations using a developmental framework (Salt et al 2006). Monitoring behaviour over time and intervening with developmental or visual promotion (Sonksen et al 1991, Salt et al 2006) enables the parent or caregiver, in partnership with professionals, to establish how the child is responding to the learning opportunities presented. In addition to these observations, adapted standard materials can be introduced once the child is able to show some predictable and organized behavioural output, e.g. eye-pointing, 'yes/no' responses, purposeful manipulative skills, or definite verbal responses. The psychologist of the team works closely with the paediatrician to determine whether visual or cognitive constraints may account for a child's difficulty in completing a task. Through joint decision-making, we reach a clearer picture of what the child currently can achieve, thereby permitting a confident interpretation of the current level of abilities. Assessment integrated with an intervention model allows careful chronicling of the child's development in vision and cognition, motor development over time, and how the child responds to attempts to promote each area of development and the child's rate of learning.

Case histories
The following case histories of three children attending our clinics have been presented to show how we may use this functional assessment approach to identify functional visual and/ or cognitive deficits and plan habilitation and intervention.

CASE 1
Ann, aged 5, had a generalized motor disorder with no functional speech. She was registered partially sighted. However, her local team required clarification of her 'visual impairment', and asked:

• How severe is her visual impairment?
• How does her visual impairment influence choice of expressive communication methods?

Previous ophthalmology reports noted a normal eye examination, 'some' fixation and following ability, no significant refractive errors, but no acuity measures – these were 'difficult to obtain'.

Her parents commented, 'you cannot tell she can see, because she doesn't look as if she does', but were certain that she could recognize books. Communication at home was effected through asking closed questions and awaiting a 'yes/no' response (*smile/no smile* response to indicate *yes/no* respectively).

Cognitive assessment
Using the verbal comprehension scale of the Reynell–Zinkin scales (as she was unable to fully manipulate objects with her hands), Ann was found to give repeatable motor responses to several action commands. She showed reaching (not directed gaze) towards a named object presented in an array. She was unable to speak, but gave yes/no responses (smile/no smile) reliably.

Functional visual assessment

Visual Attention
Ann's eyes and head showed frequent movements. Directed visual gaze did not predictably follow stimulus presentation.

Eye Movements
Pursuit movements were jerky. Some directed saccadic shifts of gaze were noted.

Visual Acuity
She showed preferential looking responses to Keeler grating acuity cards, down to card size 11 (2.1 cycles per degree at 38cm – approximate Snellen equivalent 6/90) on two testing occasions. She could not perform optotype matching.

Vision for Pictures
Using a selection of unfamiliar coloured pictures of single objects, Ann was able to confirm or reject a picture label given by the assessor, using her yes/no responses.

Conclusions
It was concluded that Ann had significant difficulties with maintenance and control of visual attention, severely reduced near visual acuity, and visual tiring with attenuation of directed visual behaviours after sustained effort. She did not show the same fatigue responses to auditory information. She showed language comprehension skills around the level of a 2-year-old (partially sighted norms).

Habilitation and intervention advice
Ann had sufficient acuity and visual recognition ability to recognize large visually simple objects and pictures at near distance and these could be used at close distance for learning purposes. Her educational programme should be geared at the learning goals and methods appropriate for a child functioning at the developmental level of a 2-year-old.

She had insufficient functional control of gaze to use directed gaze (eye-pointing) for selection of object/picture vocabulary for communication output. Instead, it would be appropriate to make her yes/no responses more specific and to use these with listener-assisted auditory scanning (listener reads out vocabulary, and Ann selects with yes/no). Ann had sufficient cognitive ability to develop basic switch use skills and this could allow her, in the future, to independently scan and select vocabulary using auditory scanning. Picture material can continue to be used as an adjunct to auditory input; this should use single images presented against a well-contrasted plain background, with enhanced bold outlines.

CASE 2

A 10-year-old female, Sara, with a motor disorder, was progressing slowly with reading. She was wheelchair dependent for mobility, but could manipulate objects and speak. She was reported as having visual impairment and visual–perceptual problems. Her father asked:

- Do her 'visual–perceptual' problems explain her poor reading progress?
- How can her 'visual–perceptual' skills be improved?

Her visual history was as follows: early strabismus, no refractive error, optic atrophy, acuity 6/30, stable. At age 4 years, she began peering at objects and the television, and at 5 years her school reported her as 'reluctant to look at and name pictures' and 'visually distractible'. At 6 years, an optometry assessment identified 'poor visuomotor and visuospatial skills', and at 6.5 years an occupational therapy assessment concluded that she suffered from 'significant visual–perceptual problems'. With respect to cognitive skills, she was described as working well below the curriculum level expected for her age. Her reading skills were at the level of early sight vocabulary. Educational achievements on the national curriculum assessed by teaching staff were at the level of a 4- to 5-year-old for speaking and listening, reading and writing, and mathematics.

Cognitive assessment

Non-verbal assessment using the Wechsler Intelligence Scales – 3rd version UK (WISC-III UK) revealed scores in the exceptionally low range. She had no visual difficulties using the non-verbal material. Mathematical reasoning test showed skills at a 4.5-year level. Phonological processing and literacy test showed skills at a 4-year level. Language assessment using the Clinical Evaluation of Language Fundamentals showed language comprehension and expressive skills around a 4-year level.

Functional visual assessment

VISUAL ATTENTION AND BEHAVIOUR

Sara showed visually directed search for target objects and held her gaze steadily on target objects. She did *not* show peering on searching or during sustained visual inspection. She used eye contact effectively for social interaction and communication.

VISUAL ACUITY

Sonksen–Silver acuity system: 3/18. There was no significant difference between her acuity for single letters and for a linear array. Near acuity was N18 at her usual working distance of 40cm.

She followed moving targets with jerky horizontal pursuit movements. Saccadic movements were slightly hypometric.

VISION FOR PICTURES
Sonksen Picture Guide to Visual Function: she was able to identify some, but not all, visually complex pictures, as expected from her acuity measures. She was able to identify accurately numerous components in a detailed picture presented at near distance.

Conclusions
It was concluded that Sara had a moderate acuity impairment, but sufficient acuity to resolve letters. She showed no obvious impairments of attention and no crowding phenomenon. Her language skills, reading ability, and non-verbal and phonological processing skills were all at the same, approximately 4- to 5-year-old, level. Her overall cognitive level was likely to be the best explanation of slow progress with formal reading skills and of previous scores on motor-free tests of visual perception. The continuing use of the diagnostic description of 'visual–perceptual difficulties' was not justified since this diverted attention from her core difficulties, which fall into the category of severe intellectual disability.

Habilitation and intervention advice
It was recommended that Sara continue a general learning programme aimed at supporting her slowed learning, with curriculum focused on a 4- to 5-year skill level, and including the teaching of basic literacy and pre-literacy skills.

Picture material is helpful as visual support for her learning. Symbol use may also be useful as an augmentation for literacy.

CASE 3
Tina is an 11-year-old female with microcephaly, epilepsy, a motor disorder, intellectual disability, visual impairment, and no speech. Her mother wanted to know whether Tina could learn to 'talk' by eye-pointing to pictures in her choice/communication book.

Her vision history included poor visual behaviour noted within the first year, normal ophthalmological examination with light awareness only, leading to blind registration. A trial of glasses to correct hypermetropia had been suggested, but Tina had never tolerated wearing these. Her parents reported that she was currently able to 'watch' television (maintains steady head and eyes) and follow moving people. Her history of communication revealed that she could not convey her wishes clearly through a consistent yes/no response, but her parents could identify her preferences through body movements. Her school staff used a 'choice' book with large pictures, where options were read out but not shown to her.

Cognitive assessment

Tina's ability to respond to familiar phrases in context was seen to be emerging, but not yet fully established (less than 12 months age equivalent for blind and sighted norms, Reynell–Zinkin scales). She had no reliable yes/no responses to use in response to closed questions. She was unable to manipulate the toys of the Reynell–Zinkin scales, so the language subscales were used to establish developmental level.

Functional visual assessment

Visual attention tests revealed slow head movements towards visual lures. Fixation was of poor quality and not sustained.

Detection vision and visual acuity

Tina showed directed swiping movements of her left arm when presented with standard lures suspended at eye level at 30cm distance. The smallest size of lure to elicit a response was 6.25cm in diameter. No preferential looking movements were seen to either Keeler grating acuity cards or Cardiff cards.

Eye movements

She showed some slow-turning movements of her head, but no accurate saccades, between two static objects. She showed following movements to a variety of visual lures moved both horizontally and vertically, in contrast to poor maintenance of gaze on a static object. On spinning, there was no locking of eye gaze (which would indicate impairment of initiation of saccades) and some sluggish beats of optokinetic nystagmus were seen. Frequent spontaneous eye movements were seen at other times, which did not appear to have the quality of systematic inspection or searching behaviours.

Vision for objects

Tina was shown two items considered to be within her experience by her mother. Although she was able to reach out, she was not able to show any definite evidence of selection by name.

Conclusions

We concluded that Tina had some limited visual detection ability (shown through motor responses). Her frequent eye movements could not be confirmed as purposeful. She showed a predictable visual following ability for moving objects, which is likely to be most consistent with her immature level of visual development rather than evidence of selectively better vision for moving objects. Overall, she showed a very reduced range of responsive and directed visual behaviours, arising from her reduced visual acuity and low cognitive interest in visual stimuli.

Habilitation and intervention advice

Eye-pointing is not a realistic goal in light of her general visual and developmental level and visual impairment. She has a continuing need for familiar routines, phrases, and interactions to build on situational understanding of familiar routines, everyday objects, and recognition of familiar phrases in everyday contexts. Early communication of preference can be encouraged through developing choice-making between two options. Provision of multisensory clues, including vision, to aid recognition of objects and their functions, actions, and events is appropriate. Visual material should consist of brightly coloured objects presented within her arm's reach.

Summary

This chapter presents the case for, and demonstrates the importance of, a comprehensive functional assessment, drawing on a functional visual and cognitive assessment, for children with disorders of the peripheral or cerebral visual system or multidisability. Three case studies showed how functional assessment can be used to identify visual and cognitive strengths and difficulties in children with complex profiles, and interpret them within a developmental framework, as a basis for greater understanding of the child's vision and development. The findings from the assessment shape an individualized habilitation programme which focuses on the child's current developmental and visual needs and how to promote development and vision (where relevant), and suggests appropriate adaptations to the child's learning environment. This assessment framework can be applied by specialist paediatric health teams, and the benefits from integrated multidisciplinary input have been highlighted. Although we have discussed the challenges and limitations of current testing material, a creative use of current resources can lead to very helpful understandings for children and their parents and educators.

12
VISUAL IMPAIRMENT IN CEREBRAL PALSY

Elisa Fazzi, Sabrina G. Signorini, and Paolo E. Bianchi

Introduction

Visual disorders are a main symptom in the clinical picture of cerebral palsy (CP), and there is currently strong evidence that they are not just associated problems but rather – on a par with the motor disorders – intrinsically related to the underlying cause of CP. The spectrum of visual problems in children with CP is extremely broad and includes both peripheral problems related to the anterior part of the visual system, such as strabismus, refraction disorders and retinopathies/funduscopic anomalies, and visual problems of central origin, such as amblyopia, delayed visual maturation, and cerebral visual impairment (CVI).

Briefly, CVI can be defined as 'a visual deficit caused by damage to, or malfunctioning of the retrogeniculate visual pathways' (Good et al 2001), thus emerging as an expression of damage to the central nervous system at the different levels at which visual information is gathered and processed (the optic radiations, the occipital cortex, and the visual associative areas). Although the aetiology of CVI can vary (cerebral malformations, embryogenic and fetal infections, cranial traumas, degenerative encephalopathy, etc.), the most frequent cause is pre-perinatal hypoxic–ischaemic damage, which involves not only the descending motor pathways (leading to the development of neuromotor disorders, as in CP), but also the geniculate and extrageniculate visual pathways and the visual associative areas. Hence, CP and CVI share a common origin. Schenk-Rootlieb et al (1994) and Ipata et al (1994) studied visual function in two cohorts of children with CP and found that 70% showed a reduction in binocular acuity that could not be linked to an ocular disorder. Having said that, low vision is often associated with other visual disorders, such as strabismus, oculomotor and visual field deficits, and asymmetrical optokinetic nystagmus. In both these studies, the distribution of the visual deficit was found to correlate with the type of CP. Impaired visual acuity is, in fact, more common in children affected by quadriplegia or dyskinesias than in diplegic children, whereas children with hemiplegia often have normal visual acuity. In the study by Schenk-Rootlieb et al (1994), an improvement in vision over time was noted in a significant proportion of the participants; only a small percentage showed a worsening of their visual acuity. Other literature data (Cioni et al 1997, Lanzi et al 1998) also show that 60–70% of children with CP also have CVI. Indeed, hypoxic–ischaemic encephalopathy is now the main cause of CVI, in which different brain areas may be affected depending on the gestational age of the infant:

the grey matter tends to be more vulnerable in children born at term and the subcortical white matter is more vulnerable in preterm infants (Brodsky 2002).

Periventricular leucomalacia (PVL) is the lesion that – more than any other – explains the relationship between CP and CVI. It can be taken as a paradigm of the anatomical–pathological substrate in which the contemporaneous involvement of the visual system and the adjacent corticospinal tracts explains the coexistence of motor and visual symptoms. Clinical neuroradiological studies have previously demonstrated a correlation between visual deficit and reduction of periventricular white matter where the optic radiations run (Uggetti et al 1996, 1997, 2001, Jacobson et al 1996, 1998a, Cioni et al 1997, Lanzi 1998, Jacobson and Dutton 2000, Fazzi et al 2004).

With regards to the anatomical vulnerability of the preterm brain, Madan (2005) has recently suggested that another structure is involved in CVI, hypothesizing that the subplate neurons could provide a site of synaptic contact for axons ascending from the thalamus and other cortical sites between roughly 22 and 34 weeks of gestational age. At this age, the cortical plate has not even developed and so the subplate neurons function as a holding region for these afferent ascending pathways. This region is in close proximity to the germinal matrix and is vulnerable to the same ischaemic effects that damage the periventricular white matter.

Thus, damage to subplate neurons is thought to disrupt the development of the cortical architecture. For example, ocular dominance columns fail to develop in the visual cortex when subplate neurons are damaged at this crucial developmental time (Madan 2005).

Thus, there is evidence that visual disorders, peripheral and/or central, fall very much within the spectrum of CP comorbidity (Lanzi 1998, Fazzi et al 2004). In particular, the signs and symptoms characteristic of CVI can be linked to the involvement of the posterior visual pathway (reduction in visual acuity and/or visual field, alteration of contrast sensitivity, alteration of stereopsis, asymmetrical or absent optokinetic nystagmus), and of the oculomotor control systems (alteration of fixation, smooth pursuit and saccades, strabismus, abnormal eye movements). Furthermore, Good (2001) has also suggested that the clinical spectrum of CVI should be extended to include disorders of complex visual abilities deriving from impairment of the ability to analyse and process visual information (cerebral visual dysfunction). In the literature, these disorders are termed 'visuoperceptual disorders' or 'cognitive visual dysfunction' (Dutton 1994, Dutton et al 1999), and they would seem to constitute the main expression of CVI in patients with normal or only slightly reduced visual acuity (who are thus said to have 'higher-functioning CVI'); these pictures can go unnoticed during follow-up in the first few years of life, manifesting themselves clearly only when children reach school age (Abercrombie 1964, Koeda and Takeshita 1992, Fedrizzi 1998, Stiers 2002, Fazzi et al 2004).

The assessment of visual function in cerebral palsy

The assessment of visual function and the early identification of a visual deficit in children with CP is thus particularly important from the point of view of rehabilitation, as it allows the development of personalized treatment programmes. We also stress the importance, in the follow-up of children with CP, of constantly monitoring their visual abilities; in this way, any changes in their clinical picture or, indeed, the appearance of new signs or symptoms can be detected promptly and the rehabilitation programme of the developing child adjusted accordingly.

We would draw particular attention to the considerable difficulties involved in assessing very young and poorly collaborating children, and also to the fact that the assessment of visual function in these children is both very time-consuming and very costly, demanding specialist skills. In the past few years, several new diagnostic instruments have emerged, improving diagnostic–clinical competences.

Recently at our institution, we have established a specialized centre of child neuro-ophthalmology, which represents a new experience, both in our country and abroad. Here, the members of an interdisciplinary team (child neurologists, ophthalmologists, optometrists, and rehabilitation therapists specializing in low vision) work together to assess all aspects of visual disorders in childhood, the relationship of these disorders with neurological problems, and the impact of these problems on development. This clinical assessment forms the basis of a tailored rehabilitative intervention which takes into account the child's inter-related visual, cognitive, and motor problems.

All children with CP who are referred to our centre are submitted to the following neuro-ophthalmological assessment protocol, which is described in detail in a recent paper (Fazzi 2007).

Briefly, it involves the following:

1   clinical history and neurological examination.
2   developmental (Griffiths Mental Development Scales) and/or cognitive assessment (Wechsler Scales of Intelligence).
3   neuro-ophthalmological evaluation.

Neuro-ophthalmological evaluation comprises:

*   Observation of spontaneous visual behaviour.
*   Ophthalmological examination including assessment of refraction in cycloplegia and ophthalmoscopy.
*   Visual acuity. This is evaluated with the maximum possible dioptric correction, and using different tests depending on the child's age and on the severity of the clinical picture. Children up to the age of 2 years are evaluated using the Teller Acuity Cards (Teller et al 1986), which give resolution acuity in cycles per degree (c/deg) in all children able to collaborate. Several tests are used (Lea symbols, letter optotypes), which give recognition acuity expressed in tenths. We consider binocular visual acuity since monocular investigations are difficult to perform owing to both the young age of the children and the frequent presence of associated neurological impairment. Visual acuity is categorized as follows: very low vision (<0.05 tenths, or <1.6c/deg); low vision (0.05–0.3 tenths, or between 1.6 and 9.6c/deg); near normal vision (0.3–0.8 tenths, or between 9.6 and 26.0c/deg); normal vision (≥0.8 tenths, or >26.0c/deg). In children whose vision is not assessable, we look for signs of visual perception, both direct (object localization, movement

of the limbs and/or head towards the visual target, pursuit of a moving stimulus) and indirect (postural reactions, alteration of respiratory frequency, avoiding reactions, and smiling and other changes of facial expression).

- Contrast sensitivity, evaluated using the Hiding Heidi Low Contrast 'Face', coded as not assessable, reduced, or normal.
- Optokinetic nystagmus (absent, asymmetrical, or present), evaluated using a semi-rigid screen covered with black and white square patterns bent to form an arc or using a computer-generated random dot pattern positioned in front of the infant's face (Atkinson 2000).
- Visual field (normal, reduced). Because of the often young age of the children with whom we work and their frequent associated motor and/or mental disabilities, traditional methods cannot always be used to define with precision the extent of their visual field. Thus, we assess, using kinetic perimetry and on the basis of behavioural reactions (e.g. movements of the head, eyes, or a limb towards the target), the child's ability to locate targets presented in the different areas of the visual field. The perimeter consists of two perpendicular black metal strips bent to form two arcs, each with a radius of 40cm, with the infant in the centre of the arcs (Schwartz et al 1987).
- Stereopsis (not assessable, absent, partial, present) evaluated using the Lang Stereotest (Lang 1983).
- Oculomotor assessment: fixation (absent, sporadic, unstable, stable); smooth pursuit (absent, discontinuous, normal); saccadic movements (abnormal, normal, absent) using highly contrasting or bright objects, illuminated by a direct light source that does not dazzle the child (halogen lamps, for example, are ideal).
- Visual axis alignment to detect strabismus, using the Hirschberg test of corneal reflexes, the Cover test and the Paliaga test, and extrinsic and intrinsic ocular motility. We also look for abnormal ocular movements, such as nystagmus and paroxysmal ocular deviations.
- Visual–perceptual assessment. Here, it is worth pointing out that in children over the age of 4 years with an intelligence quotient (IQ) >55 and visual acuity greater than 3/10, visual–perceptual abilities can be assessed using the Developmental Test of Visual Perception, which allows the definition of a general visual–perceptual quotient (GVPQ), a non-motor visual–perceptual quotient (NMVPQ), and a visual–motor integration quotient (VMIQ). Patients with a GVPQ of <90 are considered to have a deficit of visual perception and are categorized as follows: 80–89, below average; 70–79, poor; <70, very poor visual–perceptual abilities (Fazzi et al 2004). Recently, we developed a more accurate protocol for assessing visuocognitive aspects in children with CP for which normative data are available in a recent article (Bova et al 2007).

The evaluation also includes neuroradiological examinations (brain magnetic resonance imaging [MRI], studying the optic pathways, or brain computed tomography [CT]/transfontanellar ultrasound). We have developed a protocol specifically to investigate visual pathway involvement and we look for the following signs: optic nerve thinning, lateral geniculate body

(LGB) gliosis, gliosis or interruption of the optic radiations, atrophy of the calcarine cortex, and white matter alterations at the level of the occipitoparietal lobe (Uggetti et al 1997).

Neurophysiological investigations are also performed (pattern and flash visual evoked potentials and electroretinogram; electroencephalogram; brainstem auditory evoked potentials).

Aspects of visual disorders in the different forms of cerebral palsy

We will now look briefly at the peculiar patterns of expression of the visual disorders in the various forms of CP. Indeed, in the same way as different motor patterns are associated with the different forms of CP, it is also possible to identify neurovisual characteristics typically associated with each form and linked to the site and extent of the damage as well as to the timing of the insult.

NEURO-OPHTHALMOLOGICAL FEATURES IN SPASTIC DIPLEGIA

In spastic diplegia we can find involvement of all the components of the visual system (eye and optic nerve, oculomotor system, primary and associative visual pathways) showing different levels of severity. The clinical manifestations of CVI frequently include ocular involvement, such as strabismus and refractive errors, but also fundus oculi abnormalities, optic atrophy, or pale temporal optic disc, with or without large optic disc cupping (Jacobson and Dutton 2000, Fazzi et al 2007a). This explains the wide range and complexity of the visual symptoms observed in children with CP. Reduction of visual acuity is often present, usually mild or moderate. Visual field deficits are described, typically characterized by reduction of the lower part of the visual field (Jacobson and Dutton 2000).

In addition, there are two further aspects that seem, in particular, to characterize the neuro-ophthalmological picture in spastic diplegia: oculomotor disorders and visuocognitive disorders.

The role played by abnormal eye movements in the clinical picture of spastic diplegia is an interesting question but one that has received little attention in the literature. Abercrombie (1964) highlighted markedly irregular slow pursuit movements and slow saccadic movements in children with CP, pointing out that eye movements play a significant role in the development of visuoperceptual and explorative abilities. Katayama and Tamas (1987) also evaluated saccades in children with CP and reported a high incidence of slow saccades and corrective saccades used to return the gaze to the target.

Hood and Atkinson (1990), considering a sample of healthy infants (aged 1 and 3 months) and a group of children with neurological deficits, assessed the children's ability to use saccadic movements as a means of shifting their gaze from a central target to a target in the peripheral visual field: this ability was found to be more impaired in the second group, and the authors suggested that this may reflect a visual attention disorder of central origin.

Fedrizzi et al (2001) analysed the role of eye movement disorders in children with spastic diplegia using an adaptation of the 'Animal House' subtest of the Wechsler Preschool Primary Scale of Intelligence (WPPSI). The children with diplegia performed less well than the healthy comparison children, taking longer to perform the task and recording a higher number of omissions. They also had considerable difficulty following the sequential scanning order needed to perform the task and in performing anticipatory saccadic movements to evaluate the position and characteristics of the next target. It is possible that this difficulty is related to a central disorder of selective visual attention. These children's inability to perform anticipatory saccadic movements could be an expression of impaired eye movement coordination, spatial selective attention, and integration of sensory information.

The inability to process different inputs contemporaneously, through frequent and rapid shifting of attention from the central to the peripheral visual field, is probably one of the key factors in the pathogenesis of the visual–perceptual impairment in diplegic children and could be explained by lesions at the level of the pathways linking the striate and parietal cortices.

The second main aspect of visual impairment in preterm children with spastic diplegia is visuoperceptual impairment (VPI), a neuropsychological pattern, detectable at preschool age (Abercrombie 1964, Koeda and Takeshita 1992, Stiers 1999, 2002, 2004, Fedrizzi 2001) and characterized by difficulty processing and analysing complex visual information. This is reflected, in particular, in impairment of visuospatial abilities (e.g. constructional apraxia, impaired visuomotor integration). This impairment derives from a malfunctioning of the parietal–occipital system (dorsal stream) and it also seems to be associated with impaired visual object recognition and difficulty attributing meaning to objects, suggesting involvement of the occipital–temporal system (ventral stream). Our experience (Fazzi et al 2004) reinforced the suggestion of a dysfunction of the parietal–occipital system (dorsal stream), a hypothesis supported by the neuroradiological finding of a signal alteration in the deep parietal white matter, in addition to the MRI signal alteration of the peritrigonal white matter and involvement of the optic radiations that are considered typical of children with spastic diplegia and PVL (Goto 1994, Ito 1996, Fedrizzi et al 1998, Uggetti et al 2001). Correlations have also been reported between VPI and the amount of peritrigonal white matter reduction (Koeda and Takeshita 1992), involvement of the optic radiations, and thinning of the posterior corpus callosum (Fedrizzi et al 1998).

Even though the visual–perceptual difficulties become more apparent when children reach school age – also on account of the increased availability of assessment instruments in this age group – they can be suspected in preschoolers too; indeed, a discordant profile of psychomotor development, with lower scores on the eye–hand coordination scales and poorer performances on the Griffith scales, may be considered an early indication of a future VPI (Stiers 2004), which will subsequently be reflected not only in a discrepancy between verbal and performance IQ but also in difficulty in specific tests assessing complex visual abilities (Stiers 2002, Fazzi et al 2004).

NEURO-OPHTHALMOLOGICAL FEATURES IN CONGENITAL HEMIPLEGIA

The visual problems encountered in congenital hemiplegia are, in general, less severe than those seen in the other forms of CP, even though there are few systematic studies on this topic in the literature. Severe visual impairment is rare, whereas there are descriptions of involvement of other aspects of visual function, e.g. optokinetic nystagmus and visual field. Mercuri et al (1996a), for example, evaluating 14 children with congenital hemiplegia aged between 6 and 12 years, found a high percentage (78%) presenting abnormalities in at least one of the visual parameters considered. Although visual acuity was the parameter most frequently impaired, abnormalities were also found in stereopsis and/or visual field.

Guzzetta et al (2001) reported a high incidence of CVI in children with congenital hemiplegia, and in particular that the aspects of vision affected were visual acuity, stereopsis, optokinetic nystagmus, which was asymmetrical, and visual field. The presence and type of the visual disorders in the above study did not appear to be related either to the severity of the motor picture or to the type and extent of the brain lesion as documented on brain imaging: a high incidence of visual disorders was, in fact, found in association with all the different patterns of brain lesion, and no constant association was found between the involvement of the different parts of the visual system (optic radiations and primary visual cortex) and visual function, as shown by the significant incidence of false-negative and false-positive results. Sparing of the optic radiations and primary visual cortex does not, in fact, exclude the possibility of a visual impairment, just as their involvement is not invariably associated with a visual dysfunction. This finding conflicts with observations in adults with acquired hemiplegia, in whom there is a correlation between involvement of the optic radiations and of the visual cortex and the presence of visual impairment, in particular visual field deficits. The presence of false-negative results could derive, in part, from the difficulties involved in studying the mesencephalon and other parts of the visual system using standard imaging techniques, whereas the false-positive results (MRI evidence of visual pathway involvement in the absence of functional abnormalities) could be an expression of the plasticity of the brain following an early insult – the suggestion being that other structures, through a hemispheric reorganization of visual function, may compensate for damage to the optic radiations or visual cortex.

Abnormal optokinetic nystagmus can, as mentioned, take the form of asymmetrical binocular optokinetic nystagmus, which shows impairment in the direction of the most damaged hemisphere. These features are in accordance with the findings of previous studies which have reported asymmetrical binocular optokinetic nystagmus in children with hemispherectomy and in children with unilateral brain lesions (Atkinson 2000). The optokinetic nystagmus abnormality in the direction of the damaged hemisphere can be interpreted in the light of experimental studies in monkeys. In these animals, lesions of the medial superior temporal (MST) area interfere with visual pursuit in the direction of the affected side, this area being the one that provides the input to the ipsilateral nucleus of the optic tract, which is responsible for the directional responses.

In man, the MST area is located in the superior temporal cortex; fibres that originate from this area run through the parietal lobe. Lesions affecting these lobes thus cause abnormalities in the slow phase of the optokinetic nystagmus. In the study by Guzzetta et al (2001), visual field deficits were found in 56% of the children evaluated. It is interesting to remark that, although 90% of the children with damage to the optic radiations and occipital cortex presented visual field deficits, damage restricted to the optic radiations was not always correlated with a contralateral visual field deficit (unlike what is usually observed in adult stroke patients and in preterm children with PVL).

Furthermore, visual field deficits were observed (Guzzetta et al 2001) in a small percentage of participants presenting with normal optic radiations and visual cortex but a parietal lesion. Similar findings have also been reported in a population of children with focal cerebral lesions (Mercuri et al 1996b).

The fact that assessment of visual field in very small children demands a shift of attention from a central target used to attract the child's attention to a laterally presented target could explain the appearance of visual field deficits in young children with parietal lesions. Other authors (Gunn et al 2002) have reported impaired performances on visual–spatial tasks in children with hemiplegia that are attributable to 'dorsal stream' malfunctioning, hypothesizing that early lesions are associated with a vulnerability of this system. The results obtained in this study indicate that subsequent difficulties in visuomotor tasks are due not only to a motor control deficit but also to impaired processing at the level of the visuospatial systems which provide information for the controlling of actions.

Gunn et al (2002), in form and movement coherence studies, showed that children with congenital hemiplegia, of whatever aetiology, perform worse than age-matched comparison children in movement coherence tests, thereby indicating an increased vulnerability of the 'dorsal stream' functions. Indeed, the tests of form and movement coherence provide a measure of global visual processing by, respectively, the 'ventral' and 'dorsal streams'.

Visual deficits are thus frequent in children with congenital hemiplegia, and the severity of these disorders cannot always be established on the basis of neuroradiological investigations. All children with hemiplegia should be submitted to a detailed visual assessment protocol, regardless of the severity of their motor deficit and the type and extent of their brain lesion.

NEURO-OPHTHALMOLOGICAL FEATURES IN SPASTIC QUADRIPLEGIA
In spastic quadriplegia the visual disorder is often more severe than that observed in the other two types of CP. Affected children present a marked reduction in visual acuity associated with major impairment or absence of the basic visual functions such as fixation, slow pursuit, and saccades, which, as a result, are often impossible to evaluate. Refractive error and impaired accommodation are common (Mackie 1998; Ross et al 2000; McClelland et al 2006).

From the neuroradiological point of view, too, there is extensive involvement of the visual system; indeed, it is possible to observe involvement of the periventricular white matter, both anterior and posterior, and of the optic radiations, gliosis of the lateral geniculate nuclei and thinning of the optic nerves – these last features being expressions of the phenomenon of retrograde trans-synaptic degeneration (Uggetti 1998, Jacobson and Dutton 2000).

The visual deficit in spastic quadriplegia is difficult to quantify using traditional methods and this makes it important, in the diagnostic assessment phase, to look particularly carefully for evidence of direct and indirect signs of visual perception, also called neurobehavioural adaptations, that may confirm the presence of some residual visual function. Direct signs are behaviours that are clearly related to the visual target (e.g. location of light, turning of the head or movement of the limbs towards a visual target), whereas indirect signs (postural reactions, altered breathing rate, avoiding reactions) support the impression that the child has perceived the visual target (Porro 1998).

We studied (Signorini et al 2005) 30 children with spastic tetraplegia (12 females and 18 males; mean age at first clinical observation 34.8mo, range 2–132mo) with visual acuity not quantifiable using Teller Acuity Cards (visual acuity below 1.6c/deg). None of them presented with severe visual deficit secondary to abnormalities of the anterior segment, inadequate correction of refractive errors, or sequelae of retinopathy of prematurity.

Strabismus was present in 25 out of 30 patients (83%): 5 out of 30 (16.7%) had esotropia and 20 (66.7%) had exotropia.

Refractive errors were present in 22 out of 30 (73.3%) patients: hypermetropia in 5 out of 30 (16.7%), astigmatism in 4 out of 30 (13.3%), myopia in 4 out of 30 (13.3%), and associated refractive errors in 9 out of 30 (30%) (hypermetropia and astigmatism in eight, myopia and astigmatism in one).

Fundus oculi abnormalities were present in 25 out of 30 patients (83%), and optic subatrophy was present in 20 out of 30 (66.7%).

Binocular visual acuity was not quantifiable in these children (this was, indeed, a criterion for their inclusion in the study); fixation, smooth pursuit, and saccadic movements were absent and contrast sensitivity, optokinetic nystagmus, visual field, and stereopsis could not be assessed because of the severity of the visual deficit. Erratic eye movements were present in 7 out of 30 children (23.3%); 9 out of 30 (30%) children had paroxysmal ocular deviations, and 9 out of 30 (30%) had nystagmus.

Neurobehavioural adaptations were documented in all the participants in various combinations.

As regards the direct signs of visual perception, light localization was found in 21 out of 30 (70%), object localization in 17 out of 30 (56.6%), movement of the head and/or a limb towards the visual target in 16 out of 30 (53.3%), and pursuit of a moving stimulus in 2 out of 30 (6.7%).

Indirect signs of visual perception were present too: avoiding reactions in 10 out of 24 (30%), postural reactions in 14 out of 30 (46.6%), alteration of respiratory frequency in 15 out of 30 (50%), and smiling and other changes of facial expression in 19 out of 30 (63.3%).

Even though reduced visual acuity is the most frequent and evident symptom in individuals with quadraplegic CP, our study documented the presence of some residual vision even in the most severely affected of these children. In fact, in spite of the overall severity of the neurological and neuro-ophthalmological picture in these patients, in whom visual acuity could not be quantified using standard measures and fixation and smooth pursuit were absent, prolonged clinical observations in appropriate settings nevertheless made it possible to demonstrate the presence of neurobehavioural adaptations, confirming their conservation of visual perception. Although this residual vision can be difficult to demonstrate, it is crucial to persevere in the endeavour because these signs have considerable value and important repercussions, not only on these children's diagnosis but also on their habilitation. Indeed, by making them aware of their residual vision, we can help them to exploit it to further their own psychomotor development and relationship with the world.

Conclusions

The spectrum of visual dysfunction associated with CP is very broad. It can emerge as a predominantly oculomotor disorder or a disorder of the functions of the primary or associative visual pathway. We have also seen that the ophthalmological abnormalities are frequently present in association with one another. A full investigation of all the different aspects of visual function is thus mandatory in order to arrive at a precise definition of the clinical picture and consequently of the programme of rehabilitation.

In our experience, the clinical pictures of the main forms of CP (diplegia, hemiplegia, and quadriplegia) can be defined not only by specific motor patterns but also by specific neuro-ophthalmological profiles. In fact, we have seen that visual impairment in children with CP can include peripheral problems, such as ocular disorders (refractive errors, fundus oculi abnormalities), central problems covering the spectrum of CVI, which, more than the other aspects, characterize their visual picture (reduction in visual acuity, contrast sensitivity, and visual field), and oculomotor dysfunction (i.e. impairment of oculomotor abilities). The final component is visual–cognitive dysfunction, which seems to be linked more to diplegic CP than to the other two groups and is more evident in school age in those with good visual acuity and/or visual field.

The degree of the visual impairment reflects the severity of the visual pathway involvement, as confirmed by the different pictures associated with each of the motor patterns. In fact, we found particularly severe visual dysfunction in children with tetraplegic CP, in whom visual acuity was very reduced or not assessable, oculomotor abilities were severely impaired or absent, and abnormal eye movements, such as paroxysmal ocular deviations, were frequent; there was also a high presence of fundus oculi abnormalities. In these children, neurobehavioural adaptations were recurrent.

The visual profile of diplegic CP was characterized mainly by cerebral visual symptoms such as absent stereopsis, altered contrast sensitivity, asymmetrical optokinetic nystagmus, and moderate reduction in visual acuity. Impaired oculomotor abilities, especially saccadic movements, were characteristic. Ocular involvement was expressed by refractive errors, particularly hypermetropia, and strabismus. Impairment of visuocognitive functions was found to be typical of this motor pattern, as confirmed by the literature and by our previous studies (Stiers et al 2002, Fazzi et al 2004).

The neuro-ophthalmological profile in hemiplegic CP is characterized by a slight reduction in visual acuity, frequently monolateral, reduced visual field, and altered stereopsis. We also found oculomotor impairment, with altered smooth pursuit and saccades and, in about 40% of children, the presence of nystagmus. Ocular involvement seemed to be characterized by refractive errors in about 80%.

Visual impairment has a crucial influence on locomotor and cognitive performances in CP. We conclude that identification of visual disorders is crucial for rehabilitation purposes and that children with CP must receive an early and accurate assessment in order to detect visual disorders. In the more severely affected individuals, in whom the residual vision may be negligible, the identification of neurobehavioural adaptations becomes particularly important not only for diagnostic purposes, but also for the planning of an adequate, personalized programme of intervention.

Summary

Any part of the visual system can be affected in children with cerebral palsy.

Optical error and impaired focusing are common and may need to be sought and corrected if the correction will improve vision. Opacity of the lens (cataract) is seen occasionally. The retina and anterior visual pathways can also be affected in some cases. The posterior visual pathways, visual processing, and higher visual function can all be affected, particularly when white matter next to the lateral ventricles is affected.

Full expert ophthalmic history-taking, examination, and refraction, including a search for perceptual visual disorders, is warranted in every child.

Spastic diplegia is associated with lower visual field impairment and impaired visual guidance of movement and visual search (dorsal stream dysfunction), which is also associated with disordered ability to make searching eye movements. Impaired recognition due to ventral stream involvement can also be seen.

Hemiplegic children tend to have normal visual acuities. However, impaired vision on one side due to impaired visual field or attention may be seen. Impaired fast eye movement in the direction of the hemiplegia may give a false impression of hemianopia in young children because lack of eye movement to look at a target is used to infer the presence of a visual field problem.

Spastic quadriplegia is associated with poor visual function and squint (strabismus) in most cases. When they can be measured, visual acuities are commonly reduced. Visual fields are difficult to assess, but can be inferred from visual behaviour in some cases. Behavioural observation and history-taking from parents adds considerably to the interpretation of visual function. Impaired focusing is common and may also be associated with the use of hyoscine skin patches.

Habilitational strategies need to be designed to optimally employ the elements of intact visual function.

Acknowledgements

I would like to thank all our friends and collaborators from the Centre of Child Neuro-ophthalmology at the IRCCS 'C. Mondino Institute of Neurology' Foundation, University of Pavia, Italy, for their contribution to our ongoing work with visually impaired children and their families. Particular thanks are due to Professors W. Misefari and C. Bertone, to A. Luparia and C. Achille (therapists specializing in children with low vision), and to M. E. Antonini (optometrist).

13

CHILDREN WITH INTELLECTUAL DISABILITIES AND CEREBRAL VISUAL IMPAIRMENT: PROBLEMS WITH DETECTION AND DIAGNOSIS

Heleen M. Evenhuis

Introduction

This chapter has been written from the perspective of children with a developmental delay or an intellectual disability. All children with an intellectual disability, mild or severe, have some kind of brain dysfunction. This may have been caused by a genetic or metabolic problem, or by a problem during pregnancy or delivery. At a later age, an accident or a brain disease may lead to an intellectual disability. Among children with intellectual disabilities, there are many children with motor disabilities (cerebral palsy) and preterm children, who are known to have an increased risk of cerebral visual impairment (CVI). However, nothing is known about the risk of CVI in children with intellectual disabilities by other causes. There may be many children with unidentified visual problems in this group because all children with brain dysfunction probably are at risk for CVI. These problems may go unidentified because in these children it may be difficult to distinguish functional problems due to a developmental delay or behavioural problem from those resulting from a visual impairment.

So, in this chapter, we consider all children with intellectual disabilities as one large at-risk group. After giving a definition of intellectual disability, we will describe what little is known about the frequency of visual impairment in children with intellectual disabilities, and specifically of CVI. Subsequently, we will address the problems hampering early detection and further diagnostic assessments of visual dysfunction in this group. Finally, we will propose a systemic approach, for this group as well as other at-risk groups, for which we may improve detection and diagnosis, as a basis for timely and optimal rehabilitation.

Definition of intellectual disability

The term 'intellectual disability' was internationally agreed upon in the 1990s by the International Association on the Scientific Studies of Intellectual Disabilities (IASSID). At the request of parent organizations, the previous terms, 'mental retardation' or 'mental handicap', were discarded. However, the term 'mental retardation' is still used in medical literature. Locally, English-speaking countries continue to use their own terminology: 'intellectual disability' or 'learning disability' in the UK and 'developmental disability' in the USA and Australia.

Intellectual disability is generally defined as an intelligence quotient (IQ) below 70, and can, for children, roughly be estimated by dividing their functional age by their real age, and multiplying this by 100. For example, a 5-year-old child functioning at the level of a 3-year-old has an IQ of 3/5×100=60. An IQ between 70 and 55 is considered a mild intellectual disability, whereas an IQ between 55 and 35 is called a moderate intellectual disability, and an IQ below 35 a severe intellectual disability. But these cut-off values may vary in different countries. Mild intellectual disabilities are most frequent, followed by moderate intellectual disabilities, and children with severe intellectual disabilities are a relatively small group.

Current state of epidemiological knowledge

VISUAL IMPAIRMENT IN CHILDREN IN GENERAL

First, information will be given on all visual impairment, caused by ocular abnormalities as well as by brain damage in children.

Valid information on the frequency of visual impairment in the general population of children is relatively recent (Table 13.1). We found scientific reports of four epidemiological studies in large, unselected child populations in Scandinavia, France, Northern Ireland, and the USA, all applying criteria for visual impairment and blindness as proposed by the World Health Organization (WHO) (Rosenberg et al 1996, Cans et al 2003, Flanagan et al 2003, Bhasin et al 2006). These criteria do not address functioning in daily life, but just visual acuity (lower than 0.3) and restricted visual fields. These studies were based upon national or regional registers and reported prevalence. 'Prevalence' refers to the percentage with visual impairment or blindness that, at a certain moment (e.g. in the year 2000), is present in a population. In 1993, the prevalence of visual impairment and blindness among children aged 0–17 years in five Scandinavian countries varied between 0.05% and 0.1% (Rosenberg et al 1996). The authors supposed that the lower prevalences were a result of under-registration. The prevalence reported from a French county remained stable between 1980 and 1991 and was 0.06%. This lower figure is probably explained by the fact that this registry includes only disabled children who apply for specific financial support or special education (Cans et al 2003). In Northern Ireland, the prevalence among children younger than 19 years in 2000 was 0.16% (Flanagan et al 2003). In metropolitan Atlanta, GA, USA, a disabilities surveillance programme is ongoing. For the years 1996 and 2000, prevalences of 0.14% and 0.12%, respectively, were reported for visual impairment and blindness among children aged 8 years (Bhasin et al 2006).

It is increasingly recognized that in high-income countries CVI is now the most frequent cause of childhood visual impairment (Jan and Freeman 1998). The risk of CVI is increasing as a result of survival of children after very preterm or severely complicated birth. Improved recognition might also play a role. This is different for low-income countries, where vitamin A deficiency, measles, retinopathy of prematurity, and lack of glasses are still major causes of visual impairment and blindness in children (WHO 1999).

TABLE 13.1
Reported frequencies of all visual impairment (World Health Organization criteria)

	Prevalence
General children's population	
Scandinavian countries 1993 (Rosenberg et al 1996)	0.05–0.1%
French county 1980 – 1991 (Cans et al 2003)	0.06%
Northern Ireland 2000 (Flanagan et al 2003)	0.16%
Atlanta, US 1996, 2000 (Bhasin et al 2006)	0.14%, 0.12%
Overall	~0.1%
Children with intellectual disabilities	
Profound intellectual disability (Hong Kong) (Kwok et al 1996)	25% (acuity <0.1)
Down syndrome (US) (Tsiaras et al 1999)	31% (acuity <0.4)
Young adults with mild intellectual disabilities and no Down syndrome (Netherlands) (Splunder et al 2006)	2.9% (acuity <0.3)

Risk of visual impairment and blindness in children

In high-income countries, around 0.1% of children have a visual impairment or blindness, according to World Health Organization criteria. The most frequent cause is CVI. The situation is different in low-income countries.

VISUAL IMPAIRMENT IN CHILDREN WITH INTELLECTUAL DISABILITIES

It has been known for several decades that children with intellectual disabilities have a higher risk of visual impairment than other children (Table 13.1). This was easy to conclude because in special schools and institutes for children with severe visual impairments and blindness, and in disability registers, a large proportion have additional intellectual disability (Blohmé and Tornqvist 1997b, Mervis et al 2002). In the metropolitan Atlanta disability surveillance programme, 58% of 6-year-olds with a visual impairment had an intellectual disability (Mervis et al 2002).

However, the question as to how many children with an intellectual disability have a visual impairment has yet to be answered. A study in Hong Kong reported a risk of 25% for severe visual impairment in a subgroup with very severe intellectual disabilities (IQ <25), which is extremely high (Kwok et al 1996). It is also well known that children with Down syndrome have an increased risk of ocular problems. Tsiaras et al (1999) diagnosed visual acuities below 0.4 in 31% of American children with Down syndrome aged 5–19 years. The most frequent diagnoses were strabismus, nystagmus, and refractive error; an incidental case of untreated congenital cataract was also found.

In a population-based epidemiological study of visual impairment in Dutch *adults* with intellectual disabilities (Splunder et al 2005), we found that young adults with mild intellectual disabilities with causes other than Down syndrome had a risk of visual impairment or blindness (3%) that was similar to the risk in the *ageing* Dutch population (Klaver et al 1998). In young adults with moderate intellectual disabilities the prevalence was 6%, and in those with severe intellectual disabilities the prevalence was 23%, with the majority of cases originating in childhood. It was found that 40% of cases of visual impairment and blindness had not been recognized prior to the study! Unidentified visual impairments were identified as frequently in those with mild or moderate intellectual disabilities as in persons with severe intellectual disabilities.

Increased risk of visual impairment in children with intellectual disabilities
Children with intellectual disabilities have an increased risk of visual impairment, but this risk has not been quantified. Children with severe intellectual disabilities and with Down syndrome can be considered to be most at risk. The diagnosis may have been missed in a number of cases.

CEREBRAL VISUAL IMPAIRMENT IN CHILDREN
Published reports on CVI in children (Table 13.2) usually concern preterm children and children with cerebral palsy. Although many of these children have normal intelligence, children with mild or more severe intellectual disabilities can also be found among them. Exact figures on the prevalence of CVI among preterm children and children with cerebral palsy are not known because reported numbers mostly come from child neurology, psychiatry, or ophthalmology hospital departments. It is to be expected that the more severely affected children, who have the highest risk of visual impairment, visit these departments.

TABLE 13.2
Reported population-based frequencies of childhood cerebral visual impairment

Risk group	Prevalence (%)
Visual acuity <0.3	
Swedish preterm children (Jacobson et al 1998b)	0.07
Danish adults with intellectual disabilities (Warburg 2001)	9.6
All visual acuities	
At least one visual–perceptual task abnormal	
Dutch children preterm or birth asphyxia (Stiers et al 2001)	68
Belgian school children with cerebral palsy (Stiers et al 2002)	37.5

The first step in the diagnosis of CVI in children at risk has been, since the 1970s, identifying a visual impairment according to the WHO definition: a visual acuity below 0.3. This may be done through vision screening. Subsequently, the ophthalmologist assesses whether this low vision can be explained only by an ocular abnormality or if the visual impairment may also have a cerebral origin. Typical visual behaviours and findings of neurological assessment and cerebral imaging (computed tomography [CT] or magnetic resonance imaging [MRI]) may support the diagnosis.

We found two studies of CVI that were based not on hospital series, but on complete populations, in which CVI was diagnosed in the above way by specialized ophthalmologists in 0.07% of Swedish preterm children (Jacobson et al 1998b) and 9.6% of Danish adults with intellectual disabilities (Warburg 2001). We assume that this adult CVI mostly will have been present since childhood. In both groups, combinations with ocular abnormalities were frequently found. Population-based studies in children with intellectual disabilities have not been published.

Screening with standardized neuropsychological tests to assess higher visual functions has revealed that these figures represent only the tip of the iceberg. Subtle or more severe problems with visual perception could be demonstrated in 68% of 5-year-old Dutch children with a history of preterm birth or birth asphyxia (Stiers et al 2001), and in 37.5% of Belgian children with cerebral palsy attending a special school for disabled children (Stiers et al 2002). A majority of these children had visual acuities better than 0.3. It appears that CVI is a continuum from subtle to very severe impairments.

Unidentified visual problems in risk groups

Unidentified visual problems, which may profoundly influence psychosocial development, daily functioning, and school achievement, may be present in more children than we are aware of, especially in those with a developmental delay, intellectual disability, cerebral palsy, or preterm birth.

Barriers to detection and diagnosis in children with intellectual disabilities

MISSED DIAGNOSES

Visual impairment, that is a visual acuity below 0.3, may be frequently overlooked in children with intellectual disabilities. It is to be expected that CVI without ophthalmological abnormalities, which is even more difficult to diagnose, will be missed in a majority. Indeed, a colleague working as a school healthcare physician in a Dutch special school for 270 children with intellectual disabilities recently found that in none of the medical files was a diagnosis of CVI reported. One of our investigators, an orthoptist working in a low-vision team, was recently investigating the feasibility of a draft screening questionnaire for CVI in a similar school. There was an unexpected outcome: answers given for 17 out of 40 questionnaires (completed by the parents) gave reason to advise diagnostic assessment for both ocular and cerebral visual problems. This was in spite of the fact that, in the Netherlands, a public youth healthcare vision screening programme for 0- to 19-year-olds has been in place for many years.

WHAT ARE THE OBSTACLES TO DETECTION OF OCULAR AND CEREBRAL VISUAL IMPAIRMENT?

In the summer of 2006, we addressed this question with a small working party of specifically interested Dutch physicians and orthoptists in the fields of intellectual disability, paediatrics, youth health care, and paediatric ophthalmology. Our combined experience was that many young children with intellectual disabilities who are treated and followed by paediatricians do not visit the regular mother and child healthcare teams. As a result, they do not participate in preschool vision screening by these teams. At school age, not all children with intellectual disabilities may be able to cooperate with the visual acuity test (Landolt C) which is advised in the standard Dutch screening programme. As a result, visual impairments may remain unidentified in this group. Because the screening protocol does not address the possibility of CVI, and youth healthcare physicians are often not aware of its existence, children from at-risk groups with (sub)normal visual acuities will not be referred for further diagnosis. Moreover, a screening test to identify children with a suspicion of cerebral visual problems is currently not available to these physicians.

OBSTACLES TO DIAGNOSTIC FOLLOW-UP

Many ophthalmologists, paediatricians, and child neurologists do not recognize, for example, the specific visual behaviours indicative of cerebral visual problems. As a result, children tend not to be referred for specialist diagnosis and rehabilitation.

Internationally, most specialized low-vision teams have now developed the expertise to diagnose CVI in children and to offer habilitation. However, most diagnostic tests for higher visual functions, as are now applied in low vision services and academic departments around the world, have yet to be validated for children.

The number of staff members with specific expertise with very young children and children with intellectual disabilities may be limited. Assessment in these children may be hampered by difficulties with understanding, communication, and active cooperation, whereas most neuropsychological tests can be reliably applied only in children with a functional age of 4 years or over.

Further, in children with both ocular and cerebral abnormalities, it can be difficult to distinguish visual problems as a result of ocular abnormalities from those caused by CVI. As a result, in some groups of children the diagnosis may remain tentative, specific visual–perceptual problems may be missed, and advice concerning habilitation may be only global and not specific.

Obstacles to detection and diagnosis of CVI

There are multiple obstacles to detection and diagnosis of ocular and CVI in children with intellectual disabilities:

- Participation in youth healthcare vision screening is not guaranteed.
- No validated screening instrument or protocol is available for CVI.
- Referral for specialized diagnostic assessments is not guaranteed.
- For young or intellectually disabled children, assessment of higher visual functions requires adapted tests.
- Internationally, district low-vision teams may need more specific diagnostic expertise and more capacity than are currently available.

Is there a case for screening at-risk groups?

Generally, before deciding on population screening, for example for breast cancer, investments and gains are weighed against each other on a governmental level. Costs are usually high, so the yield – on a population level – should be satisfactory and should be supported by scientific evaluation. The 'disease' should occur frequently enough and be enough of a burden. Detection at an early stage should be feasible with methods that are easily applicable in the community. Effective treatment should be available to, and accepted by, the population concerned (Wilson and Jungner 1968). Target conditions to be detected in preschool vision screening include visual impairment, strabismus, refractive errors, and amblyopia. After an extensive review of the scientific literature, investigators at the University of Oxford concluded, in 1997, that there was insufficient scientific evidence of the benefit of preschool vision screening (Snowdon and Stewart-Brown 1997). The authors advised against the start of new screening programmes, as long as no more evidence of their benefits had been collected. How is the situation with screening of visual impairment in at-risk groups?

Before deciding on a screening programme, the extra burden of visual impairment in children who already have a motor or intellectual disability has to be assessed. However, no scientific studies have been published on (extra)developmental delay or functional disability caused by visual impairment in these at-risk groups, or on effects of treatment and rehabilitation. Moreover, we have no figures to hand to illustrate the size of the problem, i.e. the number of affected children. As we have already mentioned, there is no screening instrument for CVI, and diagnostic follow-up is difficult in young and intellectually disabled children. It can therefore be concluded that, in spite of the increased risk, investments in active screening of CVIs in children with intellectual disabilities are as yet insufficiently supported by scientific evidence.

> **Insufficient scientific support of screening**
> At this moment, there is insufficient scientific evidence supporting the benefits of screening children with intellectual disabilities for ocular and CVIs.

A safety net for children with intellectual disabilities

To support our clinical impression that screening for visual impairments in children with intellectual disabilities is necessary, we need to investigate the benefits of such screening. In the Netherlands, a youth healthcare vision screening organization exists with a network of trained screeners. The working party mentioned earlier proposed that, within this organization, a 'safety net' construction might be designed and evaluated for children with intellectual disabilities who do not participate in the regular screening programme. We have outlined such a safety net construction in such terms that it might be applicable in countries with different care systems (Table 13.3). First, costs and gains of the safety net should be scientifically evaluated in a test region.

CONTENTS OF SCREENING AROUND AGE 1 YEAR

Refractive errors (need for glasses) and ocular abnormalities are frequently encountered in children with intellectual disabilities. Refractive errors should be detected and treated as early as possible, but not before the age of 12–14 months because in the first year refractive errors are not yet stable (this excludes large refractive errors). For refraction measurement, but also for diagnosis of ocular abnormalities, referral to an ophthalmological team (ophthalmologist and orthoptist) is indicated in all cases. Orthoptists do not always possess tests to measure

TABLE 13.3

Safety net for preschool vision screening in at-risk groups

For whom?	Children of at-risk groups (who do not participate in public preschool screening programme):
	preterm
	developmental delay or intellectual disability
	cerebral palsy
Aims	Early detection of:
	refractive errors
	ocular abnormalities
	suspicion of cerebral visual impairment
Requirements	Limited number of screening moments to advance participation
	More extensive assessment than in regular screening → orthoptic/ophthalmological referral
Contacting	Link to vaccinations around age 1 and 4 years → direct referral by the vaccinating professional (physician, nurse, health visitor) or paediatrician

212

visual acuity in infants, but are usually able to obtain sufficient information on visual functioning by other methods. As long as youth health professionals do not have a screening test for CVI, orthoptists in ophthalmological teams seem to be best equipped to identify children with possible problems of higher visual functioning. Based on structured clinical history-taking and/or specific visual behaviours, they may suspect cerebral visual problems and advise referral to a specialized centre.

CONTENTS OF SCREENING AROUND AGE 4 YEARS

Around the age of 4 years, the screening should consist of assessment of fixation and following, strabismus, visual acuity, and visual fields (confrontational method). In principle, this can be done by youth healthcare physicians or nurses. Adapted visual acuity tests with matching cards, such as LH (L. Hyvärinen Pediatric vision tests: Lee Tests Ltd, Helsinki) and Stycar (Sheridan 1976) tests, are often the tests of choice for children with not too severe intellectual disabilities, and they are not too expensive for regular use. Referral to an ophthalmological team is indicated in case of abnormalities or when visual acuity is not measurable.

Routine assessment of refractive errors again may be indicated at this age because of the risk of amblyopia as a result of severe refractive errors. These should be corrected before the age of 6 years. However, the gain of routine referral at age 1 year and the added gain of referral at age 4 years should be scientifically evaluated first (Table 13.4).

At the age of 5 or 6 years, most children, including those from at-risk groups, are screened at their schools. In special schools, screening for CVI should ideally be added to the regular screening protocol. Initiatives for screening tests are described in the following paragraph.

Our working party stressed that other at-risk groups for ocular and CVI may be confronted with similar barriers to early detection as children with intellectual disabilities. In our experience, this specifically concerns children with cerebral palsy and children born preterm. Therefore, other at-risk groups might also take advantage of the proposed safety net construction.

TABLE 13.4
Contents of safety net preschool vision screening in at-risk groups

Screening around age 1 year	Refraction
	Ocular abnormalities
	?Visual behaviour → CVI
	?Screening questionnaire for CVI
Screening around age 4 years	Fixation and following
	Strabismus
	Visual acuity (adapted test)
	Visual fields with confrontation techniques
	?Refraction
	?Screening questionnaire for CVI

213

Tests for screening and diagnosis

A central question for research concerns the development and evaluation of screening tests and tests for diagnostic follow-up, which are applicable to all at-risk groups. Although fundamental insights into the functioning of the visual brain and possibilities of functional magnetic resonance imaging (fMRI) of the brain are developing rapidly and are most promising, at the moment fMRI has only a supportive role in the diagnosis of higher visual functioning.

The development of a screening tool for CVI in young or intellectually disabled children is a challenge which has yet to be met. This is understandable because of the multiple appearances of CVI and the varying character of symptoms in time. A tool that would enable us to distinguish between 'not suspicious' or 'suspicious' in risk groups would be satisfactory. In this respect, two initiatives are interesting. Both concern standardized checklists for CVI, based on observations by the parents.

After first evaluation of a 22-item checklist, originally designed as a help for structured history-taking, the Scottish ophthalmologist Gordon Dutton designed a 10-item screening checklist, which has yet to be validated (Houliston et al 1999).

We have already mentioned a draft screening questionnaire, which is being developed by our research team: the SCAN questionnaire for CVI in children. Based on collected data on test–retest reliabilities and differences between case and comparison groups, item reduction is in progress. After this, the SCAN's capacity to distinguish between 'not suspicious' and 'suspicious' will be tested in a new study group.

As these questionnaires are based on observable behaviours in daily circumstances, they may appear insufficiently sensitive to detect subtle problems and problems in very young children. Despite this, Dutch paediatricians and youth healthcare physicians appear eager to use these questionnaires. Indeed, after a recent postgraduate training session for paediatricians in our university hospital, which also addressed CVI, a Dutch translation of Dutton's 10-item checklist is now being completed for each child who visits the paediatric clinic for aetiological diagnosis of developmental delay or for follow-up. Paediatricians mentioned that, before this, they were hardly aware of the existence of CVI. So, even before their proper scientific evaluation, such questionnaires may increase the awareness of physicians, help them ask about visual problems, and advance referral of suspicious cases for specialist diagnostic assessment. If a valid screening test were to become available, parties other than those involved in youth health care might also contribute to detection of suspicious cases and referral, such as paediatricians, rehabilitation and intellectual disability physicians, orthoptists, and teachers.

A well-evaluated diagnostic protocol for CVI that is also applicable to young and disabled children is urgently needed. It has been shown in earlier chapters that a range of research projects into diagnosis have been completed or are in progress around the world. However, development of a complete and generally applicable protocol will take some time because of the multiple aspects to be addressed.

Steps to take

Guided by the criteria for screening proposed by Wilson and Jungner (1968), we recommend the following steps be taken to improve the detection and diagnosis of ocular and CVI in children with intellectual disabilities and other at-risk groups.

1   Show epidemiologically that ocular and CVI in at-risk groups are an important problem with respect to prevalence, disability, and natural course.
2   Develop a suitable and acceptable screening test or examination for CVI.
3   Estimate costs and gains of a screening programme that reaches all target groups and has guaranteed continuity.
4   Guarantee adequate referral and assessment by means of guidelines for, and education of, involved disciplines.
5   Develop a valid diagnostic battery applicable to all at-risk groups, for expert assessment of higher visual functions.
6   Evaluate which interventions are effective in which subgroups, by means of well-designed intervention studies.
7   Come to an agreed policy on who to screen.
8   If screening proves effective, organize more capacity in low-vision teams.

Summary

Children with intellectual disabilities have an increased risk of visual impairment, caused by both ocular and cerebral abnormalities. However, this risk has hardly, or not at all, been quantified. As far as we are aware, no country has a structured programme to detect and diagnose cerebral visual impairment in at-risk groups. Indeed, in countries with a preschool vision screening programme, participation by children with intellectual disabilities is not guaranteed. As a result, many cases may go unidentified. Although at the moment there seems to be a case for screening, there is insufficient scientific evidence supporting such a claim. Moreover, validated diagnostic instruments for screening do not exist, whereas disciplines involved in medical care for these children are insufficiently aware of the existence of cerebral visual impairment and do not recognize possible signs. As a result, probably only the tip of the iceberg is referred to low-vision teams. Specialist diagnostic assessment of higher visual functions may further be hampered by the use of tests that are insufficiently validated for children, or are hardly applicable to children with a real or developmental age below 4 years.

Using current expertise, we have presented a safety net construction for vision screening to identify both ocular and cerebral visual impairment in children with intellectual disabilities. Preterm children and children with cerebral palsy might also take advantage of this model. Costs and gains should be scientifically evaluated, at first in a pilot study. The evaluation might stimulate the development of instruments for screening and diagnosis, and result in estimates of the size of the problem.

Acknowledgements

We thank members of the Dutch working party on vision screening in risk groups for sharing their expertise and ideas, and for their comments on the manuscript. This includes Helen Ennema (mother and child healthcare team physician), Maria van Genderen (child ophthalmologist), Karen de Heus (paediatrician), Kathleen Lantau (orthoptist and coordinator, vision screening 0–19 years), Hans Limburg (coordinator, Vision 2020 Netherlands), Nelleke Meester (school youth healthcare physician), Nicolien Schalij-Delfos (child ophthalmologist), Marleen Verhoeff (intellectual disability physician), and Lien Wienen (school youth healthcare physician).

14
PRACTICAL APPROACHES FOR THE MANAGEMENT OF VISUAL PROBLEMS DUE TO CEREBRAL VISUAL IMPAIRMENT

Gordon N. Dutton, with Debbie Cockburn, Gillian McDaid, and Elisabeth Macdonald

Introduction

The limitations of the human visual system are well recognized. Visual acuity limits the size of the detail which can be seen, contrast sensitivity limits how faint something can be before it becomes invisible, the visual fields limit the extent of the area over which one can see, and the speed of visual processing limits the speed at which a moving object can be seen and identified.

At a higher level of visual processing, both dorsal and ventral stream functions have their limitations. Dorsal stream functions limit whether something can be seen in a visually crowded environment and also determine the accuracy of visual guidance of movement. Ventral stream functions limit whether what is being viewed – be it people, objects, or the environment (for route-finding, which is also likely to be served in the right frontal area [Pavlova et al 2007]) – can be recognized.

Pathology of the visual system can interfere with any of these functions, in any combination and degree, and knowledge of which aspects of vision are affected, and to what extent, can assist in determining how they interfere with daily living and education.

Characterization of each element of visual function allows matched habilitative strategies to be designed and implemented to ensure that an affected child is not inappropriately disadvantaged by being expected to function in a visual world in which crucial elements cannot be seen or appreciated. Visual perceptual dysfunction can manifest variation owing to fatigue, distraction, or stress. The resultant variability in visual performance can be misunderstood and misinterpreted as being due to behavioural difficulties.

Children who have profound visual impairment caused by cerebral damage may show little or no evidence of visual function. However, many show evidence of reflex visual function in response to a moving stimulus, which is known as 'blindsight' (Boyle et al 2005). A small proportion of such children may be mobile and able to move freely despite no apparent visual function. This has been termed 'travel vision' (Jan et al 1986).

Cerebral visual impairment (CVI) of a lesser degree can occur in many guises. Impaired visual acuities and visual fields are the best recognized and understood manifestations. Dorsal stream dysfunction, in particular, is common, and if it is not recognized it can easily be misinterpreted. The resultant inability to find things, combined with lack of attention, may be perceived as bad behaviour, and the impaired visual guidance of movement may be attributed to 'clumsiness' and inappropriately punished. The adverse effects of such misinterpretation upon a child with CVI, who is doing his or her best, can be profound. It is therefore essential to be able to identify and characterize CVI in all its guises and to implement appropriate habilitative strategies, matched to the age of the child and the nature and degree of the deficits identified.

Careful, structured clinical history-taking combined with clinical examination of functional vision assist in making a diagnosis and characterizing the visual deficits, and the everyday difficulties that they cause. Age-appropriate matched strategies, designed to ameliorate these problems, can then be implemented. The approaches described below have been assembled from a combination of discussions with colleagues internationally, the literature, audits of our clinical service, and information collected at parent conferences (McKillop et al 2006).

The principles of functional vision
Vision is used for many aspects of daily living. There are three principal elements:

1   *Gaining access to information.* Both the near and distant surroundings are monitored and analysed. Distant information, for example the presence of trees or the names of shops, is constantly being assimilated, while prolonged use of near vision is, for example, required to access information from the printed page and for play.
2   *Social interaction* is reliant upon vision to a significant degree. The ability to identify people in a group and the ability to recognize them are necessary to make contact, while social interaction requires the ability to see, recognize, and understand the linguistic elements of facial expression, gesture, and body language.
3   *Visual guidance of movement* not only facilitates reach and manipulation but is also required for movement through the visual world, whether by walking, cycling, or driving.

The normal limitations of each of these three elements are intuitively recognized in the design of our visual environment, in our social interactions, and in our everyday lives. There is no point in printing advertisement hoardings or material with too much information; similarly, with print or images which are too small to be made out. The age at which print size and crowding can be accessed is empirically recognized by printers, with print size diminishing and print crowding increasing progressively as the targeted age increases. The size of a crowd in which it is difficult to find someone, or the distance at which it is not possible to recognize someone, are also understood at an intuitive level. When it comes to moving through the visual world, it is necessary, for example, to slow down to drive through a narrow gap, on account of both the spatial and temporal limitations of visual processing. In children with CVI, any of these aspects of daily living can be impaired owing to any of the thresholds for perception being exceeded. Once these thresholds have been determined, a matched set of strategies needs to be devised, which is aimed at ensuring that such limitations have as little adverse impact as possible.

Strategies related to specific visual dysfunctions

IMPAIRED VISUAL ACUITIES AND CONTRAST SENSITIVITIES

Impaired visual acuities and contrast sensitivities limit access to information, for both near and distance. Assessment of these functions is carried out while the child is viewing with both eyes open, to determine what can be seen at maximum speed. This is required to ensure the provision of optimal materials, at both home and school, and to inform families of what can and cannot be seen on a day-to-day basis.

Access to information

Figures 14.1 and 14.2 provide a simulation of the degree of image degradation brought about by different levels of acuity and contrast sensitivity. Low acuity dictates the amount of detail that can be seen. Low contrast sensitivity diminishes the overall accessibility of the information.

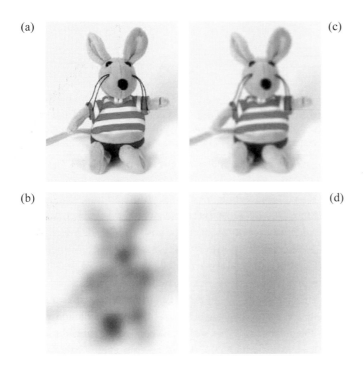

Fig. 14.1 Image of a toy mouse which is degraded to simulate reduced visual acuities. The visual acuities equate with (a) 6/6, (b) 6/18, (c) 6/120, and (d) 6/500. As the image degrades, the amount of detail which can be discriminated diminishes so that 6/18 affords access to detail, the 6/120 image allows only the largest details to be seen, while the 6/500 image is commensurate with perception of form and movement, but not detail. Produced using Sight-Sim™, courtesy of Drs Michael Bradnam, Aled Evans, and Ruth Hamilton, Department of Clinical Physics and Bioengineering, NHS Greater Glasgow and Clyde.

(a) (c)

(b) (d)

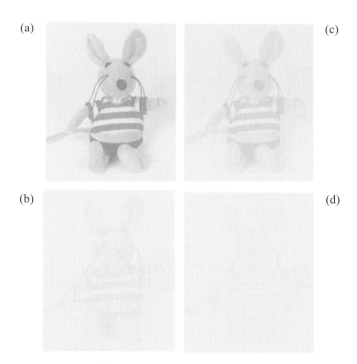

Fig. 14.2 Image of a toy mouse which is degraded to simulate reduced contrast sensitivity. The contrast sensitivity values equate with (a) 2.0, (b) 1.5, (c) 1.0, and (d) 0.5 log units of contrast. As the contrast sensitivity decreases, the mouse does not lose detail (as in Fig. 14.1), but becomes progressively less visible. Produced using Sight-Sim™, courtesy of Drs Michael Bradnam, Aled Evans, and Ruth Hamilton, Department of Clinical Physics and Bioengineering, NHS Greater Glasgow and Clyde.

The strategies required to assist children with low visual acuities and impaired contrast sensitivities are well recognized. Many families have found that sharing the screen of a digital camera and zooming in to look at a distant target together can be an effective aid. Additionally, the provision of high-contrast enlarged educational material is common practice – using books with large, clear illustrations in bold contrasting colours in which the elements of detail within the pictures can all be seen and recognized. Using low-vision aids for both near and distance can also help. Young children can use magnifiers as part of play and everyday life. Children who are short-sighted may choose to take their glasses off and to hold books and objects close to their eyes, as this affords magnification. However, children who are long-sighted are afforded magnification by their spectacle correction. Computing equipment with software designed to enlarge text and images and to present them with the requisite minimum crowding can also prove helpful, as can digital camera devices linked to the computer.

Social interaction
The 'facial expression recognition distance' can easily be elicited. The examiner adopts different facial expressions at progressively increasing distances from the child, until they cannot be identified. The same approach applies to the 'face recognition distance'.

Mobility
Reduced visual acuity and contrast sensitivity impair the ability to identify obstacles and variation in the height of the ground. Good lighting enhances contrast and the ability to navigate independently by means of vision. A bright, wide-angle torch beam facilitates mobility in the dark. Bright, high-contrast markings for step and floor boundaries facilitate safe mobility, particularly in areas which are not well known to the child. Early training in the use of a cane is warranted in those with very low vision.

VISUAL FIELD DEFICITS AND INATTENTION
The most common visual field deficits in children with damage to the brain comprise hemianopia and lower visual field impairment. The lower visual field impairment found in children with periventricular white matter pathology may be either absolute or diffuse, with reduced sensitivity of vision in the lower fields (Jacobson et al 2006).

Table 14.1 outlines the principles of the approaches which can be taken to circumvent the problems described above.

IMPAIRED PERCEPTION OF MOVEMENT
There are no routine tests available to assess movement perception in children. However, history-taking provides a means of identifying visual difficulties consistent with impaired perception of movement. Affected children commonly have a set of problems which provide corroboration for the diagnosis. These include the following:

1   inability to see moving animals when adjacent static animals are seen (Ahmed and Dutton 1996);
2   aversion to fast-moving television and films, with preference for watching programmes in which there is limited movement;
3   difficulty seeing from a moving car, with no such problems when the car is stationary;
4   older children are able to describe a football disappearing immediately after it is kicked, but reappearing as it slows down part-way through its flight path; and
5   small, fast-moving animals may be distressing because they appear 'out of nowhere' when they stop moving.

Recognition and understanding that an affected child has such difficulties is the first step, combined with careful selection of programmes and films in which content can be seen and appreciated. Ball games may need to be modified by using large, light, slow-moving balls.

TABLE 14.1
**Principles of the approaches to cater for the visual field deficits
in children with cerebral visual impairment**

Hemianopia and unilateral visual inattention

Access to near information

Text on one side can be missed. Right hemianopia impairs access to the next word, left hemianopia impairs access to the next line

Give training using tactile guides

Some children (especially those with acquired hemianopia) choose to read vertically downwards for right hemianopia and vertically upwards for left hemianopia (in this way, the text which is about to be read is not obstructed by the blind hemifield)

For visual inattention on one side, the effect of displacement of the salient text to the sighted side of the workstation is worth evaluating

If food is left on one side of the plate, consider placing the 'favourite food' on that side, to encourage search. Rotation of the plate to bring the food into view is commonly employed

Access to distant information

Training to scan the visual scene warrants consideration

Social interaction

Friends and relatives are informed that they may not be seen if they are on the affected side

For group activities, sit near the front of the class to one side, with the teacher on the sighted side

Team sports are difficult. Athletics and swimming are easier

Mobility of upper limbs

Train to search play area/workstation to find and reach for things in the hemianopic area

Mobility of lower limbs and overall mobility

Traffic approaching from visually impaired side may not be seen. Train the child to turn completely to the affected side to seek traffic before crossing road. (Parents teach by example, by doing the same.) Orientation and route-finding difficulties may necessitate mobility training

Lower visual field impairment

Access to near information

Food on the near side of the plate may be missed. Train the child to search near side of plate and to turn the plate around

Text at the bottom of the page may be missed. If so, provide a sloping workstation

Finding items on the floor, such as shoes, can be difficult. Store shoes and other possessions in a known location, possibly on a shelf at a height where they can be seen

Access to distant information

This is commonly impaired owing to associated visual crowding (see below)

Social interaction

A hand, which is proffered to shake hands, may not be seen. Train the child to look down at the appropriate moment

Visual guidance of the hands in the lower visual field cannot be achieved because they are not seen

TABLE 14.1 (continued)
**Principles of the approaches to cater for the visual field deficits
in children with cerebral visual impairment**

Changing shoes is difficult and is typically carried out by sitting on the floor with the foot elevated to a height where it is seen. Changing shoes with one foot up on a bench or a step allows the foot to be seen. Children with a degree of spastic diplegia and lower visual field impairment can, however, find this difficult

Mobility of lower limbs

Keep the floor clear of obstacles

Involve the child when low furniture is moved

The feet and the ground ahead are not seen when walking. The child naturally seeks a tactile guide to the height of the ground ahead. Examples include:

* holding on to the clothes of an accompanying adult while pulling down (this is encouraged rather than discouraged)

* using banisters and handrails

* for younger children, pushing a wheeled toy (such as a toy pram) provides a tactile guide to the height of the ground ahead

* when holding hands, the adult straightens the arm and extends it slightly backwards to provide the required tactile guide (with advance warning) of steps, pavements, and uneven ground

* providing a stick (e.g. telescopic hiking pole or long cane) and training to probe and give a tactile guide to height of the ground ahead

DORSAL AND VENTRAL STREAM DYSFUNCTION

The structured history-taking strategy described in Chapter 9 provides not only guidance towards the diagnosis but also the basis for identifying day-to-day problems and seeking solutions. Children with cognitive and perceptual visual disorders due to dorsal and ventral stream dysfunction can be at a particular disadvantage, especially if their visual acuities are near normal. This is because visual behaviour is normal in some contexts, but in other situations there may be profound visual difficulties which go unrecognized or are ascribed a behavioural cause.

Access to information

Dorsal stream dysfunction impairs visual search, which is significantly improved by keeping background pattern to a minimum (by avoiding patterned carpets, bedspreads, and wallpaper) and minimizing foreground clutter (by keeping everything tidied away). As print size decreases and print crowding increases with age progression through school, some children who have problems with visual crowding may reach a threshold and become progressively less able to read. Access to text can be enhanced by masking surrounding text or covering over the text which has just been read. For some children, increased spacing between words and lines is required, and presentation of numbers on squared paper can help with maths.

It is much easier to find a book on a library shelf than it is to find one among piles of books on the floor. This is because the library shelf provides a one-dimensional search, in contrast to the three-dimensional search among piles of books. Children with dorsal stream dysfunction commonly discover, or can be taught, that keeping their possessions in a tidy manner that facilitates one-dimensional search can make life much easier. Impaired recognition and visual imagination for two- and three-dimensional shapes can be helped by tactile methods.

The further away things are, the smaller they appear and the more there is to see. The majority of children with dorsal stream dysfunction take a long time to see something pointed out in the distance (visual acuity permitting). Again, sharing the screen of a digital or video camera, while zooming in to what is being shown, has been found by many parents to be particularly helpful.

Nearly all children with dorsal stream visual problems like to get very close to the television, presumably to minimize visual crowding and give attention to single elements. An explanation of this option, and allowing the child to sit near the television, may be warranted.

Difficulty naming colours can be helped by applying an appropriate noun to the colour for a period of a few weeks (e.g. sky blue, lemon yellow, and grass green).

Social interaction

Impaired recognition of faces owing to ventral stream dysfunction is commonly associated with the impaired ability to recognize the language within facial expression. Approaches which help a child to learn alternative strategies, such as voice recognition and memorizing other aspects of appearance (e.g. the design of spectacles), can prove helpful. Verbal explanations of one's feelings and emotions may be required to assist the child.

Inability to find a person, such as a parent, in a group is common. Imagine what it must be like in the playground. Nearly all parents of affected children describe having to always stand at a specific place along with waving and calling their child's name when meeting them from school. It is, therefore, not surprising that such children are unable to see their friends in the playground, which is, of course, socially ostracizing, and such children commonly stand at the side unable to join in. Teaching the unaffected children at an early stage that it is poor vision which is causing the problem, and adoption of appropriate social strategies, may be required.

Difficulty maintaining visual attention is another element of CVI. Some children can become distressed and angry when other restless children cause distraction, and this can be misinterpreted simply as bad behaviour. This problem can be addressed by sitting the child next to a calm, less restless, individual.

(Lack of ability to recognize faces and facial language, along with lack of social integration in the context of CVI, may lead to an alternative diagnosis, such as autism. This diagnosis may be reinforced by observing the behaviour of arranging toys and possessions in a line. Some children with CVI may indeed have additional autistic behaviours, but there may be others for whom such a diagnostic label may not be appropriate.)

Mobility and navigation

Inaccurate visual guidance of the upper limbs and/or the lower limbs (optic ataxia) as a result of dorsal stream dysfunction needs to be recognized and acted upon appropriately by occupational therapy and mobility training.

Profound difficulty in route-finding (topographic agnosia) commonly accompanies difficulty in recognizing faces (prosopagnosia), or may occur in isolation in those with ventral stream dysfunction. This condition is rare. Strategies such as setting well-known routes to song and colour-coding doors, along with repeated training, can reap dividends.

On the other hand, difficulty route-finding in crowded environments is a common feature of dorsal stream dysfunction. Training in focusing upon and remembering the sequence of landmarks on the horizon employs the principle of one-dimensional search. Practice and training in navigation from an early age, and allowing the child to lead (when there is time), is warranted.

Visual fatigue

Perceptual and cognitive visual problems in children with CVI manifest both variation and fatigue. This can explain why parents occasionally describe such visual problems but the teachers do not, because it is only when the child is tired that the problems become apparent. Children with more profound visual difficulties can have days when they appear to see well and other days when they do not. Opportunities may need to be given for a well-earned rest, when required, in a quiet and calm environment.

CEREBRAL BLINDNESS AND BLINDSIGHT

Children with occipital damage who have no detectable vision by means of formal testing may intermittently react to silent-moving objects, particularly at the side, and may manifest oculokinetic nystagmus (Boyle et al 2006). Adults with damage to the occipital lobes often have a degree of perception of movement, which may be either conscious or subconscious. This form of vision has been called 'blindsight' (Weiskrantz 1998). Soldiers who sustained occipital injury during the First World War were found to be aware of movement in the 'blind' visual field (Riddoch 1917). This is known as statokinetic dissociation, or the Riddoch phenomenon. Adults with blindness due to cerebral damage may have a relatively subconscious awareness of moving targets, lights, and colours (Weiskrantz 1998), and rocking to and fro may generate a visual image (Dutton 2003). Similarly, such children may rock to and fro. Whether this generates an image is difficult to know. The brain structures that may be responsible for blindsight include residual striate cortex, light scatter from the seeing hemifield, the extrastriate cortex, and the superior colliculus and pulvinar (Cowey and Stoerig 1991, Braddick et al 1992, Payne et al 1996, Stoerig et al 1998, Stasheff and Barton 2001). Blindsight can be difficult to elicit in young children and in those with cognitive and physical impairment. Therefore, it may not be possible to accurately determine whether or not a child has true blindsight. However, it is not uncommon for carers of children with CVI to observe the child reacting to movement in the peripheral visual field but not in the central visual field. It appears that the phenomenon is fatiguable and may be present only intermittently. Movement in the peripheral visual field may elicit a smile in the blind child with quadriplegia and profound intellectual disability.

Some children with blindsight who are fed with a spoon may intermittently open their mouths to receive food when the spoon is moved in an arc from the peripheral visual fields, but not when it approaches the mouth from straight ahead.

For those children who understand language, stating what is being seen as the child reacts to it may enhance both visual and language development.

'Travel vision' rarely accounts for the slow movement of mobile children with cerebral blindness around obstacles (Jan et al 1986).

Conclusion

It is essential to build up and maintain self-esteem and confidence in all children. As those with CVI develop, they can become painfully aware that they are unable to interact socially in the same way as others, and are unable to perform a wide range of tasks with the same competence as their contemporaries. It takes considerable skill on the part of parents, carers, teachers, and friends to integrate children in such a way that they build up the self-confidence that they need for long-term secure integration into the community.

The establishment of long-term friendships with school colleagues who support and understand is fundamental to achieving this goal, and the skill with which the primary teachers include and integrate the child into the class environment without stigmatization is critical.

In conclusion, the above descriptions constitute our current approaches to a complex topic. Further refinement will need to include defining the best strategies for each age group and ensuring that recommendations are matched to the specific visual difficulties of each child. Approaches need to be imaginative and adaptable, with experimentation to find out what works for the individual child.

15
STRATEGIES TO SUPPORT THE DEVELOPMENT AND LEARNING OF CHILDREN WITH CEREBRAL VISUAL IMPAIRMENT AT HOME AND AT SCHOOL: COMMUNICATION, ORIENTATION, AND MOBILITY

Marianna Buultjens, Lea Hyvärinen, Renate Walthes, and Gordon N. Dutton

Introduction

This section builds on previous chapters of this book in which the causes, diagnosis, measurement, and management of cerebral visual impairment (CVI)/disability have been discussed. This background of information is used to develop ideas on how parents and professionals can work, individually and together, to support the development of children with CVI.

Research into the development and structure of perception shows that activity and self-performed movement play an important role in shaping perception and making interaction and structural ties between the individual and his or her environment possible: 'The way we perceive the world around us makes us as adults forget that we have contributed to this kind of perception, since our body is involved in an exceptional circular process of action' (Varela 1985).

Today, we know that the processes of differentiation between 'self' and the world are not genetically determined but are learned. Learning begins immediately after birth, and presumably even in the womb, when the fetus becomes sensitive to the surrounding tactile environment.

'If, for example, he touches himself and then the things around him, his brain learns the fundamental difference between the body and the world. As for the body he gets a double sensory response, as for the world just a single one' (Roth 1994). The so-called double sensation (to touch and be touched at the same time) can be experienced only by movement and touching. This initial experience is the basis for all further perception- and activity-related differentiations and is considered to be the foundation for each perception ever made (Palágyi 1924).

For those involved in education, understanding perception as an active, 'circular' process of movement, perception, and learning integrates tactile, visual, and auditory perceptions with motor activity. Isolated visual or auditory stimuli are of less educational value than integrated experiences which encourage and allow a child to move as independently as possible. The development of perception and understanding results from and is reinforced by self-motivated experience and requires, for example, the child with limited mobility to move autonomously (Hoffman 1998). When movement is limited as a result of brain pathology, play situations, which afford such opportunities despite limited movement, as in a ball pool, need to be created.

Assessment of vision for education and development

Several specialists may be involved in the assessment of a child's visual functioning: the ophthalmologist and optometrist determine causation and degree of visual dysfunction, while the vision rehabilitation specialist may provide information and training in the use of devices to enhance, or substitute for, impaired visual function. The results of assessment need to be explained to parents clearly and simply, accompanied by reports (in plain language) for the child's teachers and therapists. This information is used to guide reassessment of functional vision in the familiar and non-threatening environment of the home, nursery, or school. This ensures that the habilitational strategies applied match the child's visual abilities. Specialist teachers and therapists for visual impairment have the opportunity to observe each child in different situations, and to relate visual performance to age-related norms. If teachers, thera- pists, and classroom assistants observe systematically, and apply basic evaluations of visual function as a part of their work, they can respond appropriately to the day-to-day variations in function that are common in children with brain damage.

The heterogeneity of expression of visual disorders means that, despite having a diagnosis, it is often only with the passage of time, as the child grows and matures, that the impact of the disorder on the child becomes apparent. What are the implications for relationships with family and others? How will the child find his or her way around? How will he or she get on with studies at school? Will the child be independent? The World Health Organization (WHO) documents *Management of Low Vision in Children* and the *International Classification of Functioning, Disabilities and Health – Children and Youth Version* provide the framework for considering these questions. The four main areas where vision is used for – *communication, orientation and mobility, sustained visual tasks*, and *activities of daily living (ADL)* – which are depicted in the four-leafed clover in Figure 15.1, provide a practical framework to report functional vision (Hyvärinen 2008).

COMMUNICATION

Failure to make eye contact can provide the first clue to the family that an infant's vision is poor. Ideally, all infants known to have damage to the brain require assessment of accom- modation and refraction to determine whether spectacles will enable the infant to see the parents' faces better and to start to develop the skills for visual communication. For infants with poor vision, parents and family can receive assistance to learn how to appreciate the ways their infant responds to the warmth and tenderness of their touch, the sound and tone of

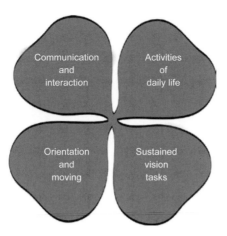

Fig. 15.1 A practical framework to assess and report functional vision. The four-leafed clover of visual functioning was designed as a symbol of the four main areas of visual functioning that are present in all cultures and at all ages (Hyvärinen 1985). The four main functional areas were, in 1992, included in the WHO document *Management of Low Vision in Children.*

their voices, and the day-to-day scent of the home environment, all of which makes the infant feel loved and secure. A video of the interactions between infant and family members can be helpful as it is often easier to observe such interactions at a later stage, rather than at the time of the interaction. If impaired communication and bonding at this early stage is cause for concern, it is important to arrange contact with a psychologist who has experience of children with visual impairment, including CVI, and who has skills in analysing and enhancing communication behaviours.

Contrast sensitivity for communication can be quickly assessed from the age of 3–4 months. If the response is similar to the response of the infant in Figure 15.2, then important observations of numerous brain functions have already been made: the infant has followed the picture with combined movement of eyes and head, which is age appropriate; has recognized a smiling face; and has responded with a normal social smile. In less than 10 seconds, visual, oculomotor, emotional, and social skills, and control of body and head movements have all been evaluated.

The human face has low contrast. The importance of low contrast information in communication is not widely appreciated. Nobody whispers to a person with hearing impairment. Why is it, then, that we regularly 'whisper' visually to people with visual impairment? Facial expressions are transient, rapidly moving, low contrast events. They are low contrast information in motion. Therefore, both the contrast sensitivity and motion perception abilities of each child should be known and the faces of teachers and all other persons rendered as clearly visible as possible. Teachers could put on their make-up when coming to, rather than leaving, school. Moustaches hiding the upper lip and teeth do not allow perception of lip movements. Speech reading, finger spelling, signs, body language, and facial expressions should all be considered in the individual educational programmes.

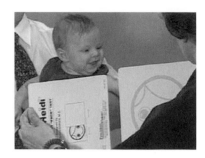

Fig. 15.2 Using preferential looking with Hiding Heidi cards (Good-lite Co., Elgin, IL, USA) to estimate contrast sensitivity.

Face recognition is a function that develops quite early. Infants aged 8 months follow their parents' movements and keenly study their faces when they are talking with their friends and relatives, as if to understand the social situation. They can recognize their parents by facial features at a distance of several metres. This can be tested if the parent leaves the room and comes back wearing a different sweater or coat. Hair is an important detail for recognition, even for children who have normal face recognition. Therefore, a radical change in a person's haircut may render him or her a stranger until he or she speaks and surprises the infant with a familiar voice. Face recognition is such a socially important function that it should be considered during the healthcare visit at the age of 1 year as well as in the neurological assessment of all 5-year-old children.

Face recognition can be difficult if a child has poor visual acuity or ventral stream dysfunction. In some cases, information from facial structures cannot be processed at all. Most children with poor face recognition have a good enough perception of facial features to enable them to *match* photographs correctly (and find pictures in which faces are the same), although they do *not recognize* familiar faces in those photographs. This is called *prosopagnosia*. In testing for prosopagnosia, it is important to first test if the child can match the photographs. Therefore, two or three similar photographs of each person's face are needed. If matching is possible, but naming is incorrect, then there is specific loss of face recognition.

During testing, the identities of people in the photographs are not revealed, because the photographs cannot then be used with the same child at a later stage. Children use small unrelated details in the photographs to remember whose face is in the picture in the same way as they use shoes, clothing, jewellery, etc. to recognize people. Poor face recognition can make a child insecure in a playgroup, where children's voices may be quite alike.

Dorsal stream dysfunction, with impaired visual search, impedes the ability to identify a parent from a group and is another cause of impaired social integration, despite an intact ability to recognize individuals on a one-to-one basis.

The play situation can be structured by making the decision, with the agreement of the other children's families, that each child always has or wears something that can be used for recognition. The 'good morning' sessions that are held in most nurseries and playgroups provide an opportunity for children to tell their names to the child with recognition problems. If the child's problem is not recognized or taken seriously, playing in a group of children may be so stressful that the child prefers to talk to adults or to play alone, which may be incorrectly ascribed a label of autistic-type behaviour. It is very important that these issues are explained to staff in nurseries and schools so that there can be no misunderstanding, such as staff believing that the child has no problems but is simply spoiled and badly behaved. If such misunderstandings persist, it is important for the health and well-being of the child that he or she should be moved to a different school or nursery that has an environment with a better structure in communication and interaction.

Facial expressions may not be perceived normally by some children with CVI, even if facial features can be perceived and recognized. In addition, problems in perception and recognition of facial expressions often accompany prosopagnosia. Training in the linguistic significance of facial expressions using a magnifying mirror and tactile and kinaesthetic information can be started quite early. Parents and teachers can reinforce this training by expressing their emotions verbally at the same time as adopting the appropriate facial expression.

Chrissie (aged 6) and her mother enjoy their session at the magnifying make-up mirror. Chrissie watches mum putting on her make-up, then they have a game, with mum making faces and Chrissie trying to copy. Mum will make a happy face and say 'Look, I'm happy!'. Chrissie has a go at copying what mum has done. Their favourite expression is when mum wrinkles her eyebrows, pouts her lips, and says 'I'm annoyed and fed up!'. Both of them burst out laughing, as they know they each feel like that quite often!

Dual sensory training like this appears to be effective in helping the child both develop a variation in facial expressions and 'understand' the facial expressions of other people. The child learns to listen carefully to the tone of voice and react accordingly, which may sometimes mislead us into believing that visual perception has improved. Tests that require description of facial expressions in photographs also test language, and children also quickly learn to recognize the pictures by heart. Observations of responses to facial expressions that are *not* combined with simultaneous auditory cues or speech are the best way of following the development of training. Clear, prolonged facial expressions seen 'face on' need to give way to more subtle, quicker expressions viewed from different orientations.

The use of pictures in communication is often considered as an alternative for children who are unable to develop spoken language. However, on occasion, such pictures are introduced without either vision having been assessed or reference to the known functional visual acuity. The smallest detail in such pictures must be visible and matched to the measured acuity. The thickness of lines seen by preferential looking can be used as an initial guide for choosing the thickness of lines and details for use in pictures for communication. It is important to know if a child can match colours and perceive and match forms (shapes). Optimal picture perception is affected by a variety of factors: optimum spectacle correction for refractive error and accommodative dysfunction; intact visual pathways and image processing to perceive colour and detail; and the ability to match and recognize. A child has to progress from recognizing the three-dimensional object to its two-dimensional representation – from the concrete to the abstract and symbolic.

A simple way to assess this is to use the Lea Puzzle (www.lea-test.fi/). Sometimes children can match colours and seem to match shapes, but in fact they are using colour cues. This test identifies such visual dysfunction.

See Chapter 16 for further discussion concerning pictures for communication.

Amy wanted to help her little boy, Kevin, who is 5 and has cerebral palsy, to learn about pictures. She knew that he liked looking at the pictures in the books she read him, but she wasn't sure what he was seeing in the pictures. She started with a simple object, Kevin's red ball. She said, 'Kevin, where's the ball? It was on the tray with a cup and a spoon. He eye-pointed to it and Amy picked it up. She said, 'Let's draw the ball together'. Amy put a fat red crayon in Kevin's good hand and they had great fun drawing a circle together and colouring it in. Amy hung the drawing up in the kitchen so that the rest of the family could admire it. The next morning she took Kevin over to the drawing and asked, 'What's that?'. Kevin laughed. Amy took it off the wall and over to Kevin's tray, where he eye-pointed to the ball. Amy put the ball beside the drawing. She was so proud of Kevin's achievement.

Orientation and movement

If the visual (or acoustic) world feels irritating and confusing, and appears to offer little information, then one's own body and movements become a focus of attention and potentially provide an important starting point for habilitation. This may be the case for many young children with severe CVI. It is important to help young children to take their hands and (if possible) their feet to their mouths if they do not do it spontaneously themselves; it is important to help the child touch his or her knee, elbow, head, or jaw, and feel his or her own movement. This helps the child to learn to distinguish between himself or herself and the environment. Simple language and song can be used to describe what is happening. This potentially helps the child to give meaning to his or her own actions and the actions of others. Independent movement, with its related sensations, plays a much more important role in learning and development than being led by another. The bodies and the movements of parents are also important areas of experience. By participating in movements and activities, such as being rocked in the parent's arms, the young child gains a range of experiences, yet feels safe and protected.

The hand can lead the eye, and visual experiences need to be cross-referenced through touch. By frequently touching and dealing with objects, the visual perception of them may be enhanced. If visual information becomes disturbing, it can be helpful to switch to relying on touch for short periods.

Experience of movement is the key for the perception of space and the use of vision to guide movement through it. From about 8 months of age, children need to gain a lot of experience of 'direction' – up and down, forward and back, this side and that side (and, later, left and right). Using language (and songs) to describe the child's movement complements learning. To be able to see how high a room is, and to learn how far away something is, and to estimate a distance is founded on prior experience. A child learns to estimate the distance between a table and a chair by crawling around, or by walking with a toy brick trolley or pushchair. What is important is that the child is moving independently and not 'being moved'. For children who have additional disabilities, such as cerebral palsy, the experience of bringing about movement can be assisted, but this should be done in the security of the parent's arms or lying against the parent's body where the child will not be afraid to try to reach out and touch. Adults should, of course, offer protection, but most importantly support the child in his or her own exploration, movement, and activities.

Profoundly impaired vision discourages exploration. The 'Little Room' can also provide a safe environment, which encourages the young child in movement and exploration. This can be made from a box. Objects can be hung from a heavy-duty rubber band, and textures can be attached to the sides so that if a child moves his or her hands he or she will encounter something of interest to feel, hear, grasp, and bring to the mouth for exploration. This kind of little room for infants and children with some useful sight differs from the 'Little Room' for blind babies described by Lilli Nielsen (1989) because it has visual and tactile boundaries, not a see-through upper side. Other small spaces can be created in corners, behind sofas, or under tables. These safe environments encourage children to explore and also to make sounds such as squealing for joy and laughing.

Trusting in their own movement and activities contributes considerably to the development of a child's self-confidence and helps the child to deal with unfamiliar or disturbing situations. Like any other movements, spastic and athetoid movements potentially convey a meaningful tactile and proprioceptive input and should be supported, with advice from a physiotherapist, and not stopped or inhibited.

We believe that, from its very first breath, each child finds his or her own specific way of dealing with his or her surroundings. If these surroundings are not compatible with the needs of a child with CVI, then we cannot simply make the child 'compatible', but must create surroundings and experiences that are suitable for the child. The challenge for all educational and therapeutic work is to provide the optimal context that freely allows meaningful communication and interaction to develop amongst all who are concerned.

The ability to use vision to guide movement and the ability to see moving objects are rarely considered in clinical examination. Impaired motion perception may not be evident before the child starts to walk independently, but may later be recognized if the child walks faster than other children of the same age and frequently *collides with large obstacles,* such as dustbins. The older child may also ride a bike straight into large obstacles. Young children cannot analyse their visual world and describe how they see the surrounding objects. From adults who perceive motion only at low frequencies, and cannot see fast-moving targets, we have learned that walking at a normal pace may make nearby objects blur, which is unpleasant. When the speed of walking is increased, the blurred objects disappear and objects further away (with low relative speed) become more visible. However, the risk of bumping into objects on either side becomes a safety problem. Using a push toy on wheels can help a toddler to move more safely, and older children can be taught by a mobility specialist to use a mobility cane for their specific needs.

Peter's teacher thought he had attention-deficit–hyperactivity disorder (ADHD) because he kept walking quickly and bumping into things. His parents knew this wasn't the case, and obtained advice from a mobility specialist, who identified that Peter was unaware of his surroundings when walking and had difficulty perceiving the quality of surfaces. Once Peter was given a cane to run over the surface of the ground ahead, he was able to slow down and become calm when moving. The provision of side shields to his spectacles eliminated peripheral moving blur and made movement much more pleasant for him.

These strategies may also prove useful when a child has an impairment of the lower field of vision or has difficulty making out the quality and depth characteristics of a surface, not knowing whether a darker surface is a hole, a raised surface, or just a mark on the ground. (Such children can be seen to walk around a large pattern in the carpet as if it is an obstacle.) It is important to explain to staff at nursery or school why the child experiences these difficulties so that they can understand and help.

Difficulty processing fast movement can cause unexpected problems.

When taken to visit her mother's friend, Debbie started screaming uncontrollably when the lady's small dog ran into the room to greet her. Debbie later told her mother that all she could see was 'this blurry ball' coming towards her, then disappearing and popping up elsewhere. The fast movement, which Debbie could not perceive, made the dog 'disappear' and then 're-appear' suddenly somewhere else. When the dog was made to sit quietly and Debbie could stroke it, she gradually lost her fear of it.

Use of the children's other senses can help children deal with information in motion.

Jim's dad loved taking him to the park. Like all parents, he was afraid that Jim might run into a moving swing, but he knew that it was even more important for Jim to be aware of the swings, because Jim can't see fast movement. His dad spent a lot of time pointing out landmarks around the swings to his son, so that he would know when they were near. He also got Jim to listen very carefully to the sound of the swing, the swoosh becoming louder as it came towards him and quieter as it went away, as did the sounds of the children's voices on the swings. Jim became good at knowing when it was safe, but his dad still kept an eye on him, just in case.

Difficulty handling visual and other information at the same time is a symptom which can be observed in quite young children and can be taken as a sign of a limited capacity of the function of handling incoming information. It is most obvious in children who cannot use vision when walking – they stop, look, then walk, stop, look, and walk. It does not mean that they need to rest after a few steps, but that it is difficult to see when moving.

Children using wheelchairs independently need to learn to move, stop, look and take in what they can see, and have it explained to them by the accompanying adults. Constantly describing where the child is and what the child is doing can be a great help, as children with CVI may process what they see and hear more slowly, before they become familiar with it. Once children have learned familiar routes they no longer need this approach, but new details warrant description. This helps the child to learn, then seek out a critical number of details, such as landmarks on the route, and to remember the order in which they come.

Tactile landmarks are often used by children with CVI without the adults noticing. If tactile landmarks are provided along the routes, such as a tactile border along the wall that children can use to 'trail' their hand along, the need to look carefully is reduced and the visual overload decreases. In some children with CVI the analysis of surrounding structures in new places is so demanding that the image sometimes blurs to a 'wall' around the child. Although the child may be aware that this is not a real structure, it may lead to him or her being afraid to walk without guidance.

The *orientation and mobility* training of these children requires careful analysis. If their visual–spatial awareness is impaired and their internal visual maps are unreliable, what visual landmark information can be used? How should the cane be used? Will memorizing routes as a sequence of landmarks help? Some children cannot remember the order of the landmarks except when they are sung to the tune of a familiar song that the child can hum to himself or herself when walking. The training in orientation and mobility for children who have poor spatial awareness and poor orientation in space is thus very different from the training of children with blurred images but normal processing of visual information. Formal orientation and mobility training needs to take into account home, school, and the known and unknown outside environment.

Road safety awareness training should start at a young age for all children, but additional skills are very important for young people such as Chris. Knowing how to use crossings safely and learning to use her long cane effectively will be high on the orientation and mobility specialist's list for Chris.

Chris is functionally nearly blind to traffic. Cars that move fast are not visible to her. They suddenly appear at the traffic lights. Sometimes she sees a car approaching but appears not to know how fast the car is travelling. She sees cars travelling in the same direction and with the same speed as the family's vehicle, but a truck coming from a side road 'appears out of nowhere'.

16

APPROACHES TO THE MANAGEMENT IN SCHOOLS OF VISUAL PROBLEMS DUE TO CEREBRAL VISUAL IMPAIRMENT

Marianna Buultjens, Lea Hyvärinen, and Renate Walthes

Introduction

When the parents of a child with cerebral visual impairment (CVI) take their child to a school for the first time, he or she may be the first pupil with CVI that the school has encountered. In this situation, the parents may find that the staff of the school find it difficult to immediately notice and acknowledge that their child suffers from CVI, as the disorder becomes apparent only when the child is watched for the way he or she uses his or her vision. The parents may advise the staff to observe the way in which the child uses his or her vision, and also explain the approaches they believe are needed to help their child benefit from school.

Parents need support from their extended family, friends, other parents, and from informed and sensitive professionals. Many parents quickly become experts in understanding how their child perceives the world, but it is good for them to know that they are not alone in this. We hope that each parent will find an understanding school for their child with imaginative staff who are willing to think long and hard on how they are teaching and presenting material to their pupils, and who are willing to try out new ways and ideas, taking into account the following:

1   The needs of the individual and those of the overall class need to be catered for, and balanced. An initial focus on delivery of the curriculum can facilitate optimal communication.
2   For older children and teenagers, acceptance by the peer group is fundamentally important and may initially precede the provision of special attention or specialized equipment.
3   The older the child, the better he or she will develop strategies to deal with the visual problems, but regular review of the strategies and the devices used for specific circumstances is warranted.
4   To talk about visual problems is difficult because we can all talk about *what* we see, but not *how* we perceive that which we know to be normal. One's frame of reference for what is normal perception is one's own vision. We have little facility to gain insight into what is 'normal perception' for others, and the same holds true for the '*alternative* normal perception' of those with CVI. In dealing with a child with CVI, professionals and parents may

be perplexed, or may have developed their own independent views about how the child sees the world. Providing an alternative interpretation of how the child sees may be very helpful but may come across as threatening. Most parents are, however, relieved when a structured explanation and set of strategies to deal with the visual problems are provided.

In this section we consider a range of issues that have arisen in the education of children with CVI. A pragmatic approach is required which combines diagnostic and observational aspects of the child's behaviour with approaches that match both the design of the environment and the educational strategies employed to deal with the visual limitations and the needs of the child. This has to be adapted with new ideas and strategies as the child develops.

Practical problems at school and some of their solutions

The following issues have to be considered in the context of school surroundings and lessons: environmental aspects; activities such as reading, copying, and drawing; and perception issues.

ENVIRONMENTAL ASPECTS

Teaching materials (e.g. illustrations in books) should have good, clear outlines, with no pastel colours blending into each other so that forms/shapes disappear for children who have poor contrast sensitivity. Whenever teaching materials are created, they ideally should be viewed through 'demonstration/simulation spectacles' that depict the lowest contrast sensitivity of a pupil in the classroom to allow the teacher to understand what that student may perceive when the picture is shown. If a student does not perceive *all* the details in the information then there is not enough information to assimilate and the child may misunderstand or incompletely access the information.

The best *lighting level* or *optimal luminance level* for the child with CVI needs to be determined as it may improve contrast sensitivity. This should be used both at home and in school. Ideally, funding should be available to schools for optimizing the quality of illumination and contrast by painting and using indirect lighting and blinds to stop glare.

Filter lenses may decrease dazzle and thus improve contrast sensitivity, so their value needs to be assessed. They need to be tested with the child both indoors (for use in classrooms) and outdoors. They can be of great help for games and sports at school and for recreational activities. Visual adaptation problems due to changing lighting conditions are not common in children with CVI, but a child may have another condition, such as a retinal disorder that causes either a delayed visual adaptation to lower luminance levels or photophobia (sensitivity to light), or both. If a child has delayed adaptation, he or she requires a torch if asked to find something in a cupboard or in a poorly lit basement. Outdoors, children with photophobia need to wear their filter lenses and a cap with a brim that is dark on the lower surface so it reflects less light than a light-coloured brim. If adaptation to the luminance level in the classroom after a break outside takes longer than a few minutes, the child should play in a shaded area of the playground, otherwise too much of the lesson is lost because of decreased vision during the slow readaptation time.

Spectacles and *magnifying devices* are difficult for school staff to understand. It is important that information is given to school staff about spectacles and optical and non-optical devices. They need to know how the child should use them, when they should be used, and when the child may choose not to use them. Schools need to have this information if a child has been prescribed spectacles. If a child does not want to use the spectacles, the situation needs to be carefully assessed again. Children will use spectacles if the lenses improve their vision and the frames fit comfortably. If the spectacles cause a small-angle strabismus or too large a change in the image quality from what the child sees without the new spectacles or sees with the old spectacles (a change in either the power of the spectacles or the form of the front surface of the lenses), this may make the spectacles uncomfortable. Children, like adults, will use spectacles only if they help them to see more comfortably!

If low-vision aids are provided, the use of each new device should be taught to the child. This is essential, and parents and teachers should insist that training is provided by either the professional who prescribes them or a specialist teacher of the visually impaired. Training a young child to use a telescope/monocular aid requires special skills. It is a good idea to let all children with CVI try out magnifiers and other aids such as closed-circuit TV (CCTV), now known as video magnifiers.

Tracy (10 years old) has periventricular leucomalacia, but normal visual acuities and normal contrast sensitivity. She has difficulty with face recognition and recognition of landmarks and has mild cerebral palsy. When she feels stressed her ability to read print deteriorates. She visited her local visual impairment centre and tried out a video magnifier. She was so delighted that it offered her the immediate choice of different sizes of text so she asked if she could borrow it to try it out. Within a day of getting it home, Tracy had worked out how to magnify a part of a page instead of a whole page and how to move the book so that she could read comfortably. She lost no time in devouring her new Harry Potter book!

We don't necessarily understand what is good or comfortable for children. They can push themselves to read 9-point (very small) text to please someone who is testing them, but won't remember anything they have read because all their energy has gone into seeing letters and words. Small hand-held magnifiers are easy to carry around and even very young children can enjoy using them to look at small objects and details in pictures.

When trying to decide what letter size and spacing will be comfortable for young children, letters can be drawn with a medium fibre-tip pen and printed with a computer using a range of different sizes and spacing. The size and spacing of print that affords greatest ease and speed of access to the information can be chosen. When a child has learned to read, a word processor can be used to identify the optimal size and spacing between letters, words, and lines for learning and comprehension. Some children with CVI and normal visual acuity and contrast sensitivity can have such poor fixation, accommodation (ability to focus), and saccades (the fast movements from one fixation to the next) that they read best by having one single large word in the middle of the computer screen and get to the next word by pressing the arrow key.

Colour vision changes are not common in children with cerebral damage. They are more common in children who have changes in the central retina or who have optic atrophy. However, colour matching can be difficult. The 'colour game' that can be copied from www.lea-test.fi may reveal confusions in matching colours. When a child has difficulty matching colours, some difficulties in classroom work will occur. Therefore, it is imperative that the teacher knows of this difficulty so that he or she can help the child by offering alternative materials that do not rely on colour matching. Naming of colours may be difficult even if a child can match colours quite normally. It is analogous to the situation of face recognition – we may recognize a person by facial features but cannot find the name of that person in our memory. One way to help children remember the names of colours is to link them with appropriate words, for example 'green grass', 'yellow lemon', or 'blue sky'.

Pictures for communication

Before deciding whether to use pictures, or which pictures to use, for communication, teachers should draw familiar objects to make sure that the picture is understood as representing the object and can be seen and recognized. Some communication pictures have more than one object represented and sometimes one object obscures part of another. Can the child make out and recognize the different objects in the picture? For some children it is very difficult to make sense of pictures where there is more than one object. It can be helpful to cover up part of a 'busy' picture so that the child gradually builds up knowledge of all the different things or people in the picture. Always make sure that any objects the child is working with are in front of or on a plain background of contrasting colour.

Always check whether the child understands that the two-dimensional drawing has an added symbolic meaning, in that it represents not just the objects depicted but also an additional concept such as 'snack time' or 'lunch'. Sometimes the child has learned what the card signifies but does not know what is in the picture!

Visual and auditory overload

Visual and auditory overload in classrooms causes tiredness and concentration difficulties. An excess of children's paintings and other decoration causes clutter and can make it harder for children to concentrate on what the teacher is saying or the work that he or she should be doing. If this is the case, these distractions should be diminished or put in an area behind the children which will not disturb the pupils. Ensure that the area of the classroom which the child is facing does not have many distracting decorations on the walls.

The movement of active children in the peripheral visual field can be especially irritating for the affected child. This can interrupt the child's writing and thinking during daily work or an examination, and it can be particularly difficult for the child to return to the work in hand. This can cause distress.

Some visually impaired children also have a hearing impairment, with or without auditory processing problems. Their experience of the classroom, and especially of the playground, is difficult to imagine, and breaks may be even more demanding than the work in the classroom.

Overload is a common problem for children with brain damage. Their total brain capacity is limited, and many functions are still conscious for them at an age when they have become subconscious and nearly automatic for their peers. If a child with CVI has to perform several demanding tasks at once, he or she may lose head control, body control, and even fall. (One of the writers of this chapter witnessed such an incident. While listening to a discussion on her vision in relation to schoolbooks, one young girl lost her balance and almost fell over.)

ACTIVITIES

Reading is the most common and often the most demanding visual task at school. Fixation of gaze and saccades are often abnormal in children with CVI. They may be the only major problems, but are often also accompanied by poor accommodation. When a child has reading problems, oculomotor functions should be observed and recorded on video if possible. If the effort of fixation causes overload, words can be presented sequentially one at a time in the middle of the screen at a size which is large enough to render exact fixation and accommodation unnecessary.

If reading and writing are ineffective through the visual mode, auditory teaching materials and tactile approaches to learning should be evaluated without delay. Children may use Braille despite 'normal' sensory functions if irregular oculomotor functions make the use of visual materials impossible or too demanding to access. A combination of reading from a screen along with writing in Braille can assist children who have profound problems in visual recognition with learning to read.

Copying and drawing single and composite geometric forms is a common task in testing whether a child is ready for school. The assessment aproach should be modified when testing children with CVI who have not been used to drawing at home before coming to nursery school. The forms/shapes to be copied should be drawn while the child is watching. This may have to be done several times if it is a completely new task for the child. You can say, 'Look, I can draw a straight line, and then I can draw another line that is parallel to the first line, that means it is beside the first line all the way. And I can draw a third line next to the second line. Now it is your turn, draw a line next to my lines in the same direction . . . now a second line in the same direction . . . and a third.' A circle, an angle, a triangle, a square, and two rectangles partially on top of each other are then drawn in a similar way along with an explanation of what is being done. If the child cannot understand these instructions, or if a child cannot draw because of motor difficulties, we can assess his or her visual functioning by using sticks that are moved by the tester while asking the child whether they form the required pattern of parallel lines, angles, triangles, squares, or two rectangles partially on top of each other.

Concepts of direction, such as 'parallel', need to be learned in play situations by placing numerous objects in the same direction before a child is ready for testing. Some children with CVI have such great difficulty with the basic concept of direction that they do not understand what is meant by it even if they have been working on it for weeks. Some children complain that the lines change their position, and therefore it is difficult to know when the lines are parallel or which angles are of the same size. Whether the difficulty is in the coding of the information (in the primary visual cortex) or in the processing of the image cannot be assessed during the assessment of visual functioning at school, and it is difficult even in laboratories when young children are concerned. Since direction and orientation are commonly used concepts in teaching, difficulties in the use of these concepts must be made known so that they can be addressed. Children with cerebral palsy (CP) and children with CVI without CP seem to have specific difficulties in the development of visual–spatial awareness and its concepts. Sometimes children start to develop these concepts and abilities when their posture improves and they have a better awareness of the height and structure of their own body. It is, therefore, very important for a teacher to work collaboratively with an occupational therapist and a physiotherapist.

Learning by touch and acoustic patterns for blind children is the given way to complete the idea of a visual form, object, or pattern. Teachers who adopt this multisensorial approach tell of the positive benefits for the whole class, including the children who are not diagnosed as having a visual problem. However, mathematics seems to be a problem area that requires new thinking. Children who have poor awareness of concrete space often also seem to have great difficulties with abstract space. Use of teaching techniques for blind children and use of mathematical programs to compensate for difficulties in visual strategies should be tried from early on. It is sometimes hard to get Abacus and Braille accepted for use by children who have 'normal' visual acuity and a wide visual field. However, these tactile methods have proved beneficial for some children whose visual world has a structure clearly different from the norm. The use of acoustic patterns, rhythm, and sonification (Csocsán 2007) is a new method that could also be investigated in teaching children with spatial problems.

PERCEPTION ISSUES
Perception of lines can be assessed with the 'Lea-Mailbox' and 'Lea-Rectangles' (http://www. lea-test.fi) tests, which are games aimed at assessing the perception of line direction and the length of lines. The test situation can be used as a purely visual task (ventral stream) and as a hand–eye coordination task (dorsal stream).

In the Lea-Mailbox game the child is asked to post cards through a slot which is orientated in different ways. Normally the turning of the wrist and the fingers starts immediately and the orientation of the card is in the same orientation as the slot by the time the child's hand is halfway to it. If the motor functions of the wrist are restricted, it is better to present the mailbox horizontally. If the child does not perceive the direction of the slot, the card will not be turned. This test situation depicts how visual information concerning the orientation of lines is used to bring about visual guidance of movement of the hand. This function is mediated through the dorsal stream. The ventral stream function of recognition of orientation is made by asking the child to detect when a narrow object, such as a stick or a pencil, is orientated in the same direction as the slot. Children with normal vision can detect a disparity of less than $5°$.

The Lea-Rectangles game can be used in a similar way to assess perception of length of lines by asking which of two or three rectangles is the longest. Some children arrange the rectangles in order of their length before one has had time to explain anything. The length of lines also needs to be assessed in simple drawings and more complex pictures to find out the effect of surrounding visual information on perception of the length.

If a child does not have the concepts of 'longer' and 'shorter' they can be taught by using visual, tactile, and kinaesthetic information. If the child learns that one rectangle is outside the other rectangle by using his or her hands to feel the difference in length, and thus develops the concepts 'longer' and 'shorter' but still does not visually perceive the difference, the child needs to be carefully tested by a paediatric neurologist and/or neuropsychologist as the child may not have this specific function in visual processing.

Visual field disorders occur in the area of both the visual field and the sensitivity of the field. Areas of decreased function, called scotomata, are difficult to map before school age, and even at school age require an experienced tester who knows what to look for because the form and size of scotomata vary in different conditions and are often important diagnostic features. Small scotomata on the right side of fixation (in countries where reading is from left to right; on the left side in countries where reading is from right to left) may fall on a few letters and disturb a child who is learning to read by sounding out the letters rather than reading whole words. If a child makes unusual, irregular errors during reading it is wise to test reading with texts of increasing size. If the errors change when the text becomes larger and disappear at a certain size then the child does not have a reading error but probably has a small scotoma disturbing spelling. In that case, the child may try tilting the text so that the scotoma is between the lines and the usual size of text can be used. If not, text may be enlarged so that the scotoma loses its effect.

Picture perception may be difficult even if visual acuity, contrast sensitivity, and colour vision have been assessed as being normal. Pictures used as optotypes in visual acuity tests, like those in Lea tests, are simplified pictures of concrete objects that are easier to perceive than pictures with a number of details partially covered by other details. 'Reading' a picture requires scanning to grasp a general structure, perception, and recognition of parts before the content of the picture is comprehensible. The direction of lines and length of lines are basic components of all pictures. These components are coded in the primary visual cortex when the information arrives there through the visual pathways (magnocellular and parvocellular pathways). If the coding is not perfect, or the further processing of the information is irregular, lines in shapes may appear to 'wiggle' or be difficult to see, which makes geometric forms much more difficult for the child to handle than we would expect based upon the child's other visual functions.

Schoolbooks are often too cluttered, or 'rich in information', and therefore confuse children who have difficulties in processing pictures. In books where there are pictures on both pages with the text printed on the pictures it is worthwhile for teachers of children with visual processing disorders to insert an additional white page between the original pages with the text written on the white page in bold, large letters with slightly increased spacing. Some schools have rescued books from the early 1970s from the backs of cupboards, and children and teachers alike have enjoyed them for their clear text and separate illustrations. We should carefully scrutinize the textbooks chosen by schools because difficulties with picture perception occur in a larger number of children than just those known to have CVI.

Limited functioning capacity should be recognised in young children and taken as a sign of a restriction in the child's total capacity to handle information. For example, children who cannot use vision when walking – they stop, look, then walk, stop, look, and walk – because it is difficult to see when moving. Similarly, a child may be functionally deaf when carefully looking at something, blind when listening, may lose head and/or body control during a demanding visual task, or drop an object if there is new sensory input, such as someone touching the child.

The child's total capacity may be so limited that several simultaneous tasks are not possible if they each require conscious planning and execution. Similar tasks are subconsciously managed in a normally developing child who often enjoys trying to do several things at once as a competition with himself or herself. Vision may disturb other functions, which is usually easiest to observe in motor functions. When a child turns his or her head away before reaching for and grasping an object, we should ask ourselves if the child is using an early neck reflex to start the movement of the arm (which is easy to see in the quality of the movement) or if it is likely that the visual feedback loop is defective. In the latter case, we can ask the child not to turn the head but to close the eyes when the hand is approaching the object. If it is easier for the child to reach for the object with the eyes shut than when looking at the object, then visual information is not giving proper maps during the movement. It is better to rely on the map that the visual system gave before the movement started.

Other sensory stimuli can be equally irritating or cause interruptions. A sound from outside or from the corridor, or a smell or fragrance, may need to be explained before a child can continue with a task. Sometimes it is difficult to remember that, for many children, the environment is an auditory environment and vision plays a subordinate role. If we close our eyes for a while and listen carefully, we experience a classroom in a very different way from when our eyes are open, or if we watch a video made in a classroom we become aware of the high level of noise in even the best-run classes! If a child does not have the capacity to process out the non-essential noise, it must be very hard to cope in those 'lively' settings.

Activities of daily living

In many special schools, subjects such as orientation and mobility, communication skills, and activities of daily life form part of the school day. In mainstream schools, skills in orientation and mobility may have to be acquired after school or at the weekend and during holidays. Activities of daily living (ADL), such as acquiring specific social skills and other independence skills, are more difficult to come by. Yet these are the very skills that teenagers feel they need most. Parents, of course, do much to help their children, but in the teenage years it is often easier if someone outside the family is involved.

Body language may not be perceived or interpreted normally. Now and then one meets children who are constantly asking classroom staff and other children 'Are you angry?', as if they are unable to read the usual movements of body language. If a child has been diagnosed as having specific loss of perception of body language, drama sessions at school can be recorded on video showing the child how he or she looks in the different situations while trying to express the feeling of the person or animal he or she is representing. For teenagers, training in front of a mirror can be effective. At that age, motivation is usually high because without the ability to read body language a teenager is lost in communication with other teenagers.

Often children are unaware that they do not have the usual social skills of their peers. 'Turn taking' in conversation is very important, but very difficult for young people who cannot see well or perceive body language.

Communication and interaction is based on mutual interpretation. If one does not react the way we are used to, we often infer that this person acts intentionally and do not consider that the behaviour is connected to the way the person may see or hear. To be able to deal with diversity requires more attention to how children with impaired vision experience us.

Cerebral visual impairment in children is still a very young field of research in which neurological discoveries predominate. The general question of how one can acquire a visual understanding of the world and learn to live with a feeling of security while coping with CVI is far from being answered. In order to develop supportive and helpful strategies for these children and young people, we need a circular process of creating new conceptual models, developing functional assessment approaches, and observation in specific settings. Interdisciplinary research and the collaboration of all special education disciplines in developing new pedagogical concepts are crucial not just to describe the strategies and patterns of behaviour of children with CVI, but to understand them.

Conclusion

The world is a wonderful, complicated place and each one of us perceives it in our own way. Children with CVI give us an insight into both how *we* perceive and how *they* perceive the same phenomena. Like all parents and professionals, our duty of care is to help our children grow and thrive. We have the additional challenge *and* reward of jointly discovering with our children a new way of perceiving, learning to live in, and enjoying our world.

The above paragraphs describe several aspects of visual functioning that constitute the 'jigsaw' pieces of CVI. A single child may learn to compensate so well for the impaired functions that no one will suspect underlying CVI, but the resultant behaviour may be erroneously ascribed a cognitive or behavioural explanation. A child with CVI or visual processing problems commonly, but not always, has other impairments and disabilities that are more obvious and thus dominate the image that we have of the child. There is also a group of children with good visual acuities and no evidence of CP with focal dysfunction of the visual brain to account for the visual behaviours described.

17
STRATEGIES TO HELP CHILDREN WHO HAVE BOTH VISUAL AND HEARING IMPAIRMENTS

Stuart Aitken

If, as has become accepted wisdom, 80%[1] of what we learn is through vision and the child is blind, what happens if the child also has a hearing impairment? In this chapter, the impact of hearing impairment in association with cerebral visual impairment (CVI) is considered. The effects of various forms of CVI on a child's access to education and learning are outlined, and the effects of CVI in association with hearing impairment are considered.

Effects of cerebral visual impairment on education and learning

The effects of CVI on visual functioning and performance vary depending on the demands of the activity, the nature of CVI, and the extent of the impairment. If we limit our discussion to the effect on educational management, a useful starting point is to consider which areas of a child's curriculum would be affected, in what way, and to what extent. Clearly, it would be an impossible task to ascertain the effects of CVI on each and every curriculum area for all possible curricula for each country in the world. However, common features do exist between many curricula whether that curriculum is based on statute, such as in England (Education Reform Act 1988), or through guidance frameworks, such as that operated in Scotland (SED 1987) or elsewhere. Examples of skills that many different curricula require of pupils include the following:

- accessing information, for example by reading text, which in turn will vary depending on whether the child is learning to read (early reading) or has learned to read and is accessing text (skilled reading);

---

[1]Although many reports cite the figure of 80%, it is difficult to determine the original source for this widely quoted figure. Subtly different interpretations can be found; for instance, the Eye Care Council states that more than 80% of learning is done visually (http://www.seetolearn.com/see-to-learn.html) as does Cincinatti Children's Medical Center (http://www.cincinnatichildrens. org/about/news/release/2005/11-sight.htm). Others refer to the 80% figure within a narrower context such as to learning that occurs in the first 12 years of life (http://findarticles.com/p/articles/mi_8174/is_20090813/ai_n50924543/) or specifically within the context of reading (http://www.ssc.education.ed.ac.uk/courses/VI&multi/vnov08i.html) or to learning that takes place in the classroom (http://www.optom.on.ca/students_and_educators/eye_see_eye_learn/what_is_eye_see_eye_learn).

- accessing information, for example by interpreting figures such as maps, diagrams, and photographs;
- expressing or recording thoughts, most commonly by writing or typing;
- understanding symbols, for example in maths, science, and drawing;
- learning foreign languages;
- participating in music by playing or otherwise appreciating it, or by the more abstract skill of understanding and interpreting musical scores;
- moving around between areas requiring both mobility skills (memories for skills, or 'how to' memory) and orientation skills or declarative memory (Baddeley and Hitch 1974); and
- applying higher-order skills such as planning, problem-solving, switching attention, social interaction, and motivation.

Rather than considering which type of CVI manifestation (e.g. hemianopia) will be associated with which particular visual dysfunction (e.g. figure–ground separation), a focus on the educational curriculum considers the effect on education skills and learning.

Table 17.1 presents, in diagrammatic form, the extent of the effect of various areas of cerebral visual dysfunction described in earlier chapters on the skills required to follow curriculum areas. Columns represent examples of CVI discussed elsewhere in this book. Table 17.1 is an oversimplification. Each area of the curriculum could be subdivided still further. For example, within 'reading processes' early reading could cover the differential effects of each manifestation of CVI on the three main stages of early reading (Frith 1985, Dodd and Carr 2003). Different types of CVI will have different degrees of effect on the following:

- logographic or visually cued reading, which involves memorizing the visual shape of words;
- phonetically cued reading or breaking words down into their letters and sounds (Ehri 1991); and
- orthographic reading, requiring the child to analyse groups of words. This is also known as sight-word reading and renders reading more automatic and fluent.

For a more detailed discussion of the development of reading see Frith (1985). Following up the example of reading, we can see from Table 17.1 that different categories of CVI will not only have different effects depending on the curricular area in question, but also may have a differential effect within any one curricular area. For example, inattention and neglect versus nystagmus may have differential effects on early reading versus skilled reading. Someone learning to read is not yet able to use the context provided by surrounding letters or words to help them decode for reading. A skilled reader, on the other hand, can rely on other elements such as 'word- or phrase-chunking' to supply that context, and thus mitigate the effects of neglect or nystagmus.

The examples of curricular areas affected differentially by CVI encompass many different skills. In the same curricular area two different aspects can be affected quite differently. In the area of music, for example, hemianopia will have a serious effect on literacy for musical scores. It may have less effect on appreciation of music.

Cerebral visual impairment and hearing impairment

Vision and hearing are often known as the two main distance senses. Through them we access most of the information beyond what we can reach out and touch. Impairment of both senses means that the possibility of one sense compensating for the other impaired sense is much reduced (Aitken et al 2000). Indeed, Helen Keller's alleged statement[2] that 'Blindness cuts you off from things; deafness cuts you off from people' presents a stark reminder of the problems faced by children with hearing and visual impairment, such as finding out information, communicating with others, and moving around in the environment.

A number of different terms have been used to describe impairments to both hearing and sight. In 1993 the term 'deafblind' came to be used in place of 'deaf/blind' or 'deaf-blind' in most countries (Lagati 1995). Combining the words 'deaf' and 'blind' to create 'deafblind' suggested a unique impairment in which deafblindness is more than just deafness plus blindness. The terms 'deaf-blind' and 'multisensory impaired (MSI)' continue to be used in some countries. The term 'deafblind' is used in this chapter.

In the general population the most common cause of impairments to both vision and hearing remains ageing, but each year a number of children are born deafblind or acquire deafblindness in childhood. Just as the causes of visual impairment in the industrialized world have changed from being predominantly infectious diseases, so too have many of the causes of childhood deafblindness. Worldwide, there has been a reduction in congenital rubella syndrome (CRS), the infectious disease which gave rise to epidemics of childhood deafblindness, such as that in the 1960s. The decline of CRS as a cause, first reported by Best in 1983, continued following the introduction of the measles mumps rubella (MMR) vaccination (Brown 1997). In parallel with this, there has been a steady increase in the numbers of identified causes and the proportion of children with additional, often complex, impairments associated with deafblindness (Brown 1997, Brown and Bates 2005). Others (Chen 1998, Miles and Riggio 1999) have noted a similar change in the population of children born deafblind, with more having additional, often multiple, impairments. Brown and Bates (2005) note that the 2003 USA National Deaf-Blind Child Count listed over 70 possible causes in 10 000 children. Of this figure, 60% had cognitive impairments and 40% had complex healthcare support needs (National Deaf-Blind Child Count Summary 2004).

The most common profile of deafblindness is now one of children with a combination of peripheral and central sensory impairments together with 'a complex array of medical and therapeutic procedures and equipment' (Brown and Bates 2005). Changes in the profile of deafblindness in children requires us to better understand the impact of neurological impairment, including CVI, on the child's education management.

Strategies for educational management

In parallel with changes in the nature of deafblindness in children, there have been marked changes to educational approaches for deafblind children. In the 1960s a more behaviourist approach was common, whereas now approaches tend to be more child centred and

---

[2]Although widely referred to, the authors of this chapter cannot find a source for this statement.

TABLE 17.1

Association between examples of cerebral visual impairments (CVIs) and areas of educational curriculum. Rows represent areas of the curriculum affected by each type of CVI

Effects/Cause	Achromatopsia	Akinetopsia	Blindsight	Dyslexia	Dyscalculia
Accessing information					
Reading processes					
– early reading	Often				
– skilled reading	Often	Small text			
Interpreting figures					
– maps					
– figures/pictures					
Expressing thoughts					
– writing					
– typing					
Understanding symbols					
- maths					
- science					
- drawing					
Foreign languages		TV aids			
Music – play, appreciate					
– interpret scores					
Mobility – procedural					
Orientation (declarative)					
'Hidden curriculum'				Often	Often
– Planning		Interpret moving figures or objects		Often	
– Problem solving				Often	
– Switching attention				Indirectly	Indirectly
– Social interaction					
– Motivation					

Each cell is either blank, shaded, or contains text. Blank cells indicate no significant problems are present in that curricular area with the condition shown at the top of the column. Shaded cells indicate that problems should be expected in that curricular area. The degree of shading approximates the severity of the effect. Text in cells usually says 'associated' or 'often associated' indicating that the CVI itself is not thought to cause that problem but is often associated with the effects.

Hemianopia	Inattention and neglect	Nystagmus	Prosopagnosia	Simultanagnosia	Topographic agnosia
Right homonymous hemi and range of reading problems					
			If faces		
				Difficulty scanning	
			Associated		
			Associated		
			Associated		
			Associated		
			Associated		
					Associated

constructive – with interaction and communication at the core of a child's curriculum (Brown and Bates 2005). Rather than introducing a one-size-fits-all approach, the emphasis is now increasingly on highly tailored and individualized approaches, with communication at the core of intervention.

The range of possible effects of hearing loss in conjunction with CVI is vast. For example, unilateral deafness (deafness in one ear) results in no, or poor, sound localization. All sound seems to come from one place, making it difficult for the person to discriminate sounds when there is background noise, resulting in the need to avoid noisy environments. For a child with almost any form of visual impairment, anything that adversely affects his or her auditory localization abilities can have a crucial effect. It can affect how the child can listen in a group setting, in a noisy classroom, and elsewhere. With such wide-ranging potential effects, it is easy to see how peripheral unilateral deafness, in the presence of akinetopsia, for example, can adversely affect mobility skills as well as confidence, motivation, and self-esteem.

A study by Porter et al (1997) illustrates the range of approaches employed in UK schools by teachers of children who are deafblind. The study looked at 82 children aged 2–19 years in three different types of schools – mainstream schools, schools for those with severe intellectual disability, and schools specializing in sensory provision (e.g. deafblind classes). They identified 145 strategies, and an interesting pattern of how the teaching setting influenced which strategies were deployed. At the risk of reducing a complex and fascinating study to the level of sound-bites, they found that teachers in mainstream settings focused mostly on how the task was presented, demonstration, and physical prompts, whereas those in schools for pupils with severe intellectual disability focused on physical prompts, positioning, and contact as well as speech. Lastly, teachers in sensory settings combined these approaches and included a much greater emphasis on both formal and individualized approaches to communication (Porter et al 1997).

Cerebral visual impairment and cerebral hearing impairment
Before discussing CVI in combination with processing disorders in hearing, a brief overview of auditory processing disorders is presented.

AUDITORY PROCESSING DISORDERS: AN OVERVIEW
Unlike the term 'CVI', the terms 'cerebral' or 'central' hearing impairment are rarely used, the preferred term being 'auditory processing disorder' (APD) – a term recently recognized as synonymous with '(central) auditory processing disorder' (CAPD) (American Speech and Hearing Association 2005). The term APD is used here to refer to difficulties in processing or making sense of auditory information that comes to the brain.

Although APD continues to be a diagnosis associated with controversy (Jerger and Musiek 2000), the American Speech and Hearing Association (ASHA) has, in a series of carefully considered publications by its task force on APD, provided clarity to practitioners (ASHA 1996, 2005). APD is associated with problems in one or more of the following areas:

- auditory discrimination, being able to tell that one sound is different from another (especially speech), and recognizing patterns in sounds (musical rhythms are one example of an auditory pattern);
- temporal aspects of audition (auditory processing relies on making fine discriminations of timing changes in auditory input, especially differences in timing between the way input comes through one ear as opposed to the other);
- auditory performance decrements with competing acoustic signals (listening in noise); and
- auditory performance decrements with degraded acoustic signals (listening to sounds that are muffled, missing information, or for some reason not clear) (ASHA 1996).

While the above list is useful for understanding what is going wrong at the level of processing sounds, it is also helpful to consider how these difficulties affect performance (Colenbrander [2005] makes a similar distinction regarding CVI). Kelly (1995) has described APD as simply 'what we do with what we hear' and 'receiving [auditory] information and acting upon it meaningfully' (quoted in Matson 2005). How does APD affect what children can do? Johnson et al (1997) point to some of the characteristics of children with APD, including poor concentration and attention span, inconsistent responses to auditory stimuli, delayed responses to verbal stimuli, often asking for things to be repeated, being easily distracted by auditory and visual stimuli, difficulty listening when there is background noise, and difficulty localizing sound sources (Johnson et al 1997).

Differential diagnosis of auditory processing disorder
A cursory glance at the list of effects of APD shows why it can be difficult to distinguish the effects of APD from other impairments and disabilities. Kelly (1995) listed 19 behavioural characteristics found in APD or in children with an intellectual disability. Of the 19 intellectual disability characteristics, only four were not associated with APD. Even then, some writers on APD would associate the first two, hyperactivity and impulsivity, with APD. Perhaps not surprisingly, APD also showed similar behavioural manifestations to dyslexia, sharing 12 of the characteristics (Kelly 1995).

In terms of its behavioural manifestations, APD overlaps to some extent with 'auditory neuropathy' (Hood 1998). However, APD includes more than disorders of the auditory nerves just as CVI would not be equated with disorders of the optic nerves. Difficulties that arise as a result of APD can appear and develop in hugely different ways between different children. APD can manifest as problems of categorizing sounds, discriminating between sounds (especially speech), remembering auditory sequences, or auditory association. The severity of these difficulties can vary between children.

APD also shares behavioural manifestations with attention-deficit–hyperactivity disorder (ADHD), autistic spectrum disorder (ASD), and other developmental disorders (ASHA 2005). Again, the ASHA position paper helps to clarify that, although APD may coexist with such disorders, it does not cause them.

One of the difficulties with diagnosing APD is being able to test for it. Unlike with many diagnostic tests of peripheral hearing impairment, the child needs to be able to participate. Some recommend a minimum mental age equivalent of 7 or 8 years (Bellis 2003). Other inclusion criteria include intelligible speech, ability to follow directions in order to complete testing, and a minimum intelligent quotient (IQ) of 85. For many with CVI, these selection criteria would be a tall order to meet.

Until the recent ASHA statement, some writers would have eschewed a diagnosis of APD in the presence of CVI. Such writers had argued that APD should be applied only when a perceptual deficit is limited to the auditory system and nowhere else (e.g. Cacace and McFarland 1998). This meant that those with auditory processing deficits who also had any other kind of sensory temporal deficits (e.g. Tallal et al 1993) would not meet diagnostic criteria for APD. Given that akinetopsia is one example of a temporal deficit occurring in visual processing such children could not, on this basis, have been considered to have APD.

In the face of mounting evidence that different areas of the brain work together, both within and across sensory modalities (see various chapters in this book), the ASHA task force regarded this position as flawed. However, even the task force's modified position, that APD is present when perceptual processing impairment is more pronounced in the auditory modality (ASHA 2005), does make it more difficult to sustain a diagnosis embracing impaired perceptual processing in both vision and hearing.

Strategies for managing cerebral visual impairment and auditory processing disorder

Given the diagnostic criteria and difficulties in diagnosis, it is not difficult to see why most children with CVI might not appear on the radar for APD. Does that mean that children with CVI should not be considered to have APD? On a first principles analysis, that would seem to be an overly restrictive position to take. Just because we cannot easily test for a disorder does not mean that it does not exist. Moreover, the likelihood of a proportion of children with CVI also having APD must be high. Given that the proportion of APD in the population of intellectual disability is high (Kelly 1995) and the proportion of those with CVI in intellectual disability is high (see Chapter 14), it would seem reasonable to infer that a proportion of the children with CVI and intellectual disability discussed in Chapter 14 will also have APD.

Does it matter if a child's impaired hearing is as a result of peripheral rather than central loss when it comes to choice of an intervention strategy? At a practical level, it can matter a great deal. Amplification using hearing aids could well damage the cochlea, which, in a child with APD and no peripheral loss, could be functioning normally even though the child's behaviour, response in particular, to speech appears to be similar to that of a deaf child. Given, too, that a blind child may not have normal orientating responses to sound, it is too easy to assume that not turning to sound is an indication of deafness. With CVI making it difficult for some to localize sound and APD compounding that difficulty, recourse to hearing aids may not be the most appropriate course of action.

Heightened awareness that APD may exist in conjunction with CVI will include consideration of risk factors for forms of APD. Shapiro (2003) notes that bilirubin toxicity can result in auditory neuropathy or other more generalized APD. As children born with multiple diagnoses may well have raised bilirubin levels, it is important to be aware of the possibility of APD. Heightened awareness also means being in a position to select from the general advice for supporting a child with APD, which can also be applied to a child with CVI. General advice to select from includes the following:

- Make sure that the child looks at you when you speak to him or her to allow easier lip-reading, often used by children with APD.
- Before that, make sure that the child is aware that you are talking to him or her.
- Speak clearly, then make sure the child has understood you (not the same as parroting the speech back).
- Seat the learner with APD at the front of the class to allow him or her to lip-read what the teacher says more easily.
- Ensure that the child has a clear view of the board for written information.
- Provide written information on the board when speaking.
- Always provide written additional instructions on paper to which the child can refer (e.g. http://www.infosheets.apduk.org/).

Kelly (1995) reports the following suggestions that teachers may find helpful:

- Seat the student towards the front of the room, with clear visual access to both the teacher and the board, and with the back to the window area
- Have the student look at the speaker's face.
- Limit background distractions.
- Present directions in short, concrete segment with visual cues.
- Rephrase directions.
- Maintain structure and schedules.
- Preview materials to be presented using a variety of media.
- Build the student's self-esteem at every opportunity.

Beyond these simple strategies, a growing number of evidence-based approaches to managing APD is emerging. These focus on remediation of auditory skills (e.g. Tremblay and Kraus 2002, Musiek 2004) as well as compensatory techniques that include introducing environmental modifications such as frequency modulated assistive listening devices (Bellis 2003). Even with the growth in evidence-based approaches, Matson (2005) reports a consensus among authorities on APD to the effect that 'Remediation continues to be an area in need of research development. It seems that professionals are frustrated by a "blanket approach" of remediation strategies for every type of auditory processing difficulty' (Matson 2005, p. 41).

For any visually impaired child the ability to discriminate sounds, to know what to listen for and attend to in background noise, and to filter out extraneous sound and keep attention focused are vital skills that can compensate for impaired vision. A child with CVI or other form of sight impairment depends heavily on being able to select out sound from background noise, to listen to audio books and tapes, and to use ambient sound to help orientate in their environment. Additional demands are placed on the auditory system to compensate for visual loss, but APD means not being able to compensate to the same extent. Referring to Table 17.1, we can infer the impact that APD may well have for children with CVI. For example, children with a visual processing disorder resulting in dyslexia will, if they also have APD, be less able to use phonological techniques to compensate for visual-based dyslexia.

Children with complex support needs

For children with more complex communication, physical, and other support needs (Aitken and Millar 2004) arising from multiple impairments including CVI, discriminating speech sounds from background noise poses a greater challenge (Durkel 2001). Rather than trying to rise to the challenge of diagnostic testing, it helps to behave towards all children with complex communication support needs, including those with CVI, as if they also have APD, unless proved otherwise. The emphasis is not on diagnosis but on determining what might be done differently to make sounds meaningful. This necessitates providing good-quality listening environments so that all sensory input is associated with meaningful activities. Speech used should be simple and direct, using two- or three-word phrases rather than sentences, attaching words that relate to what is happening to the student in the here and now. All sensory input should be connected to meaningful activities (Durkel 2001).

Complex communication support needs

Some would argue that a focus on introducing specific forms of intervention to address sensory modality concerns with children who have complex communication support needs may not be the best strategy for intervening in a child's learning and development. Instead, they argue in favour of a more holistic child-centred and functional approach based around communication.

These two views are present in different approaches recommended to support people who have CRS. Nicholas (2000) argued in favour of a neuropsychological approach based on the suggestion that the rubella virus may cause damage to the reticular system and prefrontal cortex of the brain. Observers of children with CRS often report children to have behavioural manifestations associated with reticular and prefrontal cortex damage – difficulties initiating actions, switching attention between activities, and in planning and controlling behaviour (Schanke 1992, reported in Nicholas 2000).

In contrast, Long and Hart (2009) argue that, irrespective of the area of cortex damaged by the virus, the optimum strategy for educational intervention was through a functional co-creative communication approach (Nafstad and Rødbroe 1999). Long and Hart (2009) showed that by focusing on extending communication opportunities, giving access to a range of motivating activities, and developing mutual trust and respect, many of the behaviours associated with prefrontal damage disappeared or were reduced. Neuropsychology was able to provide potential explanations for behaviour, but a focus on enhancing communication was the route to intervention.

Functional communication: levels of analysis

In what Aitken et al (2001) called a 'new medical model', an approach is taken that integrates both neurobiological explanations and analysis with intervention strategies to use with

254

children who have complex support needs. Drawing on three examples, they showed how the model can assist in improving the child's communication and interaction: an integrated approach to providing wheelchairs and communication aids; designing a suitable physical environment; and choosing a symbol system to support a child's personal communication. We will illustrate the model and its focus on communication using the latter example.

Suppose a child with CVI and hearing impairment benefits from using symbols as part of a visual environment to support personal communication. Which symbols would be optimum – those that are high-contrast black on white, or those that are colour? Visual impairment specialists will often advocate using high-contrast stimuli while speech and language pathologists will often propose using colour symbols. Which one is correct? Aitken et al (2001) looked at this question. They argued that, on the basis of maximizing availability of pre-attentive features in the visual system to enhance figure–ground information (Treisman 1986, 1987, Weissten and Wong 1986, Gouras 1991), the optimum choice would be to choose colour symbols such as picture communication symbols (McNaughton 1993). Using colour in symbols gives access to all eight pre-attentive features of colour, movement, end of line, orientation, and curvature as well as contrast, brightness, and closed areas (Treisman 1986).

The approach benefited from an analysis at several levels from the cell through to classroom and school practice. Understanding each level on its own was insufficient to bring about change. The empirical findings also went on to influence symbol redesign by the major commercial firm producing symbols used by people with a range of communication support needs in the UK (Detheridge and Detheridge 2002).

Focusing on the child's functional communication with an analysis at several levels is relevant, too, to the field of autism. Milne (2010) has suggested that low-level abnormalities in the visual system may explain some of the visual perception problems reported in children with ASD. She found that presentation of simple visual stimuli resulted in abnormal cortical activity, even at the level of the C1 component of visually evoked potentials. A number of authors support her findings on early low-level visual processing, such as figure–ground segregation – essential for face recognition and for perception of symbols (e.g. Saint-Amour 2005). It would be interesting to determine how the findings fit with evidence that many children with ASD are supported in their communication by a visual environment (Abbot 2002) and how that visual environment could be optimized for different forms of CVI.

Conclusion

Much remains to be understood about the effects of CVI in combination with hearing impairment. Detailed observation and reporting will help to reveal which intervention strategies work best in which circumstances and with which children. Interdisciplinary collaboration between ophthalmology, audiology, education, genetics, neurology, speech and language therapy, and others will help to unravel the complexity of the cause and effect and apply testable predictions. Through detailed case-by-case analysis, it will become more possible to attribute cause and association, identifying whether the problem lies in specific language impairment, ADHD, ASD, APD, or other. It is difficult enough to do this with children who do not have a visual impairment. It is all the more difficult where visual impairment is present, especially in the presence of CVI.

Summary

Both auditory input and perception can be deficient in children with CVI. Impaired auditory discrimination, recognition of sound patterns, localization of sounds, listening in noise, and extracting meaning from muffled sound can limit access to information, interfere with social interaction, and diminish academic performance. Such auditory dysfunction diminishes capacity to compensate for visual impairment.

When there is evidence of impaired hearing or auditory processing disorder (APD) in a child with CVI, clear spoken communication while facing the child is recommended to facilitate lip-reading combined with a customized programme of remediation of listening skills and compensatory strategies. Background auditory distraction needs to be kept to a minimum, particularly in children with complex needs.

Clear, slow, well-articulated, and distraction-free communication using simple, consistent vocabulary to enhance the child's experience may be required. This can be enhanced by employing high-contrast, colour-coded picture communication or symbols (matched to the child's measured functional visual acuity) with minimal surrounding visual distraction.

18
SETTING UP INTEGRATED SERVICES FOR CHILDREN WITH CEREBRAL VISUAL IMPAIRMENT

Margot Campbell and Marianna Buultjens

Introduction

The needs and well-being of individual children with cerebral visual impairment (CVI) and their families must be central when setting up services for them. This client group has complex medical, social, and educational needs necessitating the involvement of professionals from many disciplines – each with a different ethos and procedures – who often use professional terminology that is not always mutually intelligible. Under these circumstances coordination and cooperation are essential. Children's Visual Impairment Services Tayside Agencies (CVISTA) is an interagency group of professionals in Tayside, Scotland, working in a coordinated way to provide services for children with visual impairment and their families. This model of integrated services will be used to illustrate principles of good practice which are not necessarily country or system specific but which help to ensure that the services offered are easily accessible and provide for the individual needs of the child and his or her family.

It is generally internationally accepted that a range of professionals, together with parental input, are necessary to provide an accurate and useful assessment of vision in children and to ensure appropriate service delivery. How this is done will vary depending on the type of provision available and those charged with providing it. Kelley et al (1998) differentiate between interdisciplinary, multidisciplinary, and transdisciplinary approaches as follows:

> In the transdisciplinary model, a case manager is designated and carries out a program in consultation with various specialists. In the multidisciplinary team (traditional medical model) representatives of several disciplines interact with an individual and work in parallel, which can isolate the delivery of services. In the interdisciplinary team model, reciprocal interactions between and among disciplines provide independent assessment and direct service with shared planning and team meetings decreasing fragmentation and overlap.

The multidisciplinary approach has been practised for several decades, providing assessment and services/programmes for children with visual impairment and for children with CVI

(Gale and Cronin 1998). CVISTA has elements of all three approaches and has chosen the terms 'integrated services' or 'interagency' to describe its practice.

A questionnaire (Laemers and Walthes 2001) designed to provide both quantitative and qualitative information on services for multiply disabled, blind, and visually impaired children throughout Europe, and which received replies from 27 countries, found that working across the professional disciplines was generally recognized as being essential, but in some countries it was more difficult to achieve than in others because of strong professional boundaries. At an earlier conference held in 1995 in Bad Berleburg, Germany, organizational aspects of effective intervention was one of the topics examined. Presentations on the practical problems, at that time, of building up an early intervention system in Poland (Tomaszewska 1996), problems in the transdisciplinary approach in UK (Gray 1996), and consideration of what is necessary to build up functioning systems on a national level and on the level of individual facilities – drawn from the Swedish experience (Enqvist 1996) – addressed some of the complex issues involved. This led to a number of recommendations (the Dortmund Recommendations 2001). Recommendations 3 and 5 are of particular relevance: 'Vision assessment of both anterior and posterior processes (eye and brain function) should be carried out by an interdisciplinary team. The main focus should be on the visual ability for interaction and for orientation and daily living skills in natural surroundings' and 'With the permission of the parents, the functional diagnosis should be shared among all professionals concerned with the respective child. Medical and early intervention teams should have reciprocal obligation to notify each other about all children they are aware of who have multiple disabilities and visual impairment'.

These and other international studies, as well as those closer to home, have provided valuable insights and contributed to the background knowledge and understanding which have led to the developments described in this chapter.

Why do services need to be integrated?

As earlier chapters in this book confirm, most children with CVI have additional physical or intellectual disability and have complex difficulties. In Scotland, many professionals from both statutory and voluntary agencies provide services to this group of children and their families. There are local variations in exactly which professionals provide which services and which agencies are involved. However, in most areas there are local teams of health professionals who have responsibility for the medical management of children with complex disabilities secondary to neurological problems. These neurodisability teams comprise a paediatrician or neurologist along with physiotherapists, occupational therapists, and speech and language therapists. In addition, there are professionals in education who assess the child's learning needs and who identify the appropriate support in school. There are professionals who provide emotional and practical support to parents. There are those who give advice on financial matters and entitlement to the state benefits system. There are professionals who advise on specialist equipment for home and for school and on adapted housing. There are those who provide respite care. There are organizers of children's clubs and activities and those who facilitate and support access to sport and leisure.

In addition, there is an array of other professionals from health, education, social services, and voluntary agencies who specifically provide services to visually impaired children. These professionals include ophthalmologists, orthoptists, and optometrists providing eye care; specialist teachers for children with visual impairment; and rehabilitation workers who provide orientation and mobility training and teach independence skills. There are social services specifically for the blind, and local and national visual impairment agencies which provide services to visually impaired people of all ages.

Prior to the formation of the CVISTA team in Tayside in 2003, individual professionals providing services to visually impaired children and their families did so mostly independently of other agencies. There was a lack of communication between the professionals, who were not always aware of the services provided by other agencies and who did not fully understand the role of other professionals. There was, at times, overlap and duplication of work carried out, but more often there were gaps and delays in services being provided. In order to access some services, children had to be on the blind or partial sight register. However, many children who were not on the register were known to have a degree of visual impairment requiring additional support which could not be accessed. There were examples of interagency working, but these were informal and there was no agreed interagency referral pathway. The neuro-disability team and other professionals did not know which visual impairment professionals to involve for each individual child. The result was that the visual needs of these children frequently were not clearly identified and appropriate visual strategies and supports were not implemented. Failure to implement appropriate visual strategies and supports compromises the developmental progress of children with CVI, who often have multiple factors affecting their development and learning.

The Visual Impairment Scotland report (2003) suggested that the difficulties experienced in Tayside were reflected across Scotland, and the need for community-based interagency visual impairment teams was identified. The CVISTA team was set up by a community paediatrician in response to the local situation in Tayside and to the recommendations made by Visual Impairment Scotland in its report.

Integration of services

The first step towards the formation of the CVISTA team was to organize a meeting of representatives from the agencies providing services to visually impaired children and their families. In Tayside, this involved representatives from 16 different agencies. The professionals were asked to present clearly to one another the services provided by their agency and how these could be accessed, and also to describe their own roles and work practices relating to children with visual impairment and their families. Prior to this, most of the professionals had not met each other and were unclear about the services provided by others. The meeting led to an enhanced understanding and appreciation of the work carried out by different professionals.

The representatives from the agencies formed the CVISTA team, which identified the aims required to provide an integrated service for each visually impaired child, detailed below:

- achieve his or her developmental potential;
- achieve his or her educational potential;

- make friends and form relationships;
- have access to sporting and leisure activities;
- be able to develop his or her own interests;
- have equal opportunities for education and employment;
- be as independent as possible; and
- be included in society.

The next task entailed the following:

- agreeing interagency referral pathways; and
- compiling and facilitating a coordinated interagency management plan for each child.

The interagency referral pathway for children with cerebral visual impairment

The CVISTA team agreed on a single point of contact for referrals to visual impairment services. Referrals are made jointly to the core coordinating team, comprising the community paediatrician and specialist teacher for children with visual impairment, whose role is to:

- liaise closely with parents;
- organize functional visual assessments;
- involve other visual impairment specialists at the appropriate times for each child;
- instigate and coordinate interagency management plans; and
- liaise and share visual information with other professionals involved.

How is an interagency management plan compiled and implemented for each child?

First, functional vision assessment (FVA) is carried out. Functional vision is the sight available for use in everyday activities. In the CVISTA model this assessment is performed in either the child's school or a health centre near the family home. The members of the FVA team are the community paediatrician and the specialist teacher for children with visual impairment together with an orthoptist and optometrist. The orthoptist measures the visual functions. A hospital optometrist investigates accommodation and refraction and includes low-vision aid assessment and provision of appropriate low-vision aids from nursery stage onwards. Following the assessment, the community paediatrician compiles a report, written in easily understandable language, explaining the child's visual difficulties in the context of his or her medical problems and incorporating information from ophthalmology and paediatric services. This report is shared and discussed with the child's parents.

The second step in the process is to arrange a meeting of all those involved in developing strategies and in providing services to the child. These include representatives from the neurodisability team and other professionals providing services to children with complex disabilities as well as the relevant CVISTA professionals. At this meeting the outcomes of the FVA and any other recent assessments are discussed, further assessments deemed necessary are identified, and strategies for achieving progress for the child are identified.

Format of each interagency management plan

Each plan contains the following:

- a list of agencies and professionals currently involved with the child; and
- a checklist of assessments which may already have been carried out or which may be required. These may include reports on or from ophthalmology, functional vision, low-vision aids, orientation and mobility and independence skills relating to vision, developmental assessment, occupational therapy, physiotherapy, speech and language therapy, school progress, low-vision technology, educational psychology, or social work.

The key issues for each child include the following:

- communication and social skills;
- access to learning/school curriculum;
- orientation and mobility;
- independence;
- leisure and social activities;
- emotional well-being; and
- an action plan with action points and deadlines for individual professionals.

Plan review dates are set, usually every few months, to ensure that the appropriate visual strategies are being implemented and that the child has access to the services required from the visual impairment agencies.

Benefits of integrated services for children with cerebral visual impairment and their families

BENEFITS RESULTING FROM THE INTERAGENCY MANAGEMENT PLANS

The interagency management plan ensures that:

- services are provided according to the child's needs without the requirement for visual impairment registration;
- parents are supported by the core coordinating team and no longer have to find their way through the array of independent agencies;
- gaps in service are identified and rectified, for example a lack of orientation and mobility specialists for children has been addressed;
- measures are in place to assist visually impaired children to develop independence in all areas of daily living – these issues are now also being addressed throughout Scotland;
- provision of low-vision technology to support access to learning has enabled existing expertise and resources to be shared more widely (additional equipment has been obtained with grant funding);
- difficulties in accessing appropriate sport and leisure activities, especially in rural areas, are being addressed;

- management plans are now shared effectively with each child's school and voluntary organizations which provide leisure activities, holidays, and respite care; and
- an information pack for parents describing the services available has been compiled.

BENEFITS FOR SERVICE PROVIDERS

For service providers the integrated approach leads to efficient and effective working practice. Clear interagency referral pathways assist the neurodisability team and associated professionals to manage children with complex disabilities while information from the visual impairment team informs their practice. Joint working widens everyone's knowledge and expertise. For example, joint working by occupational therapists and orientation and mobility specialists leads to implementation of optimal mobility strategies for the child with CVI. Inappropriate referrals are avoided and service provision is optimized. Sharing of information prevents duplication of data collection. Overlap of work by different agencies is avoided. The time saved can be used for liaison, planning, and better service delivery.

Funding

Initial funding for the CVISTA team came from successful bids to the Scottish Executive's 'Changing Children's Services Fund' by the three local authorities in Tayside. This initiative provided short-term funding. The funding was required to set up the functional vision assessment clinic and for the community paediatrician to take on the coordinating role. Other professionals changed their way of working without cost implications. Exit strategies, to ensure that services would be maintained, were required by the local authorities before funding was granted.

Depending on the local situation in any country, extra funding may be required for specific services to meet the needs of visually impaired children. It is essential that all staff involved have adequate time factored into their job plans and that interagency working is prioritized.

In 2006 the Scottish Executive undertook a review of all eyecare services in Scotland. Following the recommendation in this review, start-up funding was made available to health boards to implement these. One of the recommendations was that the principles underlying the CVISTA model of integrated services be applied across Scotland, and this is now being implemented.

Short case study

Lisa is 15 years old and has cerebral palsy and associated intellectual disability. Lisa's visual impairment is caused by a combination of CVI and retinopathy of prematurity. She also has a myopic refractive error for which she wears glasses. Lisa attends a special school for children with intellectual disability. There are many professionals involved with Lisa and, because the process of post-school planning has begun, the professionals from adult services will also become involved.

The functional vision assessment provided information for Lisa's current social, learning, and leisure needs (Fig. 18.1). Although Lisa is visually aware of people at a distance of 4 metres, she does not recognize them by sight until they are as close as 2 metres, and for her

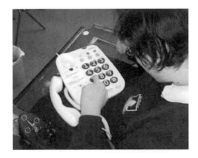

Fig. 18.1 Information on Lisa's functional vision has led to the provision of a telephone with large, high-contrast numbers that she is able to see.

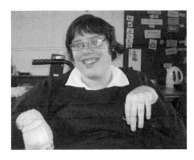

Fig. 18.2 The interagency management plan has emotional well-being of the child or young person as its ultimate aim.

to make out facial expressions they must be within 1 metre. This has implications for social interaction, and those working with Lisa on social skills now take this into account. Lisa has reduced visual acuity and contrast sensitivity and also has difficulty seeing objects against a complex or busy background. This information helped her teacher to provide reading material in the correct size and contrast and to make sure that objects were presented on her table at the correct distance and against an uncluttered background. In addition, Lisa has been provided with a video magnifier with a distance facility, which enables her to see the teacher's face, or an object, or the whiteboard. It means she is not distracted by other objects in the classroom, and can also make out the teacher's facial expressions. This visual information has also been essential for developing strategies for independence. Lisa is now, for example, learning to use the telephone (Fig. 18.1).

Lisa's visual field is not restricted and this helps with moving independently in her power wheelchair, although her depth perception problems mean that she has some difficulty knowing whether the level of the surface has changed when floor or ground surfaces change. Lisa already knows routes within the school building, and recently an independent living skills specialist from adult services has been working along with her occupational therapist in extending her use of the power wheelchair to outside the school.

Information on Lisa's visual functioning strategies is being shared with professionals and volunteers who help her to enjoy sports and leisure activities after school to ensure that she makes the most of these opportunities. Lisa carries a 'personal passport' incorporating this information so that she can easily inform people she meets of her visual abilities. By ensuring that all professionals working with Lisa have the appropriate information regarding her vision, and the strategies she uses to overcome her visual difficulties, Lisa's confidence has increased in social situations and she is better able to express her feelings and make choices. She has been helped to have appropriate independence and to join in peer group activities. All of these things contribute to achieving happiness and fulfilment in life (Fig. 18.2).

Conclusion

We believe that the principles underlying the CVISTA model described in this chapter could be transferred to other climes and cultures, provided that they can be embedded within a suitably funded structure. This ensures that the integration of services does not rely solely on the good will and enthusiasm of individual parents or professionals, but will continue to function even with a change of personnel. This continuity is essential when dealing with the lives of growing children and their families.

19

CLASSIFICATION OF VISUAL FUNCTIONING AND DISABILITY IN CHILDREN WITH VISUAL PROCESSING DISORDERS

Lea Hyvärinen

Introduction

The interpretation of visual functioning and disability in children with visual processing disorders is the subject of considerable debate. At one end of the spectrum, only children with decreased visual acuity are considered to have visual impairment and disability (International Classification of Diseases [ICD] criteria of visual impairment). At the other end, all visual functions, their strengths, deviations from the norm, and overall visual functioning are considered.

The new International Classification of Functioning (ICF; WHO 2001) should influence assessment and classification of the different forms of visual processing disorders in children. The International Classification of Functioning, Disability and Health, Children & Youth Version (ICF-CY; WHO 2007) stresses the assessment of visual functioning rather than the measurement of a few visual functions such as visual acuity and visual field, which are used for surveys of visual impairment but are insufficient for the type of assessment required to guide rehabilitation and education (McAnaney 2010). The goal of the ICF and the ICF-CY is to develop uniform concepts and terminology in health, education, and related services nationally and internationally, in order to improve interdisciplinary coordination in provision of services and documentation.

The ICF provides a classification for the purposes of early intervention, rehabilitation, education, and social service provision and suggests that each specialty should make *adaptations to the basic text*. So far, the classification of children with disability due to impaired visual processing, also called cerebral visual impairment (CVI), has not been discussed with the goals of the ICF as these relate to early intervention and education of children with impaired vision with or without other disabilities. *Participation in activities* and the *optimization of environmental factors* also need to be described as they are seen in the specialty of ophthalmology in the context of early intervention and education of children with visual impairment.

Visual processing problems are common in children with motor disabilities (especially cerebral palsy), in children with intellectual disabilities, and in children with impaired hearing or deafness. The classification of the functioning of these children is often based upon the more obvious functional problem despite the fact that their impaired vision might be the most restricting factor in the participation of many activities. This chapter is written to provide an overview of the key issues concerning visual impairment due to damage to the brain, with or without other disabilities, as a step towards the development of an international classification.

Aspects to be covered in the classification
The following issues warrant consideration in the design of a classification of visual functioning of children with brain damage-related visual disability. The classification should provide the facility to do the following:

- cover all types of vision loss;
- consider other losses of functioning;
- include objective quantitative categories; and
- include the very young, as damage is often present at birth or soon after, necessitating early intervention.

Types of Functioning Related to Vision and Affected by Vision Loss
Normally sighted children are able to see detail, and have a wide field of vision with refractive correction if required. Their working distances are comfortable in ergonomically designed activities.

Children with impaired but useful vision compensate for their decreased visual acuity and contrast sensitivity by bringing objects, texts, and pictures closer (geometric magnification) and/or by magnifying the image with optical or electro-optical devices.

Those with a narrow field of vision scan the environment (as when using long cane techniques) and luminance levels are adapted according to need. Text is printed with enlarged bold font and increased spacing when needed, and pictures are redrawn with better contrast and less detail. Orientation, localization, and mobility techniques are evaluated and compensatory strategies are taught. Communication distances at which facial expression can be seen are determined and employed. Communication is a major problem in children with impaired vision, particularly in toddlers and teenagers who depend on body language more than children in other age groups.

Blind children require strategies based on the use of the other senses, especially hearing, smell, taste, tactile, and haptic information, but also by using memory and reasoning. Children with very poor vision may inappropriately be encouraged to rely on their limited vision and not, for example, to use long cane techniques and learn the orientation methods for blind people. Such children need to employ all available techniques and strategies in order to become independent young adults (in some cultures independence is valued less than in others, particularly for girls, and this issue must be recognized).

Visual functioning of children with impaired vision due to brain damage shows variation between techniques that differ from the variation of the same techniques used by children who have poor quality of the incoming visual information but normal processing of the degraded image.

Infants and children are highly dependent on the opinions and attitudes of their family and school; thus, *participation* and *the effect of environment* should also be covered in the evaluation.

Evaluation of the degree of visual disability tends to be founded upon those visual functions that can be routinely measured and observed. For this reason, children with visual processing disorders and normal visual acuities and visual fields do not receive the help they require because many countries rely upon the ICD criteria of visual acuity and visual field to allocate resources, and the ICF criteria are not applied. With the present book, we might initiate a discussion that leads to a more holistic evaluation of visual functioning.

DOMAINS USED IN THE ASSESSMENT
The ICF and the ICF-CY describe nine functional domains to be considered in assessment:

- learning and applying knowledge;
- general tasks and demands;
- communication;
- mobility;
- self-care;
- domestic life;
- interpersonal interactions and relationships;
- major life areas; and
- community, social, and civic life.

The World Health Organization (WHO) document 'Management of low vision in children', which has been used since 1993 in the assessment of educational needs of visually impaired children, recommends a simpler version of assessment of functioning in four main areas:

- communication;
- orientation and moving;
- activities of daily life; and
- sustained vision tasks.

These four functional areas exist in all cultures, independent of economic or social status, and at all ages, and therefore serve well as the *core functional areas* to be assessed. In each of the four main areas of functioning a child's techniques and strategies need to be observed and assessed. In each area children may also have specific problems caused by impaired processing of visual information. Based on the assessment, *a child's ability to participate like his or her peers* should also be described. In the assessment of infants and toddlers, the ICF-CY list of domains is not appropriate and needs to be restricted to the core functions as defined by the WHO.

Loss of a single or a few visual processing functions, without any other changes in vision, exists in children, although it is rare. Nearly all children with problems in processing of visual information have some changes in the image quality or oculomotor functions. Therefore, the assessment should cover these three aspects of vision:

- quality of visual information used by the child for processing;
- quality of the processing of visual information; and
- quality of the oculomotor functions.

INCLUSION/EXCLUSION – USE OF TERMS
'Visual functioning' covers all visual functions, sensory functions in all parts of the visual system, and oculomotor functions. ICF does not mention motion perception and processing of visual information in the chapter 'Seeing'. These functions are integral parts of visual functioning and are included in this discussion.

'Visual disability' is present if loss or impairment of visual function(s) negatively affects any of the functional domains. Disability may be mild, moderate, severe, profound, or total. If a person has developed *compensatory functions,* these need to be considered in the assessment of functioning. Since visual disability in children is often complicated by comorbidity, the *effect of other disabilities* needs to be considered if they restrict the use of vision.

The term 'seeing' is not used in this text. Instead, the term 'vision' is used throughout, because it is the term used in clinical medicine and in basic research. The old expressions of 'eyesight' and 'ocular visual impairment' are not used. Vision is a brain function. Lesions affecting vision can be in the eyes or any part of the visual pathways and networks. The location is not the deciding factor; rather, it is how a lesion affects the quality of the inflowing visual information or its processing.

Types of visual disability in children with visual processing problems
Changes in visual sensory functions can occur in three main parts of the visual system:

- in the peripheral parts of the visual system – eyes and optic pathways;
- in the processing of visual information in the primary visual cortex, visual area 1 (V1), and other visual cortices which process and combine the parts of the incoming information so that it is perceived as an image;
- in the use of the image for recognition functions in the ventral stream and as 'vision for action' in the dorsal stream; and
- in the processing of other areas related particularly to emotions.

Changes in the quality of the oculomotor functions may alter or prevent the use of vision and should therefore be considered in the assessment and classification.

The quality of visual information transferred from the eyes to the primary visual cortex is usually described based on measurements of the size of the visual field, the scotomas in the visual field affecting visual acuity, contrast sensitivity, colour vision, motion perception, and visual adaptation to changes in luminance level. These measurements do not directly reflect the quality of the information in the pathways, but, rather, reflect the quality of the image formed after processing the information in the visual cortices.

During the transfer of visual information from the retina towards the primary visual cortex, most of the information is normally inhibited from entering the brain. In the lateral geniculate nucleus (LGN), 80–90% of synapses convey non-retinal inputs that modify the information (Sherman and Koch 1986). The most obvious difference between the retinal and LGN discharges is the significantly lower firing rate of the LGN neurons. On average, for every 10 retinal spikes, approximately only four LGN spikes are relayed to the cortex. The massive non-retinal inputs from the visual cortex and from the brainstem all suggest that the LGN could significantly modify the flow of visual signals from the retina to the visual cortex and serve as a gate, a filter, or both (Kaplan et al 1993). Therefore, changes in the *inhibitory functions* also need to be considered, especially in the assessment of children with severe or profound brain damage. If the inhibitory functions have not developed, visual information enters the brain as chaotic waves and children may keep their eyes shut except in dim light with very limited structures at which to look.

Oculomotor functions may be abnormal because of peripheral lesions or changes in the brain functions, or a combination of both types of lesion (e.g. in a child with traumatic changes in the extraocular muscles and brain). Insufficient, irregular, or spastic accommodation, unstable fixation, and irregular saccades are common and can cause severe problems. Nystagmus is less often a serious problem in visual tasks, although it may cause problems in interaction and social contacts, as does strabismus in some cases.

QUALITY OF VISUAL INFORMATION ENTERING THE BRAIN
The effect of ocular abnormalities on the quality of the visual information available for processing should be carefully evaluated before assessing the processing of visual information.

The effect of changes in the eyes and visual pathways on the quality of visual functioning is smaller than usually depicted. Rather severe losses of visual acuity, contrast sensitivity, and colour vision do not seem to affect normal processing of the visual information. Increasing size, contrast, and selecting colours that decrease confusion can partially or fully compensate for losses in these three functions.

Decrease in the size of the visual field affects functioning in communication and in moving. Visual field expanders do not function except in certain situations. Thus, techniques typically adopted by blind people are used by persons with greatly limited visual fields.

Decrease in visual information related to movement and motion perception occurs rarely in the peripheral visual system, but it is possible in diffuse retinal degenerations.

Decrease in visual adaptation to changes in luminance is often one of the most disabling factors, but its effect can be prevented by filter lenses and by planning the luminance level of the environment. The effect of luminance level on functioning needs to be assessed in standard illumination, in bright daylight, and at a low mesopic luminance level with and without optical devices.

As the visual information transferred through the optic pathways may have normal structure or may have distortions when entering the coding and processing in the cortical functions, the changes of the image quality should be compensated by increasing size or contrast, or changing colours of the test materials during assessment of the quality of processing in the ventral and dorsal stream functions.

Visual information related to motion and low contrast form is dominant in the tectal pathway and can thus be transferred to brain functions faster than through the route of the primary visual cortex. The tectal pathway is often forgotten in clinical assessment and even in some textbooks of neurology, but it is the pathway of information for fast reactions to something new in the visual field, and is thus crucial for avoidance of accidents.

Although we use clinical tests to assess vision, it should be understood that each measurement depicts also the quality of the higher processing functions. When we measure visual acuity, we measure a recognition function of abstract forms (Roman letters, numbers, other characters) or recognition of pictures of concrete objects, as in the paediatric visual acuity tests. Some clinical measurements, especially the current visual field measurements, may give misleading information of the functional quality of visual field because motion perception within scotomatous areas tends not to be assessed.

VISUAL ACUITY

Visual acuity should be measured using line tests with *logarithmic design* (WHO 2003). Young children and children with developmental delay may not be able to be tested with visual acuity charts. In these cases, visual acuity is measured with single symbol tests, knowing that the results may overestimate visual acuity. Children with problems in reading should be tested with tightly grouped line tests to reveal increased crowding phenomenon, and with texts of varying size and spacing to detect small scotomas, which may make one or two letters disappear. During the measurement of visual acuity, *increased crowding causing reduced acuity* is often the first sign of problems in processing visual information.

The visual acuity values of children with brain damage may not depict the need of magnification of texts. A child may have normal visual acuity (1.0 decimal [0.1 log MAR 6/6, 20/20]) or better, and yet prefer reading with a CCTV using 3cm-high letters when reading books. It is not understood why there is such an unusual need of magnification, especially if the child can read usual print size (12–14 point) for a short time. However, there must be an aspect of vision that we cannot yet measure if a child chooses to read books with a CCTV and has a better reading speed and a longer reading time than when reading without a CCTV.

Visual acuity tests shall use the *same optotypes in the distance and near vision tests* (WHO 2003). During testing, pointing at the optotype to be read is not allowed in the basic measurement (if the tester wants to learn how much pointing improves visual acuity, a second measurement with pointing is performed) and luminance on the surface of the tests should be between 80 and 160cd/m^2 (WHO/PBL/03.91). Such a high luminance level is difficult to arrange for vertical charts. Therefore, distance tests should preferably employ light boxes with adequate illumination. If visual acuity is best at mesopic luminance levels (in dim light), visual acuity should be measured at that level or using specific filter lenses that decrease photophobia.

Grating acuity tests as detection tests are used in examination of visual acuity of infants and children at early levels of development. Grating acuity tests (1) allow interpolation of visual information from a much larger area than optotype tests and (2) do not depict recognition function like the optotype tests but depict *detection of difference between the two surfaces presented simultaneously*. Therefore, the results shall be expressed as cycles per degree (cpd) *not* as optotype acuity values, which might be greatly misleading. The difference in optotype and detection grating acuity values, when both values can be measured, can be up to 20- to 30-fold.

Grating acuity as a discrimination test is advisable whenever there is discrepancy between optotype acuity values and the performance of the child, especially in children with difficulties in mathematics and/or in perception of geometric forms. Grating acuity values are usually higher than optotype acuity values, but they can also be lower if the island of vision used to see the optotype test is very small and is surrounded by a large central scotoma. Children can also have a *specific loss of perception of gratings* owing to the coding problems of the grating.

CONTRAST SENSITIVITY

Low contrast visual information is important in perception of many features in the environment (corners of rooms and the line between wall and ceiling being the most common low contrast line information) and in communication situations because facial expressions are conveyed by fast-moving faint shadows, especially on pale Nordic faces and on very dark faces.

Contrast sensitivity can be measured based on low contrast visual acuity tests or using grating tests at low contrast levels. Contrast sensitivity is depicted by a curve, and thus at least two additional points on the curve need to be measured after the visual acuity value as optotype or grating acuity value, the end of the curve at the *x*-axis, has been measured. In clinical work the measurement of optotype acuity at 2.5% contrast gives the upper end of the slope of the contrast sensitivity curve in most cases. If the child cannot perceive optotypes at the 2.5% level, even if the test is employed for near vision, measurement at higher contrast levels is needed. Limiting the lowest level of measurement to a 10% contrast level does not depict functioning at low contrast.

The contrast sensitivity curve based on measurement of visual acuity at low contrast levels is often different from the curve based on measurements of grating acuity at the same contrast levels. It should be noticed that *the form of the contrast sensitivity curve is a function of the size of the grating stimulus used*. In assessment of normal vision, a grating with five cycles of lines is a standard. In the assessment of central visual field of a child who may have patchy loss of visual field, measurement with a grating with 10 cycles of lines is needed. The differences between the contrast sensitivity curves measured with stimuli of different size depict the irregular losses of information in the central visual field (Hyvärinen 1981, 1983).

In a normal visual system, the slope of the contrast sensitivity curve is in the same location independent of the size of the grating stimulus between diameters 2.5 and 40 degrees. Central scotoma decreases the area of a grating as a stimulus and thus it is possible that the maximum value of contrast sensitivity is normal when a large stimulus (10–20 degrees in diameter) is

271

used but very low when a small grating stimulus (2.5–5 degrees in diameter) is used. The differences between the contrast sensitivity curves measured with stimuli of different size depict the irregular losses of information in the central visual field (Hyvärinen 1981, 1983, 2010). Clinical measurements of contrast sensitivity are often done with small grating targets without acknowledging these basic rules, and thus the reported values are misleadingly low.

COLOUR VISION

Quantitative colour vision measurement gives additional insight into the quality of vision if testing is done with large and standard-sized caps. Colour vision seems to be the most robust visual function in many children with CVI.

VISUAL ADAPTATION

Adaptation to intermediate and high mesopic luminance levels is needed in many daily activities. Therefore, measurement of the speed of cone adaptation should be included in the examination of all children with diffuse retinal disorders even if there are no observations of vision difficulties at low luminance levels. The child may avoid places with low luminance levels.

MOTION PERCEPTION

Encoding of motion-related visual information might be disturbed in the retina in diffuse retinal disorders, or its transfer may be insufficient owing to lesions in the magnocellular pathway. Pathology affecting cortical motion processing can affect the ability to see movement or to interpret its nature. On the other hand, since motion-related information can enter into the cortical functions via the tectal pathway, lesions in the optic radiation may cause absolute visual field defects, or quadrant or hemianopic losses in the Goldmann or automated perimetry, although there is perception of motion within these 'absolute' scotomas. The absolute visual field defects may not be functionally absolute; children may have useful motion information for moving and adults may be able to function in traffic.

INHIBITORY FUNCTIONS

Ongoing processing in the visual cortices and in the brainstem affects the incoming visual information, creating a filter that allows only 10–20% of the information to pass to the primary visual cortex. Inhibitory functions seem to be ineffective in children with severe brain damage. Without effective filtering, visual information is chaotic.

Quality of coding and processing of visual information in the visual cortices

When entering the primary visual cortex, the three basic components of visual information – form (contrast edges, lines), colour, and motion – are coded, and, in children who have binocular vision, information coming from the eyes is fused so that a single binocular image can be formed during further processing.

Testing of changes in the processing of visual information is a traditional part of neuropsychology. However, in neuropsychology the tests are designed with the assumption that (1) there is sufficient quality of the incoming information, (2) its encoding in the primary visual cortex is normal, and (3) the person has had normal visual experiences before the loss of vision. In visually impaired infants and children, none of these three prerequisites is usually present. Visual information may be irregular because of changes in the eyes and/or pathways. Inexact encoding of direction and length of lines, colours, and movement in the primary visual cortex is common. Most of these children have not had normal visual experiences that they can remember, although these may have been very helpful during a limited time in their early development.Tests used in neuropsychology should be specially redesigned for testing children with changes in the quality of incoming information and/or processing in the visual cortices if the quality of the child's visual information cannot be sufficiently improved with optical or electro-optical devices.

The structure of the image may be disturbed at the level of the primary visual cortex if coding of any of the basic components is irregular. *Unsteadiness of orientation of lines* seems to be more common than irregularities in perception of *length of lines*.

As stated in the section 'Visual acuity', children with CVI can have a *specific impairment of perception of gratings.* Some children do not perceive gratings at all but describe the grating as a surface with one colour – black or white. Some children perceive the grating pattern in a small area of the test surface, the rest of the test being irregularly patterned. Some other children are unable to define the orientation of the lines because the lines seem to move, probably due to irregularities in the coding of grating patterns. Some children, and also adults, immediately turn their gaze from the grating and refuse to look at it, stating that it is unpleasant, and it may even cause nausea. It is fortunate that regular grating patterns are rare in our environments, except in paintings and graphics, and sometimes in school materials, in which case they may disturb writing and calculations.

Quality of processing in the ventral and dorsal stream
Table 19.1 is a list that many teachers and therapists use as the minimum observations for understanding a child's functioning and for planning an individual educational plan (IEP). Families, therapists, and teachers make most of the observations. The functional diagnosis requires optimal inter- or transdisciplinary work.

This list does not cover all cognitive visual functions, and has been compiled on the basis of children's functioning at school. The functions are not strictly separated as functions in the ventral or dorsal stream because such description of functions omits simultaneous visual functions in numerous other parts of the brain, especially connections to the amygdala and other centres serving emotions, immediate reactions, and different types of memory, as well as information through the powerful tectal pathway for the vision in action. In children with CVI there can also be unusual combinations of the functions in the ventral and dorsal stream. For example, recognition functions may use illusory movements of fingers to perceive the form that the child does not recognize purely visually. The child imagines following the lines of an object or picture with his or her fingers, although the hand does not move. The eyes might move and thus some information may also be collected from the eye movements. Other children may have developed use of routes so effectively that they seem to have map-based orientation in space in well-known environments.

TABLE 19.1
List of the common vision-related functions to be assessed

Recognition and reading	Perception of space
Concrete objects	Perception of one's body in space
Landmarks	Depth perception
Faces (familiar and unfamiliar)	Perception of near space and far space
Facial expressions, body language	Simultanagnosia
Pictures of concrete objects	
Geometric forms	**Perception of textures and surface qualities**
Letters	Orientation in space
Numbers	Memorizing routes
Words	Vision in traffic situations and playgrounds
Crowding effect	
Reading speed	**Eye–hand coordination**
Scanning lines of text	Grasping and throwing objects
Efficiency of reading	Drawing, free hand
	Copying, from near/from blackboard
Perception of pictures	Copying, motor planning and execution
Length of lines	
Orientation of lines	**Integration problems**
Details of pictures	Vision not used when listening or exploring
Figure–ground	Vision not used when moving
Visual closure	Balance and vision
Noticing errors	
Noticing missing details	**Compensatory strategies**
Comparison with pictures in memory	Auditory information
'Reading' series of pictures	Tactile, kinaesthetic, and haptic information
Visual problems in copying pictures	Memory, reasoning
Geometric pictures depicting three-dimensional forms	
	Disturbing factors
Mathematics	Environmental noise, visual and auditory
Calculations, logical reasoning	Balance problems and motor problems
	Medications, epilepsy

When we know an older child well, we can usually say with certainty whether the child has problems in one or several of the processing functions. Young children need to be observed for years, and even schoolchildren for 2–3 years, before we have observed them enough in varying situations and activities. This list is helpful in reminding us to observe all visual functions that should develop by a certain age.

In all recognition functions the child must have seen the object, picture, or person previously and must have been able to create a template in memory, keep it there, find it during the task, match, and then *re*-cognize. Each function of a child or infant is recorded as:

- age appropriate;
- slightly delayed or weak;
- emerging; and
- present rarely in some situations, which are described carefully so that the finding can be used in further training.

Careful observation, recording, and analysis by the vision team leads to a slow increase in the understanding of the child's functioning. Observations are collected from each person who is in contact with the child.

Many, if not most, of the clinical test situations also measure prior experiences of the child. If an activity or space is familiar, even a rather poor quality of visual information is sufficient to complete a task. If a child has never been exposed to a task (e.g. drawing or copying), concept, or image, he or she may not use the information of the test like a child with normal visual development and may not function at a level typical of him or her. This is a common problem in several neuropsychological tests.

Variation of visual functioning is a typical feature of functioning in children with problems in processing of visual information and is in part related to unusual earlier experiences, but variation in brain functions themselves is likely to be the main cause of variation. Use of compensatory information may further confuse an observer to report unusually good visual performance in a task in which the child used other modalities and memory to solve and/or perform the task.

The list of functions to be observed and assessed when examining infants and children with CVI becomes much longer than we are accustomed to when examining children with poor image quality but with normal processing of the image. Many ophthalmologists oppose assessment of processing problems, claiming that they cannot perform such a time-consuming evaluation and that it belongs to paediatric neurologists. Nor can neurologists observe the child in everyday activities and tasks. As we are assessing vision for early intervention and education, it is natural to employ the expertise of therapists, teachers, instructors, psychologists, and neuropsychologists – people who work closely with these functional areas – together with parents to collect the requisite information as a transdisciplinary team.[1] Classification should not be based on ophthalmological examination only, during which the impairments' effects on activities and participation cannot be evaluated.

---

[1] 'Transdisciplinary' means that not only do the team members share their findings but they are also trained to use all basic tests when a child is in the mood for being tested.

Quality of oculomotor functions

Children with severe motor problems are a large group among children with problems in processing of visual information. Among them, oculomotor functions are rarely quite normal. Difficulties in fixation, and planning and execution of saccades and smooth pursuit movements should be carefully observed during clinical examinations and especially during reading and other demanding near-vision tasks. With the use of small digital video cameras, the recording of eye movements during reading and during scanning of pictures has become a useful tool in special education and could be used also as a part of clinical examination.

Other common problems in cerebral visual impairment

Visual functioning is affected if a child has difficulties in other brain functions such as visual memory, attention, or control of head or trunk. The majority of children with brain damage-related vision loss also have numerous other functional problems, which must be considered in both the assessment and the classification.

PROBLEMS IN COMBINING SEVERAL FUNCTIONS

The most common problem is *inability to share attention among several functions*. In communication situations, or while talking or signing, some children are unable to visually observe their counterpart. Some children are functionally deaf when watching a person or exploring something with their hands. These problems in dividing attention are common and not always understood. A child with these problems in communication may be diagnosed as having concentration difficulties or having autistic features, although the problem really is in the limited total capacity and difficulties in using several brain functions simultaneously.

Some children cannot use vision while moving. Moving may be such a demanding function that there is no capacity available to process visual information. They look, move, stop, look, and move. Some children report that the environment 'disappears' when they move. Many children realize first at school age that their strategy in moving is different from that of their peers.

Children with cerebral palsy may require so much of their attentional functions to sit straight that looking carefully at something on the blackboard or on the desk leads to loss of head control and, often, trunk control, so that the child sits tilted with the head hanging or lies flat on the desk unable to continue working. The visual ergonomics of children with cerebral palsy and other motor problems should be investigated in detail, considering the question of whether sitting is the best posture at school.

Problems in *shifting or directing attention* to a part of a complex scene are common in children with closely symmetrical lesions in the posterior parietal lobes. However, difficulties in directing attention nearly disappear in many cases when the child or adult is looking at natural scenes. As one such child said spontaneously, 'Here outside I see everything because I do not need to look'.

HYPERSENSITIVITY

Hypersensitivity shows wide variation. Tactile hypersensitivity of the mouth prevents infants and children from exploring objects by mouth. They grow without the normal exploratory confirmation by tactile and haptic information, and thus visual information remains more abstract than in the experiences of infants and children in general. They do not learn to know their hands by mouthing, and thus the hands also convey less information than in healthy infants and children. This decreases the possibilities to improve the often seriously limited abstract space of many children with motor problems and visual processing disorders.

Hypersensitivity to visual information, or visual noise, limits the educational and play situations of many children. The amount of visual noise in the periphery of the visual field can be diminished by side shields in spectacles. Noise in the central visual field is effectively decreased when teaching materials are adapted and play areas and classrooms are cleaned of all unnecessary materials. Some children with central scotoma have photophobia owing to abnormal cone–rod interaction and benefit from filter lenses that do not transmit in the blue–green part of the spectrum.

Hypersensitivity to auditory information should also be considered in both early intervention and schools. Some children may need protective ear plugs combined with a transmission system to be able to concentrate on listening to the teacher.

EFFECT OF AUDITORY AND BALANCE PROBLEMS

Children with brain damage may have loss of hearing and/or problems in processing of auditory information. Since auditory information is the most important compensating function, even slight changes in hearing may affect the functioning of a child. One feature that often is not understood by audiologists is lack of hearing in one ear, which leads to difficulties in spatial orientation.

Visual information is important in normal balance functions. Some children have changes in their inner ear and/or central pathways for balance functions combined with poor awareness of their body in space, which may lead to great difficulties in independent movement.

EFFECT OF MEDICATION, EPILEPSY, OTHER DISORDERS, AND ENVIRONMENT

One of the important weaknesses of clinical examinations is related to variation in the functioning of children with brain damage. The heading of this section mentions some of the causes of variation. The medical causes should be recorded in the documents given to parents for the school.

Epilepsy is sometimes difficult to diagnose if it is confined to visual areas causing short losses of vision and hallucinations, possibly because the electroencephalogram (EEG) often does not show any abnormal activity if the focus is in the depth of the calcarine sulcus. If epilepsy medication, used ex juvantibus, removes the symptoms, which then return if the medicine is not taken, the diagnosis is confirmed.

Environmental causes of malfunctioning are seldom apparent during clinical examination. When related to the acceptance of the child's condition, or atmosphere at day care or at school, these can play a very important role. A child may be tired, anxious, or angry without it showing, or the child may not be in the mood to perform close to threshold, which is required for clinical testing. On the other hand, a child may experience careful testing as being so positive that he or she functions at a higher level than at school. Therefore, *it is important that all basic tests are repeated in a daycare centre or at school,* both in one-to-one situations and in a group of children.

Assessment and classification of infants and toddlers
Most problems in visual processing are due to brain damage or abnormal brain structures present at birth or soon thereafter. Early diagnosis and intervention are important, and therefore the early signs should become part of the training of all doctors and personnel. These signs include the following:

- oculomotor problems, especially convergence insufficiency and exotropia;
- poor accommodation (especially in hypotonic children with motor problems or Down syndrome) with problems in visual communication and interaction;
- looking past the face of the adult (tester or parent, 'poor eye contact') owing to eccentric fixation because of central scotoma;
- delay in recognizing family members before they say something;
- difficulties in communication with other toddlers (owing to loss or difficulties in recognition of faces, facial expressions, body language) and clinging to adults;
- panic reactions to animals (dogs) and fast-moving objects;
- problems in using toys if they are cluttered or on a patterned background; and
- delays in dressing; not knowing which way clothes should be put on.

Based on the clinical measurements and observations on the infant's/toddler's functioning, it is possible to assess visual functioning in the four main domains – communication/interaction, orientation and moving, daily activities, and use of vision in demanding near vision tasks – as well as compensatory strategies.

Summarizing the findings for clinical classification of visual functioning
After assessment of the quality of visual information, of its processing and of oculomotor functions, and after considering the effect of non-visual functions, it is usually possible to understand the strategies used in each of the cognitive visual functions in the four main functional areas.

Often there is also variation in the use of techniques and strategies depending on illumination or structure of the visual information. If we use a graphic presentation, as in Table 19.2, variation in functioning is clearly depicted.

Although we describe the functional losses and techniques/strategies used, and thus the needs for (re)habilitation and special education, it may not be enough for administrators and lawyers. They may want to have numbers in the classification. Because we have three different techniques that can be used, and four different main functional areas, we can depict the functional situation with one number by giving points to the three different techniques. It is

TABLE 19.2

Variation of strategies used in the four main functional areas

This child uses...			
	Blind techniques	**Low-vision techniques**	**Sighted techniques**
in communication	←		→
in orientation and mobility		←	→
in activities of daily living		←	→
in sustained near-vision tasks	←		→

A child with loss of several recognition functions and problems in awareness of space and spatial orientation may show great variations in behaviours. The child may function like a blind child in communication situations without eye contact and with poor emotional responses to facial expressions of the other people (because the expressions are not perceived), yet he or she may be aware of some communicative visual information such as gestures. Orientation in space may be very poor and mostly based on remembering routes, street signs, and landmarks in a certain order. People find it confusing that the child uses a cane to acquire information about the surface qualities but folds the cane and runs like a sighted child in a known environment. We are accustomed to see the white cane in the hand of a blind or nearly blind person, not in the hand of a child who seems to be able to run unhindered when using visual information. In activities of daily living the child may have problems in noticing objects on a patterned background but may notice even the smallest crumbs (these are two different visual tasks). Many children have so severely disturbed oculomotor functions that in sustained near-vision tasks they prefer Braille although their visual acuity may be normal. The table shows the large variation in visual functioning, which is the most typical feature in the functioning of children with vision loss caused by brain damage.

TABLE 19.3
Crude categories for reporting and statistics

Number of points	Category
12	Functional blindness
11–10	Severe vision impairment
9–8	Moderate vision impairment
7–6	Mild vision impairment
5	Near-normal visual functioning
4	Normal sighted functions

possible to give one point to blind techniques, two points to low-vision techniques, and three points to sighted techniques (Hyvärinen 2000). Special teachers prefer giving three points to blind techniques, two points to low-vision techniques, and one point to techniques typical of normal sight to depict the need for services. The variation is in both evaluations between 12 and 4 points.

By combining the numerical classification and the description of variation of functioning (Table 19.2), we are able to give clear information about the type and degree of disability so that the need for medical and supportive services and the structure of special education can be discussed with persons who do not have schooling in these questions. The information that has been collected for assessment and classification of functioning can also be used for statistical purposes.

The condensed information in the rough summary for clinical and statistical purposes is not enough for planning of early intervention or special education. As stated in the ICF-CY, visual functions need to be measured and observed by both medical and educational personnel and each child's family members. Functioning in each of the four main areas needs to be discussed frequently during the first year of life because of the rapid development of the infant. Later assessments, and planning of services and of education, are arranged to fit the needs of each child and family, and the daycare and educational personnel. In teenagers, the demands on visual functioning increase, especially in reading and mathematics. Only experienced special needs teachers working together with a neuropsychologist, both knowing the student's visual strengths and problems, can analyse whether an error in a mathematical task is due to a visual memory problem or a spacial attentional problem, or if it is related to error in mathematical reasoning.

A child's visual functioning can be described in the four main functional areas as, for example, in the following short summary of visual functioning of a student with a rather typical loss of visual function in both anterior and posterior parts of the visual system and mild multidisability. (This is the introductory first page of his IEP.)

Communication is restricted by low contrast sensitivity, which means that the student does not see facial expressions beyond 1m, and thus everybody should remember to come close; poor motion perception prevents perception of lip movements, the student perceives the lower part of the face as unpleasantly blurred and therefore looks past the person talking to him, which is *not* an autistic behaviour; his poor accommodation makes fixation inaccurate so he seems to look through persons, which is *not* an autistic behaviour. Compensation with hearing is good except for high-pitch tones, which makes perception of some letters difficult. Good articulation and a calm pace of talking benefit this student and all other children in the classroom.

Orientation in space is close to normal in known places, and the student has learned to use the usual routes well. He follows other children, and if he loses them he gets lost and looks distressed. Training of recognition of landmarks and their internal relationships continues, as well as the use of maps. A parent or the classroom assistant trains daily the route from home to school. A path cane is used to compensate for the lack of perception of surface qualities. In ball games, participation is replaced with functioning as the teacher's assistant, or the student works in the classroom with the classroom assistant. A part of sport at school is changed to swimming in a group of boys with a trainer and with body-building exercises and swimming with his father (1–2km a week).

Activities of daily life are close to age level. Getting dressed at the same speed as the other children requires some training. Food on the left side of the plate is not noticed. Therefore, he should learn to turn the plate as a routine function when the right side is empty (neglect, not a visual field defect). This difficulty is more pronounced if he is tired or needs to hurry, so he should come to lunch among the first children. Finding and recognizing books and putting things in order in the drawer of the desk and his schoolbag requires training. The book covers are all too alike, so books need to be covered with single-colour covers, each book with a different colour.

Sustained, demanding visual tasks near to or on the blackboard (maps) require special materials because of his low contrast sensitivity. He has learned to compensate his increased crowding phenomenon by increasing spacing and using a larger font. Handwriting will be limited to training him in writing his name; in other writing he uses his computer. Instead of copying from the blackboard, information is given on a USB stick. Training of Mathcad software continues.

The underlying cause – the paediatric disorders of the brain – were thought to be stable. With new treatments and training, the development of functioning is now possible in areas where the child had no function in early childhood, and the process continues still in adulthood, which requires further improvement in the assessment and follow-up of children with visual processing disorders.

20

TOWARDS THE DEVELOPMENT OF A CLASSIFICATION OF VISION-RELATED FUNCTIONING – A POTENTIAL FRAMEWORK

August Colenbrander

Introduction

Most existing classifications of vision-related functioning are designed for adults. For children with perinatal vision problems the situation is different. Their visual deficits more commonly present a *lack*, rather than a *loss,* and deficits at lower levels can severely limit the development of higher functions in their still developing brain. To develop a classification that acknowledges these unique aspects yet, where possible, relates to other classifications is a serious challenge.

Loss of vision in the adult is fundamentally different from lack of vision from an early age. Adult classifications are often based on symptoms. Many children are not able to verbalize their symptoms; they experience their vision as 'normal' because they have no prior experience of anything different. A better picture has to be obtained by observation and by history-taking concerning visual behaviour. 'Symptoms' arise only at a later stage when children become aware that others can perform visual tasks that they cannot.

Disorders of vision in the child can be classified according to the cause and the anatomical site, or according to the developmental and functional consequences. When discussing the *causes*, ocular (and anterior visual pathway) visual impairment (OVI) can be distinguished from cerebral visual impairment (CVI). When considering the *consequences,* fully understanding the impact of various visual deficits on development, visual behaviour, and adaptive strategies is essential for providing appropriate educational and (re)habilitative services. Providing these services requires a team-based approach, which requires a common framework of thinking. The aim of this chapter is to initiate the development of such a framework.

Historical developments

In the past, children with OVI were usually identified and given appropriate schooling, whereas CVI often went unrecognized. Today, with increased recognition of brain damage-related conditions, this is changing. Internationally, many children are integrated into mainstream education and are served by peripatetic special education teachers. This desirable trend means that increased numbers of regular teachers have to deal occasionally with children with visual deficits, a task for which they are not prepared.

Increased survival of children with special needs and increased recognition of their visual problems means that today brain damage-related visual dysfunction is present in up to half of all children with visual problems. The visual problems and the impact they have upon development and behaviour can be complex and may not be completely recognized and understood. If the old visual acuity-based service criteria, developed for OVI, are applied, such children will not receive the services they need and deserve.

The traditional visual acuity-based classifications are effective for allocating resources and planning service delivery for OVI but not for CVI. As many government agencies afford benefits to those labelled 'blind', an incorrect black and white distinction between those who are deemed to be 'sighted' and those deemed 'blind' has developed. Those on the 'sighted' side of the line can be incorrectly considered not to have vision problems, whereas those on the 'blind' side can equally incorrectly be considered to have no useful vision. The fallacies of these assumptions are evident when considering children with cognitive and perceptual visual dysfunction, who for some tasks are on the 'blind' side of the line but for other tasks are on the 'sighted' side.

The general definition of 'low vision' as a grey area between normal vision and blindness remains valid. However, more detailed distinctions (especially those based on visual acuity alone) may not apply because the ability to perform may depend on the nature of the task rather than on the traditional notion of the degree of the deficit.

In 1946 the charter of the World Health Organization (WHO) defined health as a state of 'optimal mental, physical and social well-being'. It took a while for various classifications to 'catch up'. The International Classification of causes of Death (ICD) became the International Classification of Diseases. In its ninth revision (ICD-9 [WHO 1978]) the earlier distinction of *sighted/blind* was replaced by *sighted/low vision/blind* and more detailed ranges were added (best in the US adaptation, ICD-9-CM [US Public Health Service 1980]). In 1980 the International Classification of Impairments, Disabilities and Handicaps (ICIDH [WHO 1980]) was introduced. In considering disability as the consequence of a medical condition, it followed the 'Medical model of disability'. The Bangkok report (WHO 1992) highlighted that the existing WHO criteria were developed to provide population statistics for public health needs; in such statistics, averaging hides individual differences. The existing criteria did not take into account the complex developmental and behavioural impact that visual impairment has upon the growing child, let alone the additional impact of damage to the brain in all its guises. Individual assessment of the child for educational needs requires greater flexibility.

In 2001, after a decade of preparation, the International Classification of Functioning, Disability and Health (ICF [WHO 2001]) replaced ICIDH. ICF, which also is adult centred, promotes the 'social model of disability', emphasizing functioning instead of impairment, participation in a social context instead of handicap, and introducing environmental factors. The difference between the medical and the social model can be shown by the statements: 'This child is handicapped, because she is blind' versus 'This blind child is independently mobile, because she uses a trailing wall for tactile guidance of her movement'. These two models of disability serve different and complementary purposes. The first classifies the underlying disorders and disability; the second refers to the resulting needs and societal participation.

In 2002 the International Council of Ophthalmology (ICO 2002) recommended that the terms 'low vision' and 'blindness' should be based on function rather than on visual acuities alone. It advocated the term 'blindness' for adults and children whose lack of vision requires vision substitution techniques (cane travel, Braille, talking books) and the term 'low vision' for those with limited vision who can benefit from vision enhancement, for example by increasing illumination and by magnification. However, even these more practical definitions do not apply to many children with CVI, who need a wide range of habilitational strategies matched to their specific deficits. There is still a need for child-centred classifications which take into account the very different characteristics and needs of the child.

All members of the team caring for the visually impaired child need to recognize the origin, nature, and developmental and functional aspects of visual disorders. Visual acuity-based eligibility rules for service provisions on account of ocular impairments remain relevant, but in the context of CVI these need to be extended by adding the concepts of 'equivalent visual dysfunction' and 'educational needs'.

Aspects of visual functioning

The functional implications of impairment of vision due to CVI are multifaceted. Figure 20.1 highlights how vision and vision loss can be considered from different perspectives. Ophthalmologists tend to focus upon disorders of the visual system, but it is essential that they also recognize the impact that impaired vision has upon intellectual and social development and make sure that appropriate action is taken to ensure that no child is inappropriately disadvantaged on account of poor vision.

On the left side of Figure 20.1, the term 'visual function' is used to describe how the visual system functions; this is important in the context of diagnosing visual disorders. On the right side, the term 'functional vision' is used to describe how the child functions in vision-related activities (Colenbrander 2003); this is important in the context of the provision of appropriate resources.

Parents tend to describe their child's visual problems in terms of functional vision: 'Doctor, my child cannot recognize his school friends.' The physician tends to refer to 'organ function': 'This is because his visual acuity is low,' and then defines the anatomical cause.

Various activities may be considered from different points of view; each viewpoint reveals a different aspect. In the context of the child learning to read, the minimum easily accessible print size and font depend on visual acuity. Measuring reading speed (words per minute) and reading endurance (hours per day) reveal aspects of personal ability. Enjoyment of reading reflects quality of life. All of these aspects need to be considered.

Deficits in visual function are *visual impairments* (e.g. visual acuity impairment, visual field impairment, contrast sensitivity impairment). If visual function is impaired owing to higher order perceptual or cognitive impairments, the term 'visual dysfunction' is applied.

The term 'visual ability deficit' refers to lack or loss of skills due to visual impairment. The term 'visual disability' is also used; however, in the context of classification, 'disability' may mean different things to different people, which can cause confusion (see Glossary).

The term 'visual dysfunction' is used when the child's visual functioning is not just limited because of insufficient input to the brain, but is abnormal because of defective processing of visual information in the brain.

Visual dysfunctions can be further classified according to the brain areas involved. Examples are dorsal stream dysfunction and ventral stream dysfunction (see Chapter 1).

Dorsal stream dysfunction (see Chapter 1) comprises a variety of forms of disordered visual attention with impaired visual search commonly combined with impairment of visual guidance of movement (optic ataxia) of either the upper limbs, the lower limbs, or both. The severe form of this symptom complex is known as Balint syndrome, when it is a result of bilateral posterior parietal damage.

Ventral stream dysfunction (see Chapter 1) causes impaired recognition in the context of adequate visual acuities. In children, disability recognizing people may be associated with impaired interpretation of facial expression, and is commonly associated with disability recognizing objects and severe disorientation (these behavioural features need to be distinguished from difficulty finding someone in a group, which is associated with difficulty with orientation in complex scenes owing to dorsal stream dysfunction).

The symptom complex of dorsal stream dysfunction is common. Ventral stream dysfunction can accompany dorsal stream dysfunction. Ventral stream dysfunction in isolation is rare.

Unilateral posterior parietal damage results in a variety of forms of visual inattention. Left-sided pathology results in right visual inattention. Right-sided pathology results in left visual inattention, commonly with additional right visual inattention.

In children with CVI the various forms of visual dysfunction described above commonly accompany impaired visual acuities and restricted visual fields. The reduction in acuity may be relatively minor, but the accompanying visual dysfunction can be severe. In these cases, the umbrella term 'visual impairment' is applied. The term 'visual dysfunction' can also be applied as the primary descriptor when there are no additional visual impairments. In this context, dorsal stream dysfunction is more common than ventral stream dysfunction (Dutton 2009).

Assessment of visual functioning

Ophthalmological assessment principally concerns the structure and function of the visual system, as shown in the first two columns of Figure 20.1, but should not omit the consequences for the child.

Visual functions are assessed one parameter at a time for each eye in turn, with threshold performance as the end-point. Because visual acuity is measured so often, some regard it as a general measure of the quality of vision. This is not true; visual acuity is only one of many visual functions. It measures only the magnification required for the recognition of detail on a letter chart. Other visual functions include visual field, contrast, colour vision, and dark adaptation.

Disorders of functional vision tend not to be enquired about or assessed by ophthalmologists. Hence, the *measurement* of visual functions is often used as a substitute for *prediction* or *estimation* of functional vision. However, this strategy has pitfalls, particularly in the context of the child with CVI.

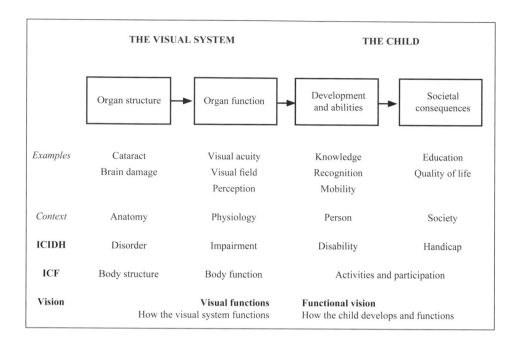

Fig. 20.1 Aspects of vision-related development and functioning. ICIDH, International Classification of Impairments, Disabilities and Handicaps; ICF, International Classification of Functioning, Disability and Health.

For direct *evaluation of functional vision* the emphasis shifts to the child's performance. Older, more able children are asked to perform standardized tasks and their performance is graded. The aim is to determine *sustainable* rather than *threshold* performance. To grade the performance, several options exist. Objective measures include the time required to perform the test or the accuracy of performance (number of errors). Description of the child's visual abilities by the parent or teacher is required in the case of young children and those whose disabilities or behaviour preclude direct assessment. Observation and documentation of the ability to recognize faces and interpret facial expressions, and the distance required for doing so, and the ability and speed of reading (if appropriate) are examples of measures which need to be taken.

In children with damage to the brain, multiple impairments, disabilities, and dysfunctions often coexist. Functional deficits in one domain may have an impact upon another.

Table 20.1 outlines some of the differences between the aspect of visual functions and their impairments and the aspect of functional vision and visual dysfunction.

MOTOR INVOLVEMENT
Most tests of visual function investigate visual recognition. In Chapter 1 these are described as functions of the ventral stream. Far fewer tests assess the dorsal stream (vision for action), which plays a role in motor abilities.

TABLE 20.1
Visual function tests versus functional vision tests

	Visual functions and their impairments (how the visual system functions)	Functional vision and visual dysfunctions (how the child functions)
Examples	Visual acuity, visual field, contrast sensitivity, dark adaptation, colour vision	Use of vision to learn: orientation and mobility, daily living skills, communication, sustained near activities, and to gain visual access to information
Measured	Separately for each eye	With both eyes open
Scale	Based on stimulus characteristics	Based on response characteristics
Tests	Single variable under controlled, usually static, conditions	Multiple variables under real-life conditions
Criteria	Threshold performance	Sustainable performance
Involves	Visual parameters only	May also reflect non-visual factors
Eligibility	Used to estimate functional vision	Matched to the child's visual needs
Cause and effect	Severe impairment (e.g. poor acuity) may cause functional limitations	Visual dysfunction can be present independent of impairment (such as poor acuity)
Education, training	Vision substitution methods when visual function is poor	Vision substitution may be needed for some functions but not for others
Motor involvement	Oculomotor functions: accommodation fixation, following, nystagmus, strabismus	Visual impact of accommodative and oculomotor dysfunction
		Impaired visual guidance of movement

Visually guided eye movements are an essential part of vision. They determine the ability to adequately scan the environment and to fixate and follow an object of interest and underlie the observation of 'fixing and following' in young children.

Visual guidance of body movements must also be considered. This includes visual guidance of hand movement for manual dexterity and visual guidance of the whole body for mobility. Persons with an ocular visual impairment may stumble because they cannot see a low contrast kerb. In this case the impairment is primary; the ability loss (stumbling) is secondary. Children who hesitate because they do not know whether a contour they can see clearly represents a flat line or a step have a primary dysfunction. In the first group the solution may be found in better contrast or better illumination (vision enhancement); in the second group the solution may involve a cane to provide tactile guidance as a form of vision substitution.

FUNCTION AND VISUAL PERFORMANCE

Visual acuity is widely used to classify visual impairment because it is reproducible and easily measured. This is justifiable for population surveys, in which statistical averages deliberately hide individual variations. However, individuals may perform better or worse than the

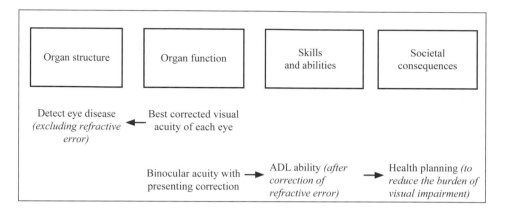

Fig 20.2 Different criteria for different applications

statistical average; furthermore, visual acuity reflects only one of many visual functions, and is not a good indicator of higher visual functioning. Population data should therefore not be used as the sole black and white determinant for planning, granting, or denying *individual* services or privileges (WHO 1992). Preferential looking and visual evoked potential (VEP) testing of visual acuity estimate the resolution of the visual system from occipital cortical activity, but this does not indicate whether this information can be employed by higher visual centres. Also, environmental factors often play a larger role for children than for adults so that visual behaviour in the clinic may not equate with that at home or at school. This means that history-taking from parents and educators can be more informative than a single visual acuity estimate in the clinic. In children these issues are of paramount importance. Vision is not only required to see, but it facilitates most aspects of learning.

Visual function tests determine the *threshold visual performance* whereas functional vision requires both *meaningful* and *sustainable* performance. Any rules for the provision of services must provide for individual adjustments for those whose functional performance is not accurately predicted by threshold measures. This also applies to the *need for services* in education and (re)habilitation. Even if visual acuity is used as an initial criterion, it should be mitigated by the additional concept of 'equivalent visual dysfunction'.

Different classifications from different points of view

For optimal communication among different professionals, all need to understand each other's point of view. This section considers the classifications for each of the four aspects discussed earlier.

CLASSIFICATION ACCORDING TO ANATOMICAL STRUCTURE

Anatomical classification of visual disorders is available in the ICD and its adaptations (WHO 1978, 1992, US Public Health Service 1980). The classification of this aspect in ICF is abbreviated and less effective. That many ocular disorders can be observed directly renders the anatomical classification of eye diseases more precise than for any other organ system,

288

including the brain. However, not all anatomical defects result in functional deficits; in some cases, major brain defects, as, for example, in a savant, may be compatible with extraordinary performance on some tasks (Treffert and Christensen 2005). Conversely, CVI can occur in the context of normal imaging and visual acuity.

CLASSIFICATION ACCORDING TO VISUAL FUNCTIONS

Visual acuity, *visual field*, and *contrast sensitivity* are the most significant measurable visual functions, but many other parameters exist, including colour vision, light and dark adaptation, and glare sensitivity. Electrophysiological measurement of visual function can also be included.

How various tests are performed and the criteria applied depends on their purpose. Figure 20.2 illustrates the difference between visual acuity measurement for the detection of eye disease and visual acuity measurement to predict the personal and societal consequences. The 2003 WHO consultation on characterization of vision loss (WHO 2003) recommended changing the emphasis of population surveys from the detection of eye disease to the burden of visual impairment.

CLASSIFICATION ACCORDING TO SKILLS AND ABILITIES

The term 'functional vision' applies to skills and abilities and, in children, to the acquisition of these skills. The term 'visual dysfunction' applies to impaired visual ability.

Visual skills and abilities are required for activities of daily living (ADL) and for orientation and mobility (O&M). The ICF provides a primarily adult-centred classification based on the *goals* of these activities, but offers less in terms of the *resources* (sight, hearing, touch) available to perform these activities. For children, a change in emphasis is required to embrace all aspects of learning for which vision is required. These include language learning (both auditory and visual, as most language is referenced to what is seen, such as a gesture or a facial expression), visual guidance of movement, and access to information both distant and near. In the context of CVI, the primary emphasis is on impaired ability owing to dysfunctions that originate in higher visual centres and not necessarily impaired ocular input. Moreover, in many cases vision cannot be considered in isolation owing to accompanying conditions such as cerebral palsy.

In the literature on adults with impaired vision, O&M are often considered together but visual deficits which impair recognition for route-finding and orientation are distinct from those that impair visual guidance of movement. Children may depend upon vision for some aspects of these tasks and upon vision substitution for other aspects. This confounds the traditional simplistic division between those who are 'blind' and those who are 'sighted'.

Chapters 9 and 15 catalogue the range of visual problems seen in children with CVI and a range of (re)habilitational strategies.

CLASSIFICATION ACCORDING TO QUALITY OF LIFE

The last columns of Figures 20.1 and 20.2 refer to *societal consequences* ('handicap' in ICIDH, 'participation' in ICF) or to quality of life. This aspect is highly subjective and depends on the effect of factors in both the human and the physical environment. In children, the use of this form of classification becomes more problematic. Useful discussions of measures of quality of life in children have recently been published (Goldstein and Bax 2009).

Severity of deficits

Mild visual impairment may manifest only when the individual is tired or under stress. Severe impairment precludes normal functioning, and there is a range in between. Various scales can be used. In the medical field, a grade 4 condition, for example, is generally considered to be worse than a grade 1 condition. For impaired ability there are two options. Like the medical model, *impairment ratings* can be applied (as in the American Medical Association *Guides* [AMA 2001, 2007]), with 0 assigned to normal and 100 to total impairment. In the spirit of ICF, however, a *scale of functioning,* in which a low score denotes poor function and vice versa, is more apposite.

The units used to measure visual acuity cannot be compared with those for visual fields let alone with those measuring other sensory disorders such as hearing impairment. However, the disabling effects of each of these deficits can potentially be compared by means of a general scale of functioning.

For older children and adults, the general scale of functioning shown in Table 20.2 can be used. For young children, such a classification needs to be set in the context of the developmental age at which various functions mature. The scale shown in this table is not vision specific. It can be applied to any domain. It can also be used for single visual functions, such as visual acuity or visual field, as described in the functional vision score (Colenbrander 1994) in the AMA *Guides* (AMA 2001, 2007). The ranges are similar to those recommended in ICF, except that ICF combines the ranges for severe and profound deficits.

Particularly from the standpoint of resource allocation for education and other services, a key issue which needs to be debated is the quantification of cognitive and perceptual visual disorders. As better classification tools are developed, special attention needs to be paid to the following points. The classifications need to (1) deal separately with each age group (e.g. infant, preschool child, school child, teenager); (2) deal with damage to the brain as a case that is separate from and different to damage to the eyes; (3) accommodate other concurrent consequences of brain damage, for example cerebral palsy, 'special needs', and intellectual functioning; and (4) quantify the severity of visual disability with respect to its effect on learning and other parameters, as well as to how it affects educational and habilitational strategies.

This approach requires expert teams to return to the drawing board. Considering the needs of a child, adult classifications (as if that child is a 'little adult') are inappropriate. No child should be disadvantaged developmentally, educationally, socially, or personally on account of failure of implementation of appropriate care. At present, children worldwide are being so disadvantaged on account of the use of adult-based criteria. We have an opportunity to change this by starting with a 'child's eye view' rather than an adult's perspective.

For the child with damage to the brain, a classification system primarily founded upon 'fingerprinting' the complex disabilities of each child and designing matched strategies for each child's needs is required. By designing sets of strategies and methods of matching each child to the strategy for his or her needs, and removing the somewhat arbitrary use of acuity and visual field as primary criteria for resource allocation, a step will be made towards the ultimate goal of preventing administrators who wish to save money from depriving children of the services they need.

Anatomical versus functional considerations

A distinction based on gross anatomy is often made between *ocular* and *cerebral* visual impairments. However, as the retina is developmentally part of the brain, and neural processing starts in the inner retina, the distinction between visual functions (and impairment) and functional vision (and dysfunction) does not fit neatly within any anatomical division because impaired central and peripheral visual functions can effectively result from damage at any location.

OCULAR VISUAL IMPAIRMENT – DESCRIBES HOW THE EYE FUNCTIONS
Conditions that fall into this category include the following:

- visual acuity problems;
- optical problems include refractive error and accommodative problems (often less obvious) as well as opacities of cornea, lens, or vitreous;
- retinal problems, including retinopathy of prematurity (ROP), malformations, colobomata, and degenerative conditions; and
- optic nerve problems, including optic atrophy and optic nerve hypoplasia.

CEREBRAL VISUAL IMPAIRMENT – DESCRIBES HOW THE BRAIN FUNCTIONS
Conditions that fall into this category include the following:

- Visual acuity problems.
- Visual field problems. Problems beyond the lateral geniculate nucleus (LGN) in the optic radiations and primary visual cortex fall under the cerebral category. This includes hemianopia or quadrantanopia associated with lateralized lesions and lower visual field problems, often associated with periventricular leucomalacia (PVL).
- Problems with motion perception, which may make the identification of moving targets more difficult.
- Problems with elements of higher visual processing, such as the perception of form, colour, and motion. Affected children may be able to sort objects by colour but not by shape. Perception of colour and contrast is reported to be more robust and less likely to manifest than the perception of form details.
- Cognitive and perceptual visual dysfunctions occurring in addition to evident visual impairment warrant inclusion in this category (e.g. when identified in the context of reduced acuity or visual field impairment). In addition, manifest damage to the brain causing profound problems arguably warrants inclusion in this category. This includes posterior parietal damage culminating in severe dorsal stream dysfunction (forms of Balint syndrome) and, more rarely, temporal lobe damage causing profound impairment of recognition.

TABLE 20.2
General scale of functioning applied to vision

Deficit ranges as in ICD-9-CM	Descriptors		Broad ranges	Function score	
Normal	Normal or near-normal visual functioning	Exceptional performance Has reserves to meet extra demands	Uses mainly sighted techniques	Excellent Reference standard	120 100
Mild deficit		Lost reserves. Problems may manifest when under stress	Uses mainly sighted techniques	Good	80
Moderate deficit		Occasionally needs low vision techniques (vision enhancement)	Uses mainly low vision techniques	Fair	60
Severe deficit	Visual functioning restricted or impossible	Frequently needs low vision aids. May use blind skills as an adjunct	Uses mainly low vision techniques	Poor	40
Profound deficit		Marginal functioning. Mainly uses blind skills with vision as an adjunct	Uses mainly blind techniques	Marginal	20
Total deficit		Cannot function visually. Must use blind skills (vision substitution)	Uses mainly blind techniques	Cannot function visually	0

- A separate category should arguably be reserved for oculomotor problems. These may include fixation problems, problems with saccades and/or smooth pursuit, problems with accommodation, and binocular alignment problems (strabismus), all of which can interfere with vision.

VISUAL DYSFUNCTION – DESCRIBES HOW THE CHILD FUNCTIONS

While the term 'impairment' describes how the eye or the brain functions, the term 'visual dysfunction' is proposed to describe disorders of visual perception that affect how the child functions in various activities of daily living. Impairments may be categorized in terms of different visual parameters (detail, contrast, colour, field, etc.) that can be assessed one at a time; dysfunction refers to more complex behaviours that are not as easily broken down into separate parameters and that are not covered by the above descriptions of CVI. Dysfunctions can occur in isolation or in association with other syndromes, such as Williams syndrome, in which the visual acuities and visual fields are normal but visual processing is abnormal and tends to be fatiguable. Dysfunctions are assessed not by varying a stimulus parameter but by determining the individual's response to a standardized task.

At the severe end of the spectrum, children whose performance is profoundly compromised on account of severe dorsal stream dysfunction (manifesting as profound disorders of attention and visual search associated with impaired visual guidance of movement [optic ataxia] owing to posterior parietal damage causing paediatric variants of Balint syndrome) need special services even if their visual acuities are normal (the impaired visual attention prevents visual field assessment). There are also rare cases of severe ventral stream dysfunction resulting in profound impairment of recognition and orientation, and cases where both are impaired but with normal acuities. These, too, require services for profound visual impairment.

The terminology proposed in this chapter separating *impairments* (how the eye and brain function) from *dysfunctions* (how the child functions as a manifestation of the brain damage) allows for the inclusion of the needs of children with cognitive and perceptual visual impairment under the category of dysfunction even if visual acuity is normal. It will hopefully satisfy those who do not want the term 'CVI' used if the visual acuity is not reduced and will hopefully facilitate discussion, especially with non-medical personnel and third parties, by clarifying that visual dysfunctions with a range of severity may exist without an underlying measurable visual impairment and that children with visual dysfunctions are as much in need of services as children with visual impairments.

Summary and recommended terminology

A framework for the classification of visual functioning is presented in Table 20.3. This framework distinguishes between *visual functions*, which describe how the eye and the basic visual system function, and *functional vision*, which describes how the person functions in vision-related tasks.

The term 'visual impairment' is used to describe deficits of measured visual functions. The term 'visual disability' (or 'visual ability defect' in countries where the term 'visual disability' has other meanings) is used when functional vision is limited as a direct result of visual impairment.

This functional classification differs from the anatomical distinction between ocular and cerebral impairments.

Ocular visual impairments are the deficits resulting from disorders of visual input. They are the most common cause of vision deficits among adults.

Cerebral visual impairments are now reported in up to 50% of children with congenital vision problems. (In adults they may also result from traumatic brain injury and from cerebrovascular accidents, for example.) This category features impairments in acuity, visual field with or without perceptual, and cognitive visual dysfunction.

Visual dysfunction is proposed to describe the condition of perceptual or cognitive deficits which may or may not be accompanied by a visual impairment. Children with visual dysfunction have the same need for services and deserve as much attention and support, matched to their disabilities, as those with visual impairments. Impairments and dysfunction commonly coexist, but the absence of an impairment should not be used to deny services to children with visual dysfunctions.

TABLE 20.3
Framework for the classification for visual dysfunction

Disorder/impairment	Effect	Abilities	Solution
Ocular disorder/ocular visual impairment (OVI)	Reduced input with normal processing of available information	Limited visual abilities	Vision enhancement and/or substitution
	Reduced input causes Reduced development	Limited and/or dysfunctional abilities	Early intervention and training
Cerebral disorder/ cerebral visual impairment (CVI)	Impaired primary processing (input may be normal)	Limited visual abilities	Early intervention and training
	Impaired perceptual processing (input may be normal)	Visual dysfunction (visual acuity may be normal)	Vision substitution to bypass the defect in visual processing

The above categories are not mutually exclusive. They may coexist.

APPENDIX

Conversion table for different measures of visual acuity

| | Measures which are independent of distance | | | | | Snellen notation indicating measure at | | | | |
LogMAR	Modified LogMAR	Decimal	Cycles per degree	Log cycles per degree		6m	5m	4m	1m	20ft
-0.3	1.3	2.00	60	1.8		6/3	5/2.5	4/2	1/0.5	20/10
-0.2	1.2	1.60	48	1.7		6/4	5/3.2	4/2.5	1/0.6	20/123
-0.1	1.1	1.26	38	1.6		6/5	5/4	4/3.2	1/0.8	20/16
0.0	1.0	1.00	30	1.5		6/6	5/5	4/4	1/1	20/20
0.1	0.9	0.80	24	1.4		6/8	5/6	4/5	1/1.3	20/25
0.2	0.8	0.63	19	1.3		6/10	5/8	4/6	1/1.6	20/32
0.3	0.7	0.50	15	1.2		6/12	5/10	4/8	1/2	20/40
0.4	0.6	0.40	12	1.1		6/15	5/13	4/10	1/2.5	20/50
0.5	0.5	0.32	9.5	1.0		6/19	5/16	4/13	1/3.2	20/63
0.6	0.4	0.25	7.5	0.9		6/24	5/20	4/16	1/4	20/80
0.7	0.3	0.20	6.0	0.8		6/30	5/25	4/20	1/5	20/100
0.8	0.2	0.16	4.8	0.7		6/38	5/32	4/25	1/6	20/125
0.9	0.1	0.13	3.8	0.6		6/48	5/40	4/32	1/8	20/160
1.0	0.0	0.10	3.0	0.5		6/60	5/50	4/40	1/10	20/200
1.1	-0.1	0.08	2.4	0.4		6/76	5/63	4/50	1/13	20/250
1.2	-0.2	0.06	1.9	0.3		6/95	5/80	4/63	1/16	20/320
1.3	-0.3	0.05	1.5	0.2		6/120	5/100	4/80	1/20	20/400

REFERENCES

Abbott C (2002) *Symbols Now.* Leamington Spa: Widgit Software Ltd.

Abercrombie MLJ (1964) Visual perceptual and visuo-motor impairments in physically handicapped children. *Percept Mot Skills* 18: 583–94.

Acers TE, Cooper WC (1965) Cortical blindness secondary to bacterial meningitis. *Am J Ophthalmic* 59: 226–9.

Accord RS (1984) Cortical blindness following bacterial meningitis: a case report with reassessment of prognosis and aetiology. *Dev Med Child Neural* 26: 227–30.

Adelson PD, Bratton SL, Carney NA et al (2003) Guidelines for the acute medical management of severe traumatic brain injury in infants, children, and adolescents. Chapter 5. Indications for intracranial pressure monitoring in pediatric patients with severe traumatic brain injury. *Pediatr Crit Care Med* 4: S19–24.

Adoh TO, Woodhouse JM (1994) The Cardiff acuity test used for measuring visual acuity development in toddlers. *Vision Res* 34: 555–60.

Adoh TO, Woodhouse JM, Oduwaiye KA (1992) The Cardiff Test: a new visual acuity test for toddlers and children with intellectual impairment. A preliminary report. *Optom Vis Sci* 69: 427–32.

Aglioti S, DeSouza JFX, Goodale MA (1995) Size-contrast illusions deceive the eye but not the hand. *Curr Biol* 5: 679–85.

Ahmed M, Dutton GN (1996) Cognitive visual dysfunction in a child with cerebral damage. *Dev Med Child Neurol* 38: 736–9.

Aitken S, Millar S (2004) *Listening to Children 2004.* Glasgow: Sense Scotland.

Aitken S, Buultjens M, Clark C, Eyre JR, Pease L (2000) *Teaching Children who are Deafblind: Contact Communication and Learning.* London: David Fulton Publishers.

Aitken S, Millar S, Nisbet PD (2001) Applying the new medical model: intervening in the environment of children who are multiply disabled. *Br J Vis Impair* 19: 74–80.

Alagaratnam J, Sharma TK, Lim CS, Fleck BW (2002) A survey of visual impairment in children attending the Royal Blind School, Edinburgh using the WHO childhood visual impairment database. *Eye* 16: 557–61.

Alford CA, Stagnos S, Poss, Britt WJ (1990) Congenital and perinatal cytomegalovirus infections. *Rev Infect Dis* 12(Suppl. 7): S745–53.

Allen D, Tyler CW, Norcia AM (1996) Development of grating acuity and contrast sensitivity on the central and pheripheral visual field of the human infant. *Vis Res* 36: 1945–53.

Altmann HE, Hiatt RL, Deweese MW (1966) Ocular findings in cerebral palsy. *South Med J* 59: 1015–18.

American Academy of Ophthalmology (2002) *Pediatric Eye Evaluations: Preferred Practice Series.* San Francisco: American Academy of Ophthalmology.

American Speech-Language-Hearing Association (ASHA) Task Force on Central Auditory Processing Consensus Development (1996) Central auditory processing: current status of research and implications for clinical practice. *Am J Audiol* 5: 41–54.

American Speech-Language-Hearing Association (2005) *Central Auditory Processing Disorders* (available at http://www.asha.org/members/deskref-journals/deskref/default).

Anderson V, Fenwick T, Manly T, Robertson I (1998) Attentional skills following traumatic brain injury in childhood: a componential analysis. *Brain Inj* 12: 937–49.

Andersson S, Persson EK, Aring E et al (2006) Vision in children with hydrocephalus. *Dev Med Neurol* 48: 836–41.

Anker S, Atkinson J, Braddick O et al (2003) Identification of infants with significant refractive error and strabismus in a population screening program using noncycloplegic videorefraction and orthoptic examination. *Invest Ophthalmol Vis Sci* 44: 497–504.

Aoki N, Oikawa A, Sakai T (1997) Isolated ophthalmological manifestations due to malfunction of a lumbo-peritoneal shunt: shortening of the spinal catheter in three pediatric patients. *Childs Nerv Syst* 13: 264–7.

Aring E, Andersson S, Persson EK et al (2007) Strabismus, binocular functions and ocular motility in a population-based group of children with early surgically treated hydrocephalus. *Strabismus* 15: 79–88.

Arroyo HA, Jan JE, McCormick AQ, Farrell K (1985) Permanent visual loss after shunt malfunction. *Neurology* 35: 25.

Ashwal S, Russman BS, Blasco PA et al (2004) Practice parameter: diagnostic assessment of the child with cerebral palsy: report of the Quality Standards Subcommittee of the American Academy of Neurology and the Practice Committee of the Child Neurology Society. *Neurology* 62: 851–63.

Atkinson J (1984) Human visual development over the first six months of life. A review and a hypothesis. *Hum Neurobiol* 3: 61–74.

Atkinson J (1989) New tests of vision screening and assessment in infants and young children. In: French JH, Harel S, Casaer P, editors. *Child Neurology and Development Disabilities*. Baltimore: Paul H. Brookes Publishing, pp. 219–27.

Atkinson J (1998) The 'where and what' or 'who and how' of visual development: an update of current neurobiological models. In: Simion F, Butterworth G, editors. *The Development of Sensory, Motor and Cognitive Capacities in Early Infancy. From Perception to Cognition.* Hove: Psychology Press, pp. 3–24.

Atkinson J (2000) *The Developing Visual Brain.* Oxford: Medical Publications.

Atkinson J (2003) Visual problems in premature infants. *Rev Neurol* 36: 569.

Atkinson J, Braddick OJ (1981) Development of optokinetic nystagmus in infants: an indicator of cortical binocularity. In: Fisher DF, Monty RA, Sender JW, editors. *Eye Movements: Cognition and Visual Perception*, Hillsdale, NJ: Lawrence Erlbaum Associates, pp. 53–64.

Atkinson J, Braddick O (2003) Neurobiological models of normal and abnormal visual development. In: De Haan M, Johnson M, editors. *The Cognitive Neuroscience of Development.* Hove: Psychology Press, pp. 43–71.

Atkinson J, Braddick O (2005) Dorsal stream vulnerability and autistic disorders: the importance of comparative studies of form and motion coherence in typically developing children and children with developmental disorders. *Cah Psychol Cognitive (Curr Psychol Cognition)* 23: 49–58.

Atkinson J, Braddick O (2007) Visual and visuocognitive development in children born very prematurely. *Prog Brain Res* 164: 123–49.

Atkinson J, van Hof-van Duin J (1993) Visual assessment during the first years of life. In: Fielder A, Bax M, editors. *Management of Visual Impairment in Childhood*. London: Mac Keith Press.

Atkinson J, Hood B, Wattam-Bell J, Anker S, Tricklebank J (1988) Development of orientation discrimination in infancy. *Perception* 17: 587–95.

Atkinson J, Hood B, Wattam-Bell J, Braddick O (1992) Changes in infants' ability to switch visual attention in the first three months of life. *Perception* 21: 643–53.

Atkinson J, Weeks F, Anker S, Rae S, Macpherson F, Hughes C (1994) VEP and behavioural measures for delayed visual development in VLBW infants. *Strabismus* 2: 42.

Atkinson J, King J, Braddick O, Nokes L, Anker S, Braddick F (1997) A specific deficit of dorsal stream function in Williams Syndrome. *NeuroReport* 8: 1919–22.

Atkinson J, Anker S, Braddick O, Nokes L, Mason A, Braddick F (2001) Visual and visuo-spatial development in young Williams Syndrome children. *Dev Med Child Neurol* 43: 330–7.

Atkinson J, Anker S, Rae S, Weeks F, Braddick O, Rennie J (2002a) Cortical visual evoked potentials in very low birthweight premature infants. *Arch Dis Child Fetal Neonatal Ed* 86: F28–31.

Atkinson J, Anker S, Rae S, Hughes C, Braddick O (2002b) A test battery of child development for examining functional vision (ABCDEFV). *Strabismus* 10: 245–69.

Atkinson J, Anker S, Nardini M et al (2002c) Infant vision screening predicts failures on motor and cognitive tests up to school age. *Strabismus* 10: 187–98.

Atkinson J, Braddick O, Anker S, Curran W, Andrew R (2003) Neurobiological models of visuospatial cognition in children with Williams Syndrome: Measures of dorsal-stream and frontal function. *Dev Neuropsychol* 23: 141–74.

Atkinson J, Anker S, Braddick O, Nokes L, Mason A, Braddick F (2004) Visual and visuospatial development in young children with Williams syndrome. *Brain Dev* 26: 506–12.

Atkinson J, Braddick O, Rose FE, Searcy YM, Wattam-Bell J, Bellugi U (2006) Dorsal-stream motion processing deficits persist into adulthood in Williams Syndrome. *Neuropsychologia* 44: 828–33.

Atkinson J, Braddick O, Nardini M, Anker S (2007) Infant hyperopia: Detection, distribution, changes and correlates – outcomes from the Cambridge Infant Screening Programs. *Optom Vis Sci* 84: 84–96.

Atkinson J, Braddick O, Anker S et al (2008) Cortical vision, MRI and developmental outcome in preterm infants. *Arch Dis Child Fetal Neonatal Ed* 93: F292–7.

Auestad N, Montalto BM, Hall RT et al (1997) Visual acuity, erythrocyte fatty acid composition, and growth in term infants fed formulas with long chain polyunsaturated fatty acids for one year. *Pediatr Res* 41: 1–10.

Baddeley AD, Hitch GJ (1974) Working memory. In: Bower GA, editor. *The Psychology of Learning and Motivation: Advances in Research Theory* (Vol. 8). New York: Academic press, pp. 47–89.

Baker-Nobles L, Rutherford A (1995) Understanding cortical visual impairment in children. *Am J Occup Ther* 49: 899–903.

Balcer LJ (2001) Anatomic rewiew and topographic diagnosis. *Ophthamol Clin North Am* 14: 1.

Bálint R (1909) Seelenlähmung des 'Schauens', optische Ataxie, räumliche Störung der Aufmerksamkeit. *Monatschr Psychiat Neurolog* 25: 51–81.

Balliet R, Blood KM, Bach-y-Rita P (1985) Visual field rehabilitation in the cortically blind? *J Neurol Neurosurg Psychiatry* 48: 1113–24.

Bamashmus MA, Matlhaga B, Dutton GN (2004) Causes of blindness and visual impairment in the West of Scotland. *Eye* 18: 257–61.

Banker BQ, Larroche JC (1962) Periventricular leukomalacia of infancy. *Arch Neurol* 7: 32–56.

Banks MS, Bennett PJ (1988) Optical and photoreceptor immaturities limit the spatial and chromatic vision of human neonates. *J Opt Soc Am A* 5: 2059–79.

Baranek GT, Boyd BA, Poe MD, David FJ, Watson LR (2007) Hyperresponsive sensory patterns in young children with autism, developmental delay, and typical development. *Am J Ment Retard* 112: 233–45.

Barkovich AJ, Kjos BO (1992) Schizencephaly: correlation of clinical findings with MR characteristics. *AJNR Am J Neuroradiol* 13: 85–94.

Barkovich AJ, Lindan CE (1994) Congenital cytomegalovirus infection of the brain: imaging analysis and embryologic considerations. *AJNR Am J Neuroradiol* 15: 703–15.

Barkovich AJ, Truwit CL (1990) Brain damage from perinatal asphyxia: correlation of MR findings with gestational age. *AJNR Am J Neuroradiol* 11: 1087–96.

Barkovich AJ, Westmark D, Rerriero DM (1995) Perinatal asphyxia: MR findings in the first 10 days. *Am J Neuroradiol* 16: 427.

Barkovich AJ, Ali FA, Rowley HA, Bass N (1998) Imaging patterns of neonatal hypoglycemia. *AJNR Am J Neuroradiol* 19: 523–8.

Barkovich AJ, Hevner R, Guerrini R (1999) Syndromes of bilateral symmetrical polymicrogyria. *AJNR Am J Neuroradiol* 20: 1814–21.

Barkovich AJ, Kuzniecky RI, Jackson GD (2001) Classification system for malformations of cortical development: update 2001. *Neurology* 57: 2168–78.

Barkovich AJ, Kuzniecky RI, Jackson GD, Guerrini R, Dobyns WB (2005) A developmental and genetic classification for malformations of cortical development. *Neurology* 65: 1873–87.

Barlow KM, Minns RA (2000) Annual incidence of shaken impact syndrome in young children. *Lancet* 356: 1571–2.

Bassi L, Ricci D, Volzone A et al (2008) Probabilistic diffusion tractography of the optic radiations and visual function in preterm infants at term equivalent age. *Brain* 131: 573–82.

Bax M, Goldstein M, Rosenbaum P et al. Executive Committee for the Definition of Cerebral Palsy (2005) Proposed definition and classification of cerebral palsy. *Dev Med Child Neurol* 47: 571–6.

Bax M, Tydeman C, Flodmark O (2006) Clinical and MRI correlates of cerebral palsy: the European Cerebral Palsy Study. *JAMA* 296: 1602–8.

Beery KE (1997) *The Beery–Buktenica Developmental Test of Visual-Motor Integration. Administration Scoring and Teaching Manual*, 4th edn. Parsippany, NJ: Modern Curriculum Press.

Bellis TJ (2003) *Assessment and Management of Central Auditory Processing Disorders in the Educational Setting: From Science To Practice*, 2nd edn. Clifton Park, NY: Delmar Learning.

Bellugi U, Lichtenberger L, Mills D, Galaburda A, Korenberg JR (1999) Bridging cognition, the brain, and molecular genetics: evidence from Williams syndrome. *Trends Neurosci* 22: 197–207.

Berezovsky A, Salomao SR, Haro-Munoz E, Ventura DF, Maffei CMA, Hortelan LR (1995) Monocular visual fields measured in eight meridians by kinetic double-arc perimetry in the first year of life. *Invest Ophthalmol Vis Sci* 36: 4185.

Best T (2003) New concepts in deafblindness. 13th Dbl Conference on Deafblindness conference proceedings [CD-ROM]. Brantford, ON: Canadian Deafblind and Rubella Association (also available from info@ nationaldb.org).

Bhasin T, Brocksen S, Avchen R, van Naarden Braun K (2006) Prevalence of four developmental disabilities among children aged 8 years: Metropolitan Atlanta Developmental Disabilities Surveillance Program, 1996 and 2000. *MMWR Surveillance Summaries* 55(SS01): 1–9.

Bieber ML, Volbrecht VJ, Werner JS (1995) Spectral efficiency measured by heterochromatic flicker photometry is similar in human infants and adults. *Vision Res* 35: 1385–92.

Bigelow AE (1986) The development of reaching in blind children. *Br J Dev Psychol* 4: 355–66.

Bigelow AE (1992) Locomotion and search behaviour in blind infants. *Infant Behav Dev* 15: 170–89.

Biglan AW (1990) Ophthalmologic complications of myelomeningocele: a longitudinal study. *Trans Am Ophthal Soc* 88: 389–462.

Billmire ME, Myers PA (1985) Serious head injury in infants: accident or abuse? *Pediatrics* 75: 340–2.

Binkofski F, Buccino G, Stephan KM, Rizzolatti G, Seitz RJ, Freund HJ (1999) A parieto-premotor network for object manipulation: evidence from neuroimaging. *Exp Brain Res* 128: 210–13.

Binyon S, Prendergast M (1991) Eye-movement tics in children. *Dev Med Child Neurol* 33: 352–4.

Birch E (1993) Stereopsis in infants and its developmental relation to visual acuity. In: Simons K, editor. *Early Visual Development: Normal and Abnormal.* New York: Oxford University Press.

Birch EE, Bane MC (1991) Forced-choice preferential looking acuity of children with cortical visual impairment. *Dev Med Child Neurol* 33: 722–9.

Birch EE, Hoffman DR, Uauy R, Birch DG, Prestidge C (1998) Visual acuity and the essentiality of docosahexaenoic acid and arachidonic acid in diet of term infants. *Pediatr Res* 44: 201–9.

Biro S, Russell J (2001) The execution of arbitrary procedures by children with autism. *Dev Psychopathol* 13: 97–110.

Birtles D, Braddick O, Wattam-Bell J, Wilkinson A, Atkinson J (2007) Orientation and motion-specific visual cortex responses in infants born preterm. *NeuroReport* 18: 1975–9.

Black P (1982) Visual disorders associated with cerebral palsy. *Br J Ophthalmol* 66: 46–52.

Blakemore C (1990) Maturation of mechanisms for efficient spatial vision. In: Blakemore C, editor. *Vision: Coding and Efficiency.* Cambridge: Cambridge University Press.

Blass EM, Camp CA (2001) The ontogeny of face recognition: Eye contact and sweet taste induce face preference in 9- and 12-week-old human infants. *Dev Psychol* 37: 762–74.

Blohmé J, Tornqvist K (1997a) Visual impairment in Swedish children. III. Diagnoses. *Acta Ophthalmol Scand* 75: 681–7.

Blohmé J, Tornqvist K (1997b) Visual impairment in Swedish children. I. Register and prevalence data. *Acta Ophthalmol Scand* 75: 194–8.

Blumenthal EZ, Haddad A, Horani A, Anteby I (2004) The reliability of frequency doubling perimetry in young children. *Ophthalmology* 111: 435.

Bova SM, Fazzi E, Giovenzana A et al (2007) The development of visual object recognition in school-age children. *Dev Neuropsychol* 31: 79–102.

Bowering ER, Maurer D, Lewis TL, Brent HP (1993) Sensitivity in the nasal and temporal hemifields in children treated for cataract. *Invest Ophthalmol Vis Sci* 36: 3501.

Bowman RM, McLone DG, Grant JA, Tomita T, Ito JA (2001) Spina bifida outcome: a 25-year prospective. *Pediatr Neurosurg* 34: 114–20.

Boyle NJ, Jones DH, Hamilton R, Spowart KM, Dutton GN (2005) Blindsight in children: does it exist and can it be used to help the child? Observations on a case series. *Dev Med Child Neurol* 47: 699–702.

Braddick OJ (1993) Orientation- and motion-selective mechanisms in infants. In: Simons K, editor. *Early Visual Development: Normal and Abnormal.* New York: Oxford University Press.

Braddick OJ (1996) Binocularity in infancy. *Eye* 10: 182–8.

Braddick OJ, Atkinson J (2007) Development of brain mechanisms for visual global processing and object segmentation. In: Hofsten C, Rosander K, editors. *From Action to Cognition (Progress in Brain Research, Vol. 164).* pp. 151–68. Amsterdam: Elsevier.

Braddick OJ, Atkinson J, Julesz B, Kropfl W, Bodis-Wollner I, Raab E (1980) Cortical binocularity in infants. *Nature* 288: 363–5.

Braddick OJ, Wattam-Bell J, Atkinson J (1986) Orientation-specific cortical responses develop in early infancy. *Nature* 320: 617–19.

Braddick OJ, Atkinson J, Hood B, Harkness W, Jackson G, Vargha-Khadem F (1992) Possible blindsight in infants lacking one cerebral hemisphere. *Nature* 360: 461–3.

Braddick OJ, O'Brien JMD, Wattam-Bell J, Atkinson J, Turner R (2000) Form and motion coherence activate independent, but not dorsal/ventral segregated, networks in the human brain. *Curr Biol* 10: 731–4.

Braddick OJ, O'Brien JMD, Wattam-Bell J, Atkinson J, Hartley T, Turner R (2001) Brain areas sensitive to coherent visual motion. *Perception* 30: 61–72.

Braddick OJ, Curran W, Atkinson J, Wattam-Bell J, Gunn A (2002) Infants' sensitivity to global form coherence. *Invest Ophthalmol Vis Sci* 43: E–Abstract 3995.

Braddick OJ, Atkinson J, Wattam-Bell J (2003) Normal and anomalous development of visual motion processing: Motion coherence and 'dorsal stream vulnerability'. *Neuropsychologia* 4: 1769–84.

Braddick OJ, Birtles D, Wattam-Bell J, Atkinson J (2005) Motion- and orientation-specific cortical responses in infancy. *Vision Res* 45: 3169–79.

Braddick OJ, Birtles D, Mills S, Warshafsky J, Wattam-Bell J, Atkinson J (2006) Brain responses to global perceptual coherence. *J Vision* 6: 426a.

Brambring M (2001) Integration of children with visual impairment in regular preschools. *Child Care Health Dev* 27: 425–38.

Brambring M, Troster H (1992) On the stability of stereotyped behaviours in blind infants and preschoolers. *J Vis Imp Blind* 4: 105–110.

Brazelton TB (1973) *Neonatal Behavioural Assessment Scale. Clinics in Developmental Medicine, No. 50.* London: Spastics International Medical Publication/William Medical Books, Philadelphia: J B Lippincott Co.

Breckenridge K, Braddick O, Atkinson J (2007) The structure of attention in preschool-age children: examining performance on a new attention battery. Society for Research in Child Development, Biennial Meeting. Boston, MA.

Brodsky MC (2001) Periventricular leukomalacia: an intracranial cause of pseudoglaucomtous cupping. *Arch Ophthlmol* 119: 626–7.

Brodsky MC (2002) Latent heliotropism. *Br J Ophthalmol* 86: 1327.

Brodsky MC, Glasier CM (1993) Optic nerve hypoplasia. Clinical significance of associated central nervous system abnormalities on magnetic resonance imaging. *Arch Ophthalmol* 111: 66–74.

Brodsky MC, Baker RS, Hamed LM (editors) (1996) *Pediatric neuro-ophthalmology.* New York: Springer-Verlag.

Brodsky MC, Fray KJ, Glasier CM (2002) Perinatal cortical and subcortical visual loss. *Ophthalmology* 109: 85–94.

Brown D (1997) Trends in the population of children with multi-sensory impairment. *Talking Sense* 43: 12–14.

Brown D, Bates E (2005) A personal view of changes in deaf-blind population, philosophy, and needs. *Deaf-Blind Perspectives* 12: 1–5.

Brown R, Hobson RP, Lee A, Stevenson J (1997) Are there 'autistic-like' features in congenitally blind children? *J Child Psychol Psychiatry* 38: 693–703.

Brown S, Schäfer EA (1888) An investigation into the functions of the occipital and temporal lobes of the monkey's brain. *Phil Trans R Soc Lond* 179: 303–27.

Buckley EG (1995) Pediatric neuro-ophthalmology examination. In: Wright KW, editor. *Pediatric Ophthalmology and Strabismus.* St Louis: Mosby, pp. 743–55.

Bunce C, Wormald R (2008) Causes of blind certifications in England and Wales: April 1999–March 2000. *Eye* 22: 905–11.

Buncic JR (1991) Normative values for visual fields in 4 to 12-year-old children using kinetic perimetry. *J Pediatr Ophthalmol Strabismus* 28: 154.

Burlingham D (1975) Special problems of blind infants. *Psychoanal Study Child* 30: 3–13.

Burton BK (1998) Inborn errors of metabolism in infancy: a guide to diagnosis. *Pediatrics* 102: E69.

Cacace AT, McFarland DJ (1998) Central auditory processing disorder in school-aged children: a critical review. *J Speech Lang Hear Res* 41: 355–73.

Cans C, Guillem P, Fauconnier J, Rambaud P, Jouk PS (2003) Disabilities and trends over time in a French county, 1980–91. *Arch Dis Child* 88: 114–17.

Cass H, Price K, Reilly S, Wisbeach A, McConachie H (1999) A model for the assessment and management of children with multiple disabilities. *Child Care Health Dev* 25: 191–211.

Cass H, Sonksen PM, McConachie HR (1994) Developmental setback in severe visual impairment. *Arch Dis Child* 70: 192–6.

Castano G, Lyons CJ, Jan JE, Connolly M (2000) Cortical visual impairment in children with infantile spasms. *J AAPOS* 4: 175–8.

Casteels I, Demaerel P, Spileers W, Lagae L, Missotten L, Casaer P (1997) Cortical visual impairment following perinatal hypoxia: clinicoradiologic correlation using magnetic resonance imaging. *J Pediatr Ophthalmol Strabismus* 34: 297–305.

Cavanagh P, Henaff MA, Michel F et al (1998) Complete sparing of high-contrast color input to motion perception in cortical color blindness. *Nat Neurosci* 1: 242–7.

Charman WN (2006) Spatial frequency content of the Cardiff and related acuity tests. *Ophthalmic Physiol Opt* 26: 5–12.

Chen D (1998) Early identification of infants who are deaf-blind: a systematic approach for early interventionists. *Deaf-Blind Perspectives* 5: 1–6.

Chen TC, Weinberg MH, Catalano RA, Simon JW, Wagle WA (1992) Development of object vision in infants with permanent cortical visual impairment. *Am J Ophthalmol* 114: 575–8.

Cioni G, Fazzi B, Ipata AE, Canapicchi R, van Hof-van Duin J (1996) Correlation between cerebral visual impairment and magnetic resonance imaging in children with neonatal encephalopathy. *Dev Med Child Neurol* 38: 120–32.

Cioni G, Fazzi B, Coluccini M, Bartalena L, Boldrini A, van Hof-van Duin J (1997) Cerebral visual impairment in preterm infants with periventricular leukomalacia. *Pediatr Neurol* 17: 331–8.

Cioni G, Brizzolara D, Ferretti G, Bertuccelli B, Fazzi B (1998) Visual information processing in infants with focal brain lesions. *Exp Brain Res* 123: 95–101.

Cioni G, Bertuccelli B, Boldrini A et al (2000) Correlation between visual function, neurodevelopmental outcome, and magnetic resonance imaging findings in infants with periventricular leucomalacia. *Arch Dis Child Fetal Neonatal Ed* 82: F134–40.

Claris O, Besnier S, Lapillonne A (1996) Incidence of ischemic–hemorrhagic cerebral lesions in premature infants of gestational age < or = 28 weeks: a prospective ultrasound study. *Biol Neonate* 70: 29–34.

Clark CA, Barrick TR, Murphy MM, Bell BA (2003) White matter fiber tracking in patients with space occupying lesions of the brain: a new technique for neurosurgical planning. *Neuroimage* 20: 601.

Clarke MP, Mitchell KW, Gibson M (1997) The prognostic value of flash visual evoked potentials in the assessment of non-ocular visual impairment in infancy. *Eye* 11: 398–402.

Cohen YE, Andersen RA (2002) A common reference frame for movement plans in the posterior parietal cortex. *Nature Rev Neurosci* 3: 553–62.

Cohen M, Roessmann U (1994) In utero brain damage: relationship of gestational age to pathological consequences. *Dev Med Child Neurol* 36: 263–8.

Colarusso RP, Hammill DD (2003) *Motor-Free Visual Perception Test*, 3rd edn (MVPT-3). Novato, CA: Academic Therapy Publications.

Colenbrander A (1994) The Functional Vision Score, a coordinated scoring system for visual impairments, disabilities and handicaps. In: Kooiman AC, Looijestijn PL, Welling JA et al, editors. *Low Vision – Research and New Developments in Rehabilitation*. Amsterdam: IOS Press, pp. 552–61.

Colenbrander A (2001) The visual system. In: Cocchiarella L, Anderson GBJ, editors. *Guides to the Evaluation of Permanent Impairment,* 5th edn. Chicago: AMA Press, Chapter 12, pp. 277–304.

Colenbrander A (2003) Aspects of vision loss – visual functions and functional vision. *Vis Impair Res* 5:115–36.

Colenbrander A (2005) Thoughts about the classification of "CVI". In: Dennison E, Hall Lueck A, editors. *Proceedings of the Summit on Cerebral/Cortical Visual Impairment: Educational, Family and Medical Perspectives. New* York: AFB Press, pp. 143–54.

Colenbrander A (2007) The visual system. In: Rondinelli et al., editors, 6th edn. *Guides to the Evaluation of Permanent Impairment*. Chicago: AMA Press, Chapter 12, pp. 281–319.

Conner IP, Sharma S, Lemieux SK, Mendola JD (2004) Retinotopic Organization in children measured with fMRI. *J Vis* 18: 509.

Connolly JD, Goodale MA, DeSouza JFX, Menon R, Vilis T (2000) A comparison of frontoparietal fMRI activation during anti-saccades and anti-pointing. *J Neurophysiol* 84: 1645–55.

Connolly JD, Andersen RA, Goodale MA (2003) FMRI evidence for a 'parietal reach region' in the human brain. *Exp Brain Res* 153: 140–5.

Connolly M, Jan J, Cochrane D (1991) Rapid recovery from visual impairment following correction of prolonged shunt malfunction in congenital hydrocephalus. *Arch Neurol* 48: 956–7.

Cornelissen P, Richardson A, Mason A, Fowler S, Stein J (1995) Contrast sensitivity and coherent motion detection measured at photopic luminance levels in dyslexics and controls. *Vision Res* 35: 1483–94.

Cowey A, Rolls ET (1974) Human cortical magnification factor and its relation to visual acuity. *Exp Brain Res* 21: 447–54.

Cowey A, Stoerig P (1991) The neurobiology of blindsight. *Trends Neurosci* 14: 140–5.

Crawford JD, Martinez-Trujillo JC, Klier EM (2003) Neural control of three-dimensional eye and head movements. *Curr Opin Neurobiol* 13: 655–62.

Cregg M, Woodhouse JM, Pakeman VH et al (2001) Accommodation and refractive error in children with Down syndrome: cross sectional and longitudinal studies. *Invest Ophthalmol Vis Sci* 42: 55–63.

Csocsán E, Klingberg O, Koskinen KL, Sjöstedt S (2002) *'Seen' with Other Eyes.* Helsinki: Schildts förlag, Ekenäs Tryckeri.

Culham JC, Kanwisher NG (2001) Neuroimaging of cognitive functions in human parietal cortex. *Curr Opin Neurobiol* 11: 157–63.

Culham JC, Valyear KF (2006) Human parietal cortex in action. *Curr Opin Neurobiol* 16: 205–12.

Culham JC, Danckert SL, DeSouza JFX, Gati JS, Menon RS, Goodale MA (2003) Visually-guided grasping produces fMRI activation in dorsal but not ventral stream brain areas. *Exp Brain Res* 153: 180–9.

Cummings JL, Gittinger JW (1981) Central dazzle: a thalamic syndrome? *Arch Neurol* 38: 372–4.

Cummings M, van Hof-van Duin J, Fulton AB, Mayer L (1987) Visual field assessment of young patients. *Invest Ophthal Vis Sci* 28(Suppl.): 202.

Dacey DM, Packer OS (2003) Colour coding in the primate retina: diverse cell types and cone-specific circuitry. *Curr Opin Neurobiol* 13: 421–7.

Dale N (2005) Early risk factors for developmental setback and autism in infants with visual impairment. In: Pring L, editor. *Autism and Blindness.* London: Whurr Publishers, pp. 74–98.

Dale N, Sonksen P (2002) Developmental outcome, including setback, in young children with severe visual impairment. *Dev Med Child Neurol* 44: 613–22.

Dalen K, Bruaroy S, Wentzel-Larsen T et al (2006) Non-verbal learning disabilities in children with infantile hydrocephalus, aged 4–7 years: a population-based, controlled study. *Neuropediatrics* 37: 1–5.

De Veber GA, Macgregor D, Curtis R, Mayank S (2000) Neurologic outcome in survivors of childhood arterial ischemic stroke and sinovenous thrombosis. *J Child Neurol* 15: 316–24.

De Vries LS, Dubowitz LMS (1985) Cystic leukomalacia in the preterm infant: site of lesion in relation to prognosis. *Lancet* 2: 1075–6.

De Vries LS, Connel JA, Dubowitz LMS, Oozeer RC, Dubowitz V, Pennock JM (1987) Neurological, electrophysiological and MRI abnormalities in infants with extensive cystic leukomalacia. *Neuropediatrics* 18: 61–6.

De Vries LS, Groenendaal F, Eken P et al (1997) Infarcts in the vascular distribution of the middle cerebral artery in preterm and full-term infants. *Neuropediatrics* 28: 88–96.

Dean P, Redgrave P, Westby GWM (1989) Event or emergency? Two response systems in the mammalian superior colliculus. *Trends Neurosci* 12: 137–47.

Dekker R (1989) *ITVIC: Intelligence Test for Visually Impaired Children, 6–15 years.* Netherlands: Bartimeus.

Delaney SM, Dobson V, Mohan KM (2005) Measured visual field extent varies with peripheral stimulus flicker rate in very young children. *Optom Vis Sci* 82: 800.

Denny-Brown D, Chambers RA (1976) Physiological aspects of visual perception. I. Functional aspects of visual cortex. *Arch Neurol* 33: 219–27.

Desmonts G, Couvreur J (1974) Congenital toxoplasmosis. A prospective study of 378 pregnancies. *N Engl J Med* 290: 1110–16.

Detheridge T, Detheridge M (2002) *Literacy Through Symbols: Improving Access for Children and Adults.* London: David Fulton Publishers.

Dobson V, Mayer D L, Lee CP (1980) Visual acuity of preterm infants. *Invest Ophthalmol Vis Sci* 19: 1498–1505.

Dodd B, Carr A (2003) Young children's letter-sound knowledge. *Lang Speech Hear Serv Sch* 34: 128–37.

Dowdeswell HJ, Slater AM, Broomhall J, Tripp J (1995) Visual deficits in children born at less than 32 weeks' gestation with and without major ocular pathology and cerebral damage. *Br J Ophthalmol* 79: 447–52.

Drummond SR, Dutton GN (2007) Simultanagnosia following perinatal hypoxia – a possible pediatric variant of Balint syndrome. *J AAPOS* 11: 497–8.

Du JW, Schmid KL, Bevan JD, Frater KM, Ollett R (2005) Retrospective analysis of refractive errors in children with visual impairment. *Optom Vis Sci* 82: 807–16.

Dubowitz LMS, Mushin J, Morante A, Placzek M (1983) The maturation of visual acuity in neurologically normal and abnormal newborn infants. *Behav Brain Res* 10: 39–45.

Dubowitz LMS, Dubowitz V, Mercuri E (1998) *The Neurological Assessment of the Pre-Term and Full-Term Newborn Infant*, 2nd edn. London: Mac Keith Press.

Duckman R (1979) The incidence of visual anomalies in a population of cerebral palsied children. *J Am Optom Assoc* 50: 1013–16.

Dumoulin SO, Jirsch JD, Bernasconi A (2007) Functional organization of human visual cortex in occipital polymicrogyria. *Hum Brain Mapp* 28: 1302–12.

Durkel J (2001) Central Auditory Processing Disorder and Auditory Neuropathy. *See/Hear* 6: 26–9. *Education Reform Act 1988* (available from: www.opsi.gov.uk/Acts/acts1988/Ukpga_19880040_en_2.htm/).

Dutton GN (1994) Cognitive visual dysfunction. *Br J Ophthalmol* 78: 723–6.

Dutton G (2003) Cognitive vision, its disorders and differential diagnosis in adults and children: knowing where and what things are. *Eye* 17: 289–304.

Dutton GN (2009) 'Dorsal stream dysfunction' and 'dorsal stream dysfunction plus': a potential classification for perceptual visual impairment in the context of cerebral visual impairment? *Dev Med Child Neurol* 51:170–2.

Dutton GN, Jacobson LK (2001) Cerebral visual impairment in children. *Semin Neonatol* 6: 477–85.

Dutton G, Ballantyne J, Boyd G et al (1996) Cortical visual dysfunction in children: a clinical study. *Eye* 10: 302–9.

Dutton GN, Day RE, McCulloch DL (1999) Who is visually impaired child? A model is needed to address this question for children with cerebral visual impairment. *Dev Med Child Neurol* 41: 212–13.

Dutton GN, Saaed A, Fahad B et al (2004) Association of binocular lower VF impairment, impaired simultaneous perception disordered visually guided motion and inaccurate saccades in children with cerebral visual dysfunction: a retrospective study. *Eye* 18: 27–34.

Dyet LE, Kennea N, Counsell SJ (2006) Natural history of brain lesions in extremely preterm infants studied with serial magnetic resonance imaging from birth and neurodevelopmental assessment. *Pediatrics* 118: 536–48.

Edmond JC, Foroozan R (2006) Cortical visual impairment in children. *Curr Opin Ophthalmol* 17: 509–12.

Ehri L (1991) Development of the ability to read words. In: Barr R, Kamil M, Mosenthal R, Peterson P, editors. *Handbook of Reading Research 2*. New York: Longman, pp. 383–417.

Eken P, van Nieuwenhuizen O, van der Graaf Y, Schalij-Delfos NE, de Vries L (1994) Relation between neonatal cranial ultrasound abnormalities and cerebral visual impairment in infancy. *Dev Med Child Neurol* 36: 3–15.

Eken P, de Vries L, van der Graaf Y, Meiners LC, van Nieuwenhuizen O (1995) Haemorrhagic–ischaemic lesions of the neonatal brain: correlation between cerebral visual impairment, neurodevelopmental outcome and MRI in infancy. *Dev Med Child Neurol* 37: 41–55.

Eken P, de Vries L, van Nieuwenhuizen O, Schalij-Delfos NE, Reits D, Spekreijse H (1996) Early predictors of cerebral visual impairment in infants with cystic leukomalacia. *Neuropediatrics* 27: 16–25.

El Azazi M, Malm G, Forsgren M (1990) Late ophthalmologic manifestations of neonatal herpes simplex virus infection. *Am J Ophthalmol* 109: 1–7.

Epstein R, Kanwisher N (1998) A cortical representation of the local visual environment. *Nature* 392: 598–601.

Eskandar EM, Richmond BJ, Optican LM (1992) Role of inferior temporal neurons in visual memory I. Temporal encoding of information about visual images, recalled images, and behavioral context. *J Neurophysiol* 68: 1277–95.

Eyre JA (2003) Development and plasticity of the corticospinal system in man. *Neural Plast* 10: 93–106.

Fantz RL (1964) Visual experience in infants: decreased attention to familiar patterns relative to novel ones. *Science* 146: 668–70.

Fantz RL (1965) Visual perception from birth as shown by pattern selectivity. *Ann N Y Acad Sci* 118: 793–814.

Farah MJ (1990) *Visual Agnosia: Disorders of Object Vision and What They Tell us About Normal Vision*. Cambridge, MA: MIT Press/Bradford.

Fausset T, Enoch J (1987) A rapid technique for kinetic visual field determination in young children and adults with central retinal lesions. Proceedings VII International Visual Field Symposium, Amsterdam, September 1986. *Doc Ophthalmol Proc Ser* 49: 495.

Fazzi E, Lanners J, Danova S et al (1999) Stereotyped behaviour in blind children. *Brain Dev* 21: 522–8.

Fazzi E, Lanners J, Ferrari G et al (2002) Gross motor development and reach on sound as critical tools for the development of the blind child. *Brain Dev* 24: 269–75.

Fazzi E, Bova AM, Uggetti C et al (2004) Visual-perceptual impairment in children with periventricular leukomalacia. *Brain Dev* 26: 506–12.

Fazzi E, Signorini G, Bova SM et al (2007a) Spectrum of visual disorders in children with cerebral visual impairment. *J Child Neurol* 22: 294–301.

Fazzi E, Rossi M, Signorini S, Rossi G, Bianchi PE, Lanzi G (2007b) Leber's congenital amaurosis: is there an autistic component? *Dev Med Child Neurol* 49: 503–7.

Fea AM, Delpiano M, Soldi A et al (1995) Photopic visual field in 2 months old infants. In: Lennerstrand G, editor. *Update on Strabismus and Pediatric Ophthalmology. Proceeding of the Joint ISA and AAPO&S Meeting, Vancouver, Canada, 19–23 June 1994.* Boca Raton: CRC Press, pp. 27–30.

Fedrizzi E, Inverno M, Botteon G, Anderloni A, Filippini G, Farinotti M (1993) The cognitive development of children born preterm and affected by spastic diplegia. *Brain Dev* 15: 428–32.

Fedrizzi E, Inverno M, Bruzzone MG, Botteon G, Saletti V, Farinotti M (1996) MRI features of cerebral lesions and cognitive functions in preterm spastic diplegic children. *Pediatr Neurol* 15: 207–12.

Fedrizzi E, Anderloni A, Bono R et al (1998) Eye-movement disorders and visual-perceptual impairment in diplegic children born preterm: a clinical evaluation. *Dev Med Child Neurol* 40: 682–8.

Fernell E, Hagberg B, Hagberg G, von Wendt L (1986) Epidemiology of infantile hydrocephalus in Sweden Birth prevalence and general data. *Acta Paediatr Scand* 75: 975–81.

Fernell E, Hagberg B, Hagberg G, Hult G, von Wendt L (1988a) Epidemiology of infantile hydrocephalus in Sweden: a clinical follow-up study in children born at term. *Neuropediatrics* 19: 135–42.

Fernell E, Hagberg B, Hagberg G, Hult G, von Wendt L (1988b) Epidemiology of infantile hydrocephalus in Sweden. Current aspects of outcome in preterm infants. *Neuropediatrics* 19: 143–5.

Ferrier D, Yeo GF (1884) A record of experiments on the effects of lesion of different regions of the cerebral hemispheres. *Phil Trans R Soc Lond* 175: 479–564.

Fetter WPF, van Hof-van Duin J, Baerts W, Heersma DJ, Wildervanck De Blecourt-Devillee M (1992) Visual acuity and visual field development after cryocoagulation in infants with retinopathy of prematurity. *Acta Pediat* 81: 25.

Field GD, Chichilnisky EJ (2007) Information processing in the primate retina: Circuitry and coding. *Ann Rev Neurosci* 30: 1–30.

Fielder AR (1993) Ophthalmic Management. In: Fielder AR, Best AB, Bax MCO, editors. *The Management of Visual Impairment in Childhood.* Cambridge: Cambridge University Press, pp. 91–8.

Flanagan NM, Jackson AJ, Hill AE (2003) Visual impairment in childhood: insights from a community-based survey. *Child Care Health Dev* 29: 493–9.

Flodmark O, Lupton B, Li D (1987) Periventricular leukomalacia: radiologic diagnosis. *Radiology* 162: 119–24.

Flodmark O, Roland EH, Hill A, Whitfield MF (1989) MR imaging of periventricular leukomalacia in childhood. *AJR Am J Roentgenol* 152: 583–90.

Flodmark O, Jan JE, Wong PK (1990) Computed tomography of the brains of children with cortical visual impairment. *Dev Med Child Neurol* 32: 611–20.

Folkerth RD (2005) Neuropathologic substrate of cerebral palsy. *Child Neurol* 20: 940–9.

Fraiberg S (1977) *Insights from the Blind.* New York: Basic Books.

Fraiberg S, Siegel BL, Gibson R (1966) The role of sound in the search behavior of the blind infant. *Psychoanal Study Child* 26: 327–57.

Freeman RD (1967) The child psychiatric home visit: its place in diagnosis and training. *J Am Acad Child Adolesc Psychiatry* 6: 276–94.

Freeman RD, Jan JE (1996) Rapid cycling affective disorders in mentally retarded children. *Semin Clin Neuropsychiatry* 1: 134–41.

Freeman RD, Goetz E, Richards DP, Groenveld M (1991) Defiers of negative prediction: results of a 14-year follow-up study. *J Vis Impair Blind* 85: 365–70.

Frisen L (1991) A child's play version of high-pass resolution perimetry. In: Mills R, Hejil A, editors. *Perimetry Update 1990–91. Proceeding of the IXth International Perimetric Society Meeting.* Amsterdam: Kugler Publisher, pp. 349–52.

Frith U (1985) Beneath the surface of developmental dyslexia. In: Patterson KE, Marshall JC, Coltheart M, editors. *Surface Dyslexia: Neuropsychological and Cognitive Studies of Phonological Reading.* London: Lawrence Erlbaum, pp. 301–30.

Gale G, Cronin P (1989) The School Years. In: Kelley P, Gale G, editors. *Towards Excellence. Effective Education for Students with Vision Impairments.* Sydney: North Rocks Press.

Gallese V, Murata A, Kaseda M, Niki N, Sakata H (1994) Deficit of hand preshaping after muscimol injection in monkey parietal cortex. *Neuroreport* 5: 1525–9.

Gamlin PD (2005) The pretectum: connections and oculomotor-related roles. *Prog Brain Res* 151: 379–405.

Gaston H (1985) Does the Spina Bifida clinic need an ophthalmologist? *Z Kinderchir* 40: 46–50.

Gegenfurtner KR, Kiper DC (2003) Color vision. *Annu Rev Neurosci* 26: 181–206.

Gerstadt CL, Hong YJ, Diamond A (1994) The relationship between cognition and action: performance of children 3 1/2–7 years old on a Stroop-like day–night test. *Cognition 53: 129–53.*

Ghasia F, Brunstrom J, Gordon M, Tychsen L (2008) Frequency and severity of visual sensory and motor deficits in children with cerebral palsy: gross motor function classification scale. *Invest Ophthalmol Vis Sci* 49: 572–80.

Gibson NA, Fielder AR, Trounce JQ, Levine MI (1990) Ophthalmic findings in infants of very low birthweight. *Dev Med Child Neurol* 32: 7–13.

Gillen JA, Dutton GN (2003) Balints syndrome in a 10 year old male. *Devel Med Child Neurol* 45: 349–52.

Girkin CA, Miller NR (2001) Central disorders of vision in humans. *Surv Ophthalmol* 45: 379–405.

Glass HC, Fujimoto S, Ceppi-Cozzio C et al (2007) White-matter injury is associated with impaired gaze in premature infants. *Pediatric Neurol* 38: 10–15.

Glickstein M, Buchbinder S, May JL 3rd (1998) Visual control of the arm, the wrist and the fingers: pathways through the brain. *Neuropsychologia* 36: 981–1001.

Goldstein M, Bax M (2009) Quality of life for the young adult with neurodisability. *Dev Med Child Neurol* 51: 665.

Good WV (1993) Ophthalmology of visual impairment. In: Fielder AR, Best AB, Bax MCO, editors. *The Managment of Visual Impairment in Childhood.* London: Mac Keith Press, pp. 30–47.

Good WV (2001) Development of a quantitative method to measure vision in children with chronic cortical visual impairment. *Trans Am Ophthalmol Soc* 99: 253–69.

Good WV, Hou C (2004) Normal vernier acuity in infants with delayed visual maturation. *Am J Ophthalmol* 138: 140–2.

Good WV, Hou C (2006) Sweep visual evoked potential grating acuity thresholds paradoxically improve in low-luminance conditions in children with cortical visual impairment. *Invest Ophthalmol Vis Sci* 47: 3220–4.

Good WV, Hoyt CS (1989) Behavioral correlates of poor vision in children. *Int Ophthalmol Clin* 29: 57–60.

Good WV, Hoyt CS, Lambert SR (1987) Optic nerve atrophy in children with hypoxia. *Invest Ophthalmol Vis Sci* 28(Suppl): 309.

Good WV, Jan JE, Desa L, Barkovich AJ, Groenveld M, Hoyt CS (1994) Cortical visual impairment in children. *Surv Ophthalmol* 38: 351–64.

Good WV, Jan JE, Burden SK, Skoczenski A, Candy R (2001) Recent advances in cortical visual impairment. *Dev Med Child Neurol* 43: 56–60.

Good WV, Hou C, Madan A, Norcia AM (2008) Effect of Grade I and Grade II intraventricular hemorrhage on visuocortical function in the very low birth weight infant. *Invest Ophthalmol Vis Sci*, submitted.

Goodale MA (1998) Vision for perception and vision for action in the primate brain. *Novartis Found Symp* 218: 21–34 and 34–39 [Discussion].

Goodale MA, Milner AD (1992) Separate visual pathways for perception and action. *Trends Neurosci* 15: 20–5.

Goodale MA, Milner AD (2004) *Sight Unseen: An Exploration of Conscious and Unconscious Vision.* Oxford: Oxford University Press.

Goodale MA, Westwood DA (2004) An evolving view of duplex vision: separate but interacting cortical pathways for perception and action. *Curr Opin Neurobiol* 14: 203–11.

Goodale MA, Milner AD, Jakobson LS, Carey DP (1991) A neurological dissociation between perceiving objects and grasping them. *Nature* 349: 154–6.

Goodale MA, Westwood DA, Milner AD (2004) Two distinct modes of control for object-directed action. *Progr Brain Res* 144: 131–44.

Goren CC, Sarty M, Wu PY (1975) Visual following and pattern discrimination of face-like stimuli by newborn infants. *Pediatrics* 56: 544–9.

Gote H, Gregersen E, Rindziunski E (1993) Exotropia and panoramic vision compensating for an occult congenital homonymous hemianopia. A case report. *Binocul Vis Strabismus Q* 8: 129.

Goto M, Ota R, Iai M, Sugita K, Tanabe Y (1994) MRI changes and deficits of higher brain functions in preterm diplegia. *Acta Paediatr* 83: 506–11.

Gouras P (1991) Colour vision. In: Kandel ER, Schwartz JH, Jessell TM, editors. *Principles of Neuroscience,* 3rd edn. New York: Elsevier, pp. 384–95.

Gray M (1996) Problems in trans-disciplinary approach. In: de Jong C, Neugebauer H, editors. *Timely Intervention: Special Help for Special Needs*. Wurzburgh: edition bentheim, pp. 107–13.

Greitz D (2004) Radiological assessment of hydrocephalus: new theories and implications for therapy. *Neurosurg Rev* 27: 145–65, discussion 166–7.

Grill-Spector K, Malach R (2004) The human visual cortex. *Annu Rev Neurosci* 27: 649–77.

Groenendaal F, van Hof-van Duin J (1990) Partial recovery in two full-term infants after perinatal hypoxia. *Neuropediatrics* 21: 76.

Groenendaal F, van Hof-van Duin J (1992) Visual deficits and improvements in children after perinatal hypoxia. *J Vis Impair Blind* 86: 215–18.

Groenendaal F, van Hof-van Duin J, Baerts W, Fetter WP (1989) Effects of perinatal hypoxia on visual development during the first year of (corrected) age. *Early Hum Dev* 20: 267–79.

Groenveld M (1990) The dilemma of assessing the visually impaired child. *Dev Med Child Neurol* 32: 1105–13.

Groenveld M, Jan JE, Leader P (1990) Observations on the habilitation of children with cortical visual impairment. *Vis Impair and Blind* 84: 11–15.

Gronqvist S, Flodmark O, Tornqvist K (2001) Association between visual impairment and functional and morphological cerebral abnormalities in full-term children. *Acta Ophthalmol Scand* 79: 140–6.

Gross CG, Rocha-Miranda CE, Bender DB (1972) Visual properties of neurons in inferotemporal cortex of the macaque. *J Neurophysiol* 35: 96–111.

Grusser O-J, T Landis (1991) Visual agnosias and other disturbances of visual perception and cognition. In: Cronly-Dillon JR, editor. *Vision and Visual Dysfunction*. London: Macmillan Press.

Gunn A, Cory E, Atkinson J et al (2002) Dorsal and ventral stream sensitivity in normal development and hemiplegia. *NeuroReport* 13: 843–7.

Guzzetta A, Mercuri E, Cioni G (2001) Visual disorders in children with brain lesions: 2. Visual impairment associated with cerebral palsy. *Eur J Paediatr Neurol* 5: 115–19.

Gwiazda J, Bauer J, Held R (1989a) From visual acuity to hyperacuity: a 10-year update. *Can J Psychol* 43: 109–20.

Gwiazda J, Bauer J, Held R (1989b) Binocular function in human infants: correlation of stereoptic and fusion-rivalry discriminations. *J Pediatr Ophthalmol Strabismus* 26: 128–32.

Gwiazda J, Bauer J, Thorn F, Held R (1997) Development of spatial contrast sensitivity from infancy to adulthood: psychophysical data. *Optom Vis Sci* 74: 785–9.

Hadenius AM, Hagberg B, Hyttnäs-Bensch K, Sjögren I (1962) Congenital hydrocephalus. II. Long term prognosis of untreated hydrocephalus in infants. *Nord Med* 68: 1515–19.

Hadjikhani N, Tootell RB (2000) Projection of rods and cones within human visual cortex. *Hum Brain Mapp* 9: 55–63.

Hambleton G, Wigglesworth JS (1976) Origin of intraventricular haemorrhage in the preterm infant. *Arch Dis Child* 51: 651–9.

Hamer RD, Mayer DL (1994) The development of spatial vision. In: Albert D, Jakobiec FA, editors. *Principles and Practice of Ophthalmology: Basic Sciences*. Philadelphia: WB Saunders Co., ch. 42.

Hammill DD, Pearson NA, Voress JK (1993) *Frostig – Developmental Test of Visual Perception*, 2nd edn (DTVP-2). Mountain View, CA: Consulting Psychologists Press.

Harcourt B, Jay B (1968) Bilateral optic atrophy in childhood. II. *Br J Ophthalmol* 52: 860–1.

Harris SJ, Hansen RM, Fulton AB (1984) Assessment of acuity in human infants using face and grating stimuli. *Invest Ophthalmol Vis Sci* 25: 782–6.

Harris SJ, Hansen RM, Fulton AB (1986) Assessment of acuity of amblyopic subjects using face, grating, and recognition stimuli. *Invest Ophthalmol Vis Sci* 27: 1184–7.

Harvey EM, Dobson V, Luna B, Scher MS (1997a) Grating acuity and visual-field development in children with intraventricular hemorrhage. *Dev Med Child Neurol* 39: 305–12.

Harvey EM, Dobson V, Narter DB (1997b) The influence of a central stimulus on visual field measurements in children from 3.5 to 30 months of age. *Optom Vis Sci* 74: 768.

Hatton DD, Schwietz E, Boyer B, Rychwalski P (2007) Babies Count: the national registry for children with visual impairments, birth to 3 years. *JAAPOS* 11: 351–5.

Hayashi N, Tsutsumi Y, Barkovich AJ (2002) Morphological features and associated anomalies of schizencephaly in the clinical population: detailed analysis of MR images. *Neuroradiology* 44: 418–27.

Heaton SC, Reader SK, Preston AS et al (2001) The Test of Everyday Attention for Children (TEA-Ch): patterns of performance in children with ADHD and clinical controls. *Child Neuropsychol* 7: 251–64.

Heersema DJ, van Hof-van Duin J, Hop WCJ (1989) Age norms for visual field development in children aged 0 to 4 years using arc perimetry. *Invest Ophthal Vis Sci* 30: 242.

Heinsbergen I, Rotteveel J, Roeveld N, Grothenius A (2002) Outcome in shunted hydrocephalic children. *Eur J Paediatr Neurol* 6: 99–107.

Hensch TK (2005) Critical period mechanisms in developing visual cortex. *Curr Top Dev Biol* 69: 215–37.

Hermans AJM (1995) Development of visual functions during the first two years of life in infants with birth weights between 1500 and 2500 gram [Thesis]. Rotterdam: CIP Printing.

Hermans AJM, van Hof-van Duin J, Oudesluys-Murphy AM (1994) Visual outcome of low birth-weight infants (1500–2500g) at one year of corrected age. *Acta Paediatr* 83: 402.

Hertz-Pannier L (1999) Brain plasticity during development: physiological bases and functional MRI approach. *J Neuroradiol* 26: 66.

Herzau V, Bleher I, Joos-Kratsch E (1988) Infantile exotropia with homonimous hemianopia: a rare contraindication for strabismus surgery. *Graefes Arch Clin Exp Ophthalmol* 226: 148.

Herzog ED (2007) Neurons and networks in daily rhythms. *Nature Rev Neurosci* 8: 790–802.

Hirsch MJ, Weymouth FW (1991) Prevalence of refractive anomalies. In: Grosvenor T, Flom MC, editors. *Refractive Anomalies.* Stoneham: Butterworth-Heinemann, p. 15.

Hodes D, Sonksen PM, McKee M (1994) Evaluation of the Sonksen Picture Test for detection of minor visual errors in preschool children. *Dev Med Child Neurol* 36: 16–25.

Hoffman DD (1998) *Visual Intelligence: How we Create What we See.* New York: Norton & Company.

Holmes G (1918a) Disturbances of vision by cerebral lesions. *Br J Ophthalmol* 2: 353–84.

Holmes G (1918b) Disturbances of visual orientation. *Br J Ophthalmol* 2: 449–68, 506–16.

Hood B (1995) Gravity rules for 2–4 year olds. *Cogn Devel* 10: 577–98.

Hood B, Atkinson J (1990) Sensory visual loss and cognitive deficits in the selective attentional system of normal infants and neurologically impaired children. *Dev Med Child Neurol* 32: 1067–77.

Hood LJ (1998) Auditory neuropathy: What is it and what can we do about it? *The Hearing Journal* 51: 10–18.

Hoon AH, Lawrie WT, Melhem ER et al (2002) Diffusion tensor imaging of periventricular leucomalacia shows affected sensory cortex white matter pathways. *Neurology* 59: 752.

Hoppe-Hirsch E, Laroussinie F, Brunet L et al (1998) Late outcome of the surgical treatment of hydrocephalus. *Childs Nerv Syst* 14: 97–9.

Horton JC (2005) Disappointing results from Nova Visions visual restoration therapy. *Br J Ophthalmol* 89: 30.

Horton JC (2006) Ocular integration in the human visual cortex. *Can J Ophthalmol* 41: 584.

Hou C, Good WV, Norcia AM (2007) Validation study of VEP vernier acuity in normal-vision and amblyopic adults. *Invest Ophthalmol Vis Sci* 48: 4070–8.

Houliston M, Taguri A, Dutton G, Hajivassiliou C, Young D (1999) Evidence of cognitive visual problems in children with hydrocephalus: a structured clinical history-taking strategy. *Dev Med Child Neurol* 41: 298–306.

Hoyt CS (2003) Visual function in the brain-damaged child. *Eye* 17: 369–84.

Hoyt CS (2007) Brain injury and the eye. *Eye* 21: 1285–9.

Hoyt CS, Fredrick DR (1998) Cortically visually impaired children: a need for more study. *Br J Ophthalmol* 82: 1225–6.

Hoyt CS, Good WV (2001) The many challenges of childhood blindness. *Br J Ophthalmol* 85: 1145–6.

Hoyt CS, Nickel BL, Billson FA (1982) Ophthalmological examination of the infant. Developmental aspects. *Surv Ophthalmol* 26: 177–89.

Hrbek A, Karlberg P, Olsson T (1973) Development of visual and somatosensory evoked responses in pre-term newborn infants. *Electroencephalogr Clin Neurophysiol* 34: 225–32.

Hubel DH (1995) *Eye, Brain and Vision.* New York: Scientific American Library.

Hughes C, Russell J (1993) Autistic children's difficulty with mental disengagement from an object: its implications for theories of autism. *Dev Psychol* 29: 498–510.

Huo R, Burden S, Hoyt CS, Good WV (1999) Chronic cortical visual impairment in children: aetiology, prognosis, and associated neurological deficits. *Br J Ophthalmol* 83: 670–5.

Hüppi PS, Dubois J (2006) Diffusion tensor imaging of brain development. *Sem Fet Neonatol Med* 11: 489.

Hyvärinen L (2000) *How to Classify Paediatric Low Vision*? ICEVI Conference 2000 (available at: http://lea-test.fi/en/assessme/cracow.html; last accessed 27 March 2010).

Hyvarinen L (2002) Vision rehabilitation in homonymous hemianopia. *Neuro Ophthalmol* 27: 97.

Hyvärinen L (2008) Cerebrale Sehschädigungen im Kindesalter. In: Leyendecker C, editor. *Gemeinsam Handeln statt Behandeln.* Munich: Reinhardt, pp. 118–126.

Hyvärinen L (2009) Probleme der Zusammenarbeit zwischen Medizen und Pädagogik bei zerebralen Sehstörungen. (Editors: Beck F-J, Drave W, Fuchs E) Kongressbericht, XXXIV Knogress, Verband der Blinden- und Sehbehindertenpädagogen, Edition Bentheim, Würzburg.

Hyvärinen L (2010) *Grating Acuity Test at Low Contrast Levels* (available at http://lea-test.fi/en/vistests/instruct/contrast/grating/grating.html; last accessed 27 March 2010).

Hyvärinen J, Poranen A (1974) Function of the parietal associative area 7 as revealed from cellular discharges in alert monkeys. *Brain* 97: 673–92.

Hyvärinen L, Rovamo J, Laurinen P, Peltomaa A (1981) Contrast sensitivity function in evaluation of visual impairment due to retinitis pigmentosa. *Acta Ophthalmol* 59: 763–73.

Hyvärinen L, Laurinen P, Rovamo J (1983) Contrast sensitivity in evaluation of visual impairment due to macular degeneration and optic nerve lesions. *Acta Ophthalmol* 61: 161–70.

Ingle DJ (1982) Organization of visuomotor behaviors in vertebrates. In: Ingle DJ, Goodale MA, Mansfield RJW, editors. *Analysis of Visual Behavior*. Cambridge, MA: MIT Press, pp. 67–109.

International Council of Ophthalmology (2002) *Visual Standards, Aspects and Ranges of Vision Loss with emphasis on Population Surveys* (available at: www.icoph.org/standards).

Ipata AE, Cioni G, Bottai P, Fazzi B, Canapicchi R, van Hof-van Duin J (1994) Acuity card testing in children with cerebral palsy related to magnetic resonance images, mental levels and motor abilities. *Brain Dev* 16: 195–203.

Ito J, Saijo H, Araki A et al (1996) Assessment of visuoperceptual disturbance in children with spastic diplegia using measurements of the lateral ventricles on cerebral MRI. *Dev Med Child Neurol* 38: 496–502.

Iwata S, Iwata O, Bainbridge A et al (2007) Abnormal white matter appearance on term FLAIR predicts neuro-developmental outcome at 6 years old following preterm birth. *Int J Dev Neurosci* 25: 523–30.

Jacobson L, Dutton GN (2000) Periventricular leucomalacia: an important cause of visual and ocular motility dysfunction in children. *Surv Ophthalmol* 45: 1–13.

Jacobson L, Ek U, Fernell E, Flodmark O, Broberger U (1996) Visual impairment in preterm children with periventricular leukomalacia-visual, cognitive and neuropaediatric characteristics related to cerebral imaging. *Dev Med Child Neurol* 38: 724–36.

Jacobson L, Lundin S, Flodmark O, Ellstrom KG (1998a) Periventricular leukomalacia causes visual impairment in preterm children. A study on the aetiologies of visual impairment in a population-based group of preterm children born 1989–95 in the county of Varmland, Sweden. *Acta Ophthalmol Scand* 76: 593–8.

Jacobson L, Flodmark O, Ygge J (1998b) Nystagmus in periventricular leucomalacia. *Br J Ophthalmol* 82: 1026–32.

Jacobson L, Ygge J, Flodmark O, Ek U (2002) Visual and perceptual characteristics, ocular motility and strabismus in children with periventricular leukomalcia. *Strabismus* 10: 179–83.

Jacobson L, Hård AL, Svensson E, Flodmark O, Hellström A (2003) Optic disc morphology may reveal timing of insult in children with periventricular leukomalacia and/or periventricular haemorrhage. *Br J Ophthalmol* 87: 1345–9.

Jacobson L, Flodmark O, Martin L (2006) Visual field defects in prematurely born patients with white matter damage of immaturisty: a multiple-case study. *Acta Ophthalmol* 84: 357–62.

Jakobson LS, Frisk V, Downie AL (2006) Motion-defined form processing in extremely premature children. *Neuropsychologia* 44: 1777–86.

James TW, Culham JC, Humphrey GK, Milner AD, Goodale MA (2003) Ventral occipital lesions impair object recognition but not object-directed grasping: a fMRI study. *Brain* 126: 2463–75.

Jan JE (1991) Head movements of visually impaired children. *Dev Med Child Neurol* 33: 645–7.

Jan JE (2001) Changing patterns of visual impairment. *Dev Med Child Neurol* 43: 219 [Editorial].

Jan JE, Freeman RD (1998) Who is a visually impaired child? *Dev Med Child Neurol* 40: 65–7.

Jan JE, Groenveld M (1993) Visual behaviors and adaptations associated with cortical and ocular impairment in children. *J Vis Impair Blind* 87: 101–5.

Jan JE, Wong PK (1988) Behaviour of the alpha rhythm in electroencephalograms of visually impaired children. *Dev Med Child Neurol* 30: 444–50.

Jan JE, Wong PKH (1991) The child with cortical visual impairment. *Sem Ophthalmol* 6: 194–200.

Jan JE, Robinson GC, Scott E, Kinnis C (1975) Hypotonia in the blind child. *Dev Med Child Neurol* 17: 35–40.

Jan JE, Freeman RD, Scott EP (1977) Stereotyped behavior. In: *Visual Impairment in Children and Adolescents*. New York: Grune & Stratton, pp. 239–55.

Jan JE, Wong PK, Groenveld M, Flodmark O, Hoyt CS (1986) Travel vision: 'collicular visual system'? *Pediatr Neurol* 2: 359–62.

Jan JE, Groenveld M, Sykanda AM, Hoyt CS (1987) Behavioural characteristics of children with permanent cortical visual impairment. *Dev Med Child Neurol* 29: 571–6.

Jan JE, Groenveld M, Sykanda AM (1990a) Light-gazing by visually impaired children. *Dev Med Child Neurol* 32: 755–9.

Jan JE, Sykanda A, Groenveld M (1990b) Habilitation and rehabilitation of visually impaired and blind children. *Pediatrician* 17: 202–7.

Jan JE, Groenveld M, Anderson DP (1993) Photophobia and cortical visual impairment. *Dev Med Child Neurol* 35: 473–7.

Jan JE, Freeman RD, Espezel H (1994a) Eye-poking. *Dev Med Child Neurol* 36: 321–5.

Jan JE, Abroms IF, Freeman RD, Brown GM, Espezel H, Connolly MB (1994b) Rapid cycling in severely multihandicapped children: a form of bipolar affective disorder? *Pediatr Neurol* 10: 34–9.

Jan JE, Freeman RD, Fast DK (1999) Melatonin treatment of sleep–wake cycle disorders in children and adolescents. *Dev Med Child Neurol* 41: 491–500.

Jan JE, Lyons CJ, Heaven R, Matsuba C (2001) Visual impairment due to a dyskinetic eye movement disorder in children with dyskinetic cerebral palsy. *Dev Med Child Neurol* 43: 108–12.

Jerger J, Musiek F (2000) Report of the consensus conference on the diagnosis of auditory processing disorders in school-aged children. *J Am Acad Audiol* 11: 467–74.

Johnson C, Kran BS, Deng L, Mayer DL (2009) Teller II and Cardiff acuity testing in a school-age deafblind population. *Optom Vis Sci* 86: 188–95.

Johnson CD, Benson PV, Seaton JB (1997) *Educational Audiology Handbook*. San Diego: Singular Publishing Group.

Kaas JH, Lyon DC (2007) Pulvinar contributions to the dorsal and ventral streams of visual processing in primates. *Brain Res Rev* 55: 285–96.

Kanwisher N, McDermott J, Chun MM (1997) The fusiform face area: a module in human extrastriate cortex specialized for face perception. *J Neurosci* 17: 4302–11.

Kapellou O, Counsell SJ, Kennea N et al (2006) Abnormal cortical development after premature birth shown by altered allometric scaling of brain growth. *PLoS Med* 3: e265.

Kaplan E, Mukherjee P, Shapey R (1993) Information filtering in the lateral geniculate nucleus. In: Shapley R, Man-Kit Lam D, editors. *Contrast Sensitivity*. Cambridge, MA: MIT Press, 183–200.

Kasten E, Poggel DA, Muller-Oehring E, Gothe J, Schulte T, Sabel BA (1999) Restoration of vision II: residual functions and training-induced visual field enlargement in brain-damaged patients. *Restor Neuro Neurosci* 15: 273.

Katayama M, Tamas LB (1987) Saccadic eye-movements of children with cerebral palsy. *Dev Med Child Neurol* 29: 36–9.

Kedar S, Zhang X, Lynn MJ, Newman NJ, Biousse V (2006) Pediatric homonymous hemianopia. *J Pediatr Ophthalmol Strabismus* 10: 249.

Keenan H, Runyan DK, Marshall SW et al (2003) A population-based study of inflicted traumatic brain injury in young children. *JAMA* 290: 621–6.

Keeney S, Adock EW, McArdle CB (1991) Prospective observations of 100 high-risk neonates by high-field (1.5 Tesla) magnetic resonance imaging of the central nervous system. II. Lesions associated with hypoxic-ischaemic encephalopathy. *Pediatrics* 87: 431.

Kelley P, Gale G, Blatch P (1998) Theoretical framework. In: Kelley P, Gale G, editors. *Towards Excellence. Effective Education for Students with Vision Impairments*. Sydney: North Rocks Press.

Kelly DA (1995) *Central Auditory Processing Disorder: Strategies for Use with Children and Adolescents*. San Antonio, TX: Communication Skill Builders.

Kelly TP (2000) The clinical neuropsychology of attention in school-aged children. *Child Neuropsychol* 6: 24–36.

Khetpal V, Donahue SP (2007) Cortical visual impairment: etiology, associated findings, and prognosis in a tertiary care setting. *J AAPOS* 11: 235–9.

King WJ, MacKay M, Sirnick A (2003) Shaken baby syndrome in Canada: clinical characteristics and outcomes of hospital cases. *CMAJ* 168: 155–9.

Kiper DC, Zesiger P, Maeder P, Deonna T, Innocenti GM (2002) Vision after early-onset lesions of the occipital cortex: I. Neuropsychological and psychophysical studies. *Neural Plast* 9: 1–25.

Kivlin JD, Simons KB, Lazoritz S et al (2000) Shaken baby syndrome. *Ophthalmology* 107: 1246–54.

Klaver CCW, Wolfs RCW, Vingerling JR, Hofmann A, De Jong PTVM (1998) Age-specific prevalence and causes of blindness and visual impairment in an older population. *Arch Ophthalmol* 16: 653–8.

Klein BP, Mervis CB (1999) Contrasting patterns of cognitive abilities of 9 and 10 year-olds with Williams syndrome or Down syndrome. *Dev Neuropsychol* 16: 177–96.

Kline LB, Bajandas FJ, editors (2004) *Neuro-ophthalmology Review Manual*, 5th edn. Thorofare, NJ: Slack Inc.

Klistorner AI, Graham SL, Grigg J, Balachandran C (2005) Objective perimetry using the multifocal visual evoked potential in central visual pathways lesions. *Br J Ophthalmol* 89: 739.

Knoblauch K, Maloney LT (1996) Testing the indeterminacy of linear color mechanisms from color discrimination data. *Vision Res* 36: 295–306.

Koeda T, Takeshita K (1992) Visuo-perceptual impairment and cerebral lesions in spastic diplegia with preterm birth. *Brain Dev* 14: 239–44.

Kogan CS, Bertone A, Cornish K et al (2004) Integrative cortical dysfunction and pervasive motor perception deficit in fragile X syndrome. *Neurology* 63: 1634–9.

Krägeloh-Mann I (2004) Imaging of early brain injury and cortical plasticity. *Exp Neurol* 190(Suppl 1): S84–90.

Krägeloh-Mann I, Petersen, D, Hagberg G et al (1995) Bilateral spastic cerebral palsy – MRI pathology and origin. Analysis from a representative series of 56 cases. *Dev Med Child Neurol* 37: 379–97.

Krägeloh-Mann I, Helber A, Moder I et al (2002) Bilateral lesions of thalamus and basal ganglia: origin and outcome. *Dev Med Child Neurol* 44: 477–84.

Krieger DT, Rizzo F (1971) Circadian periodicity of plasma 11-hydroxycorticosteroid levels in subjects with partial and absent light perception. *Neuroendocrinology* 8: 165–9.

Kupersmith MJ (1993) *Neurovascular Neuro-ophthalmology*. Berlin: Springer-Verlag.

Kwok SK, Ho PC, Chan AK, Gandhi SR, Lam DS (1996) Ocular defects in children and adolescents with severe mental deficiency. *J Intellect Disabil Res* 40: 330–5.

Lachenmayr BJ (2006) Is it possible to compensate for visual field defect? *Ophthalmologie* 103: 382.

Lachenmayr BJ, Vivell PMO (1993) *Perimetry and its Clinical Correlations*. Stuttgart: Georg Thieme Verlag

Laemers F, Walthes R (2001) Low vision in early intervention in Europe – an overview. In: Buultjens M, Fuchs E, Hyvarinen L, Laemers F, Leonhardt M, Walthes R, editors. *Low Vision in Early Intervention*. Dortmund: CD-Publication.

Lagati S (1995) 'Deaf-Blind' or 'Deafblind'? International perspective on terminology. *J Vis Impair Blind* 89: 306.

Lamb TD, Collin SP, Pugh Jr EN (2007) Evolution of the vertebrate eye: opsins, photoreceptors, retina and eye cup. *Nature Rev Neurosci* 8: 960–76.

Lambert SR, Hoyt CS, Jan JE, Barkovich J, Flodmark O (1987) Visual recovery from hypoxic cortical blindness during childhood. Computed tomographic and magnetic resonance imaging predictors. *Arch Ophthalmol* 105: 1371–7.

Lang J (1983) A new stereotest. *J Paediatr Ophthalmol Strabismus* 20: 72 [Abstract].

Lanzi G, Fazzi E, Uggetti C (1998) Cerebral visual impairment in periventricular leukomalacia. *Neuropediatrics* 29: 145–50.

Lê S, Cardebat D, Boulanouar K, Hénaff MA et al (2002) Seeing, since childhood, without ventral stream: a behavioural study. *Brain* 125: 58–74.

Leat SJ (1996) Reduced accommodation in children with cerebral palsy. *Ophthalmic Physiol Op* 16: 375–84.

Leat SJ, Gargon JL (1996) Accommodative response in children and young adults using dynamic retinoscopy. *Ophthalmic Physiol Op* 16: 375–84.

Leat SJ, Mohr A (2007) Accommodative response in pre-presbyopes with visual impairment and its clinical implications. *Invest Ophthalmol Vis Sci* 48: 3888–96.

Lebeer J, Rijke R (2003) Ecology of development in children with brain impairment. *Child Care Health Dev* 29: 131–40.

Lecanuet JP, Granier-Deferre C, Busnel MC (1989) Differential fetal auditory reactiveness as a function of stimulus characteristics and state. *Semin Perinatol* 13: 421–9.

Lewis TL, Maurer D (1992) The development of the temporal and nasal visual fields during infancy. *Vis Res* 32: 903.

Lim M, Soul JS, Hansen RM et al (2005) Development of visual acuity in children with cerebral visual impairment. *Arch Ophthalmol* 123: 1215–20.

Lim SA, Siatkowski RM (2004) Pediatric neuro-opthalmology. *Curr Opin Ophthalmol* 15: 437.

Lo Cascio GP (1977) A study of vision in cerebral palsy. *Am J Opt Physiol Opt* 54: 332–7.

Logothetis NK (1998) Single units and conscious vision. *Phil Trans R Soc Lond B Biol Sci* 353: 1801–18.

Logothetis NK, Sheinberg DL (1996) Visual object recognition. *Ann Rev Neurosci* 19: 577–621.

Logothetis NK, Pauls J, Poggio T (1995) Shape representation in the inferior temporal cortex of monkeys. *Curr Biol* 5: 552–63.

Lomber SG, Payne BR (2001) Perinatal-lesion-induced reorganization of cerebral functions revealed using reversible cooling deactivation and attentional tasks. *Cereb Cortex* 11: 194–209.

Long L, Hart P (2009) *Healthy living and the role of health detectives.* Paper presented at the conference of Health, Well-being and Congenital Rubella syndrome on 6–7 March, Crewe, UK (available at www.sense.org.uk/what_is_deafblindeness/rubella-mmr/rubella_conference).

Lowery RS, Atkinson D, Lambert SR (2006) Cryptic cerebral visual impairment in children. *Br J Ophthalmol* 90: 960–3.

Luna B, Dobson V, Scher MS, Guthrie RD (1995) Grating acuity and visual field development in infants following perinatal asphyxia. *Dev Med Child Neurol* 37: 330.

Lynch JK, Hirtz DG, DeVeter G et al (2002) Report of the National Institute of Neurological Disorders and Stroke workshop on perinatal and childhood stroke. *Pediatrics* 109: 116–23.

McAnaney DF (2010) The ICF as a framework for disability policy design and deployment. Available at: www.crpg.pt/site/documents/id/modelizacao/produtos/ICF_as_framework_for_policy.pdf (accessed 5 April 2010).

McClelland J (2004) *Accommodative Dysfunction and Refractive Anomalies in Children with Cerebral Palsy.* Faculty of Life and Health Sciences, University of Ulster, Coleraine.

McClelland JF, Saunders KJ (2003) The repeatability and validity of dynamic retinoscopy in assessing the accommodative response. *Ophthalmic Physiol Opt* 23: 243–50.

McClelland JF, Parkes J, Hill N, Jackson AJ, Saunders KJ (2006) Accommodative dysfunction in children with cerebral palsy: a population-based study. *Invest Ophthalmol Vis Sci* 47: 1824–30.

McClelland J, Saunders KJ, Hill N, Magee A, Shannon M, Jackson AJ (2007) The changing visual profile of children attending a regional specialist school for the visually impaired in Northern Ireland. *Ophthalmic Physiol Opt* 27: 556–60.

McConachie HR, Moore V (1994) Early expressive language of severely visually impaired children. *Dev Med Child Neurol* 36: 221–9.

McConachie HR, Ciccognani A (1995) 'What's in the box?': assessing physically disabled children's communication skills. *Child Lang Teach Therapy* 11: 253–63.

McCulloch DL, Mackie RT, Dutton GN et al (2007) A visual skills inventory for children with neurological impairments. *Devel Med Child Neurol* 49: 757–63.

McDonald MA, Dobson V, Sebris SL et al (1985) The acuity card procedure: a rapid test of infant acuity. *Invest Ophthalmol Vis Sci* 26: 1158–62.

McFadzean R, Brosnahan D, Hadley D, Mutlukan E (1994) Representation of the visual field in the occipital striate cortex. *Br J Ophthalmol* 78: 185.

Macfarlane A (1975) Olfaction in the development of social preferences in the human neonate. *Ciba Found Symp* 33: 103–17.

McKay KE, Halperin JM, Schwartz ST, Sharma V (1994) Developmental analysis of three aspects of information processing: sustained attention, selective attention, and response organization. *Dev Neuropsychol* 10: 121–32.

McKee SP, Levi DM, Movshon JA (2003) The pattern of visual deficits in amblyopia. *J Vis* 3: 380–405.

Mackie RT, McCulloch DL, Saunders KJ et al (1998) Relation between neurological status, refractive error, and visual acuity in children: a clinical study. *Dev Med Child Neurol* 40: 31–7.

McKillop E, Dutton GN (2008) Impairment of vision in children due to damage to the brain: a practical approach. *Br Ir Orthopt J* 5: 8–14.

McNaughton S (1993) Graphic Representational Systems and Literacy Learning. *Topics in Language Disorders* 13: 58–75.

Madan A, Jan JE, Good WV (2005) Visual development in preterm infants. *Dev Med Child Neurol* 4: 276–80. [Review].

Malach R, Reppas JB, Benson RB et al (1995) Object-related activity revealed by functional magnetic resonance imaging in human occipital cortex. *Proc Natl Acad Sci USA* 92: 8135–8.

Malkowicz DE, Myers G, Leisman G (2006) Rehabilitation of cortical visual impairment in children. *Int J Neurosci* 116: 1015–33.

Mankinen-Heikkinen A, Muostonen E (1987) Ophthalmic changes in hydrocephalus. *Acta Ophthalmol* 65: 81–6.

Manly T, Nimmo-Smith I, Watson P, Anderson V, Turner A, Roberston IH (2001) The differential assessment of children's attention: the Test of Everyday Attention for Children (TEA-Ch), normative sample and ADHD performance. *J Child Psychol Psychiat* 42: 1065–81.

Margolis LH, Shaywitz BA, Rothman SG (1978) Cortical blindness associated with occipital atrophy: a complication of *H. influenzae* meningitis. *Dev Med Child Neurol* 20: 490–3.

Marozas DS, May DC (1986) Research on effects of color reversal on the visual perceptual and visuomotor performances of spastic cerebral palsied and other exceptional individuals. *Percept Mot Skills* 62: 595–607.

Martin NA (2006) *Test of Visual-Perceptual Skills (non-motor)*, 3rd edn (TVPS-3). Novato, CA:Academic Therapy Publications.

Masland RH (2001) Neuronal diversity in the retina. *Curr Opin Neurobiol* 11: 431–6.

Mason AJS, Braddick O, Wattam-Bell J (2003) Motion coherence thresholds in infants – different tasks identify at least two distinct motion systems. *Vision Res* 43: 1149–57.

Matson (2005) *Central Auditory Processing: A Current Literature Review (Part I) and Summary of Interviews with Researchers on Controversial Issues Related to Auditory Processing Disorders (Part II) A Current Review* (available at http://dspace.wustl.edu/bitstream/1838/13/1/Matson.pdf).

Matsuba CA, Jan JE (2006) Long-term outcome of children with cortical visual impairment. *Dev Med Child Neurol* 48: 508–12.

Matsui T, Yoshitomi T, Fujita A, Mukuno K, Ishikawa S (1995) Pupil perimetry. A prototype device. *Transactions of the VIIIth International Orthoptic Congress*, Kyoto, p. 366.

Matsuo H, Endo N, Yokoi T, Tomonaga MA (1974) Visual field of the children. *Ann Ther Clin Opthalmol* 25: 186.

Matthews PM, Honey GD, Bullmore ET (2006) Applications of fMRI in translation medicine and clinical practice. *Nat Rev Neurosci* 7: 732.

May PJ (2005) The mammalian superior colliculus: laminar structure and connections. *Prog Brain Res* 151: 321–78.

Mayer DL, Beiser AS, Warner AF et al (1995) Monocular acuity norms for the Teller Acuity Cards between ages one month and four years. *Invest Ophthalmol Vis Sci* 36: 671–85.

Mayer DL, Fulton AB, Cummings M (1988) Visual fields of infants assessed with a new perimetric tecnique. *Invest Ophthalmol Vis Sci* 29: 452.

Meienberg O, Zangemeister WH, Rosenberg M, Hoyt WF, Stark L (1981) Saccadic eye movement strategies in patients with homonymous hemianopia. *Ann Neurol* 9: 537–44.

Meltzoff AN, Moore MK (1983) Newborn infants imitate adult facial gestures. *Child Dev* 54: 702–9.

Menken C, Cermak SA, Fisher A (1987) Evaluating the visual-perceptual skills of children with cerebral palsy. *Am J Occup Ther* 41: 646–51.

Mercuri E, von Siebenthal K, Tutuncuoglu S, Guzzetta F, Casaer P (1995a) The effect of behavioural states on visual evoked responses in preterm and full-term newborns. *Neuropediatrics* 26: 211–13.

Mercuri E, Atkinson J, Braddick O et al (1995b) Visual function in full-term infants with hypoxic-ischaemic encephalopathy. *Neuropediatrics* 28: 155–61.

Mercuri E, Spanò M, Bruccini G et al (1996a) Visual outcome in children with congenital hemiplegia: correlation with MRI findings. *Neuropediatrics* 27: 184–8.

Mercuri E, Atkinson J, Braddick O et al (1996b) Visual function and perinatal focal cerebral infarction. *Arch Dis Child Fetal Neonatal Ed* 75: F76–81.

Mercuri E, Atkinson J, Braddick O et al (1997a) Visual function in full-term infants with hypoxic–ischaemic encephalopathy. *Neuropediatrics* 28: 155–61.

Mercuri E, Atkinson J, Braddick O et al (1997b) Basal ganglia damage and impaired visual function in the newborn infant. *Arch Dis Child Fetal Neonatal Ed* 77: F111–14.

Mercuri E, Atkinson J, Braddick O (1997c) The aetiology of delayed visual maturation: short review and personal findings in relation to magnetic resonance imaging. *Eur J Paed Neurol* 1: 31–4.

Mercuri E, Braddick O, Atkinson J et al (1998) Orientation-reversal and phase-reversal visual evoked potentials in full-term infants with brain lesions: a longitudinal study. *Neuropaediatrics* 29: 1–6.

Mercuri E, Haataja L, Guzzetta A et al (1999) Visual function in term infants with hypoxic–ischaemic insults: correlation with neurodevelopment at 2 years of age. *Arch Dis Child Fetal Neonatal Ed* 80: F99–104.

Mercuri E, Anker S, Guzzetta A et al (2003) Neonatal cerebral infarction and visual function at school age. *Arch Dis Child Fetal Neonatal Ed* 88: F487–F491.

Mercuri E, Anker S, Guzzetta A et al (2004) Visual function at school age in children with neonatal encephalopathy and low Apgar scores. *Arch Dis Child Fetal Neonatal Ed* 89: F258–F262.

312

Mervis CA, Yeargin-Allsopp M, Winter S, Boyle C (2000) Aetiology of childhood vision impairment, metropolitan Atlanta, 1991–93. *Paediatr Perinat Epidem* 14: 70–7.

Mervis C, Boyle C, Yeargin-Allsopp M (2002) Prevalence and selected characteristics of childhood vision impairment. *Dev Med Child Neurol* 44: 538–41.

Miles B, Riggio M (1999) *Remarkable Conversations: A Guide to Developing Meaningful Communication with Children and Young Adults who are Deafblind.* Watertown, MA: Perkins School for the Blind.

Miller E, Cradock-Watson JE, Pollock TM (1982) Consequences of confirmed maternal rubella at successive stages of pregnancy. *Lancet* 2: 781–4.

Milne E, Swettenham J, Campbell R (2005) Motion perception and autistic spectrum disorder: a review. *Curr Psych Cog* 23: 3–33.

Milne, E, Scope A, Pascalis O, Buckley D, Makeig S (2010) Independent component analysis reveals atypical electroencephalographic activity during visual perception in individuals with autism. *Biol Psychiatr* 65: 22–30.

Milner AD, Goodale MA (1995) *The Visual Brain in Action.* Oxford: Oxford University Press.

Milner AD, Goodale MA (2006) *The Visual Brain in Action*, 2nd edn. Oxford: Oxford University Press.

Mirabella G, Kjaer PK, Norcia AM et al (2006) Visual development in very low birth weight infants. *Pediatr Res* 60: 435–9.

Mohn G, van Hof-van Duin J (1986) Development of the binocular and monocular visual field during the first year of life. *Clin Vis Sci* 1: 51–64.

Moller MA (1993) Working with visually impaired children and their families. *Pediatr Clin North Am* 40: 881–90.

Morad Y, Kim YM, Armstron DC et al (2002) Correlation betwenn retinal abnormalities and intracranial abnormalities in the shaken baby syndrome. *Am J Ophthamol* 134: 354–9.

Mori S, Zhang J (2006) Imaging and its applications to basic neuroscience research. *Neuron* 51: 527.

Morris KP, Forsyth RJ, Parslow RC, Tasker RC, Hawley CA (2006) Intracranial pressure complicating severe traumatic brain injury in children: monitoring and management. *Intensive Care Med* 32: 1606–12.

Morrone MC, Atkinson J, Cioni G, Braddick OJ, Fiorentini A (1999) Developmental changes in optokinetic mechanisms in the absence of unilateral cortical control. *NeuroReport* 10: 1–7.

Morrone MC, Guzzetta A, Tinelli F et al (2008) Inversion of perceived direction of motion caused by special undersampling in two children with periventricular leukomalacia. *J Cogn Neurosci* 20: 1094–106.

Mountcastle VB, Lynch JC, Georgopoulos A, Sakata H, Acūna C (1975) Posterior parietal association cortex of the monkey: command functions for operations within extrapersonal space. *J Neurophysiol* 38: 871–908.

Msall ME, Avery RC, Tremont MR, Lima JC, Rogers ML, Hogan DP (2003) Functional disability and school activity limitations in 41, 300 school age children: relationship to medical impairments. *Pediatrics* 111: 548–53.

Murshid WR, Jaralla JS, Dad MI (2000) Epidemiology of infantile hydrocephlus in Saudi Arabia: birth prevalence and Associated factors. *Pediatr Neurosurg* 32: 119–23.

Musiek FE, editor (2004) Hearing and the brain: Audiological consequences of neurological disorders. *J Am Acad Audiol* 15: 462–3.

Mutlukan E, Damato BE (1993) Computerised perimetry with moving and steady fixation in children. *Eye* 7: 554.

Nafstad A, Rødbroe I (1999) *Co-creating Communication.* Oslo: Forlaget-Nord Press.

Nagata S, Morioka T, Matsukado K, Natori Y, Sasaki T (2006) Retrospective analysis of the surgically treated temporal lobe arteriovenous malformations with focus on the visual field defects and epilepsy. *Surg Neurol* 66: 50.

Naidich, TP, Altman NR, Braffman BH et al (1992) Cephaloceles and related malformations. *AJNR Am J Neuroradiol* 13: 655–90.

Nardini M, Burgess N, Breckenridge K, Atkinson J (2006a) Differential developmental trajectories for egocentric, environmental and intrinsic frames of reference in spatial memory. *Cognition* 101: 153–72.

Nardini M, Atkinson J, Braddick O, Burgess N (2006b) The development of body, environment, and object-based frames of reference in spatial memory in normal and atypical populations. *Cogn Process* 7: 68–9.

Nardini M, Atkinson J, Braddick O, Burgess N (2008) Developmental trajectoris for spatial frames of reference in Williams syndrome. *Dev Sci* 11: 583–95.

National deaf-blind child count summary: December 1 2003 (2004) Monmouth, OR: NTAC, Teaching Research Institute, Western Oregon University.

Nelson KB (2006) Thrombophilias, perinatal stroke, and cerebral palsy. *Clin Obstet Gynecol* 49: 875–84.

Nelson KB, Lynch JK (2004) Stroke in newborn infants. *Lancet Neurol* 3: 150–8.

Nelson KB, Grether JK, Dambroisa JM et al (2003) Neonatal cytokines and cerebral palsy in very preterm infants. *Pediatr Res* 53: 600–7.

Nevin ST, Schmid KL, Wildsoet CF (1998) Sharp vision: a prerequisite for compensation to myopic defocus in the chick? *Curr Eye Res* 17: 322–31.

Newman WD, Hollman AS, Dutton GN, Carachi R (2002) Measurement of optic nerve sheath diameter by ultrasound: a means of detecting acute raised intracranial pressure in hydrocephalus. *Br J Ophthalmol* 86: 1109–13.

Newton NL Jr, Reynolds JD, Woody RC (1985) Cortical blindness following *Hemophilus influenzae* meningitis. *Ann Ophthalmol* 17: 193–4.

Nicholas J (2000) *Congenital Rubella Syndrome: Neuropsychological Functioning and Implications Illustrated by a Case Study*. Norway: Vestlandet Resource Centre (available at http://www.nordicwelfare. org/?id=118838).

Nielsen L (1989) *Spatial Relations in Congenitally Blind Infants*. Kalundborg: Refnaesskolan.

Nielsen LS, Skov L, Jensen H (2007) Visual dysfunctions and ocular disorders in children with developmental delay. I. prevalence, diagnoses and aetiology of visual impairment. *Acta Ophthalmol Scand* 85: 149–56.

Norcia AM, Tyler CW (1985) Spatial frequency sweep VEP: visual acuity during the first year of life. *Vision Res* 25: 1399–408.

Norcia AM, Tyler CW, Hamer RD (1988) High visual contrast sensitivity in the young human infant. *Invest Ophthalmol Vis Sci* 29: 44–9.

Norcia AM, Tyler CW, Hamer RD (1990) Development of contrast sensitivity in the human infant. *Vis Res* 30: 1475–86.

Olsen P, Paakko E, Vainionpaa et al (1997) Magnetic resonance imaging of periventricular leukomalacia and its clinical correlation in children. *Ann Neurol* 41: 754–61.

Palagyi M (1924) *Naturphilosophische Vorlesungen*. Leipzig: Barth.

Paryani SG, Yeager AS, Hosford-Dunn H et al (1985) Sequelae of acquired cytomegalovirus infection in premature and sick term infants. *J Pediatr* 107: 451–6.

Pavlova M, Staudt M, Sokolov A, Birbaumer N, Krageloh-Mann I (2003) Perception and production of biological movement in patients with early periventricular brain lesions. *Brain* 126: 692–701.

Pavlova M, Marconato F, Sokolov A et al (2006) Biological motion processing in adolescents with early periventricular brain damage. *Neuropsychologia* 44: 586–93.

Pavlova M, Sokolov A, Krägeloh-Mann I (2007) Visual navigation in adolescents with early periventricular lesions: knowing where, but not getting there. *Cereb Cortex* 17: 363–9.

Payne BR, Lomber SG, MacNeil MA, Cornwell P (1996) Evidence for greater sight in blindsight following damage of primary visual cortex early in life. *Neuropsychologia* 34: 741–74.

Pelak VS, Dubin M, Withney E (2007) Homonymous hemianopia: a critical analysis of optical devices, compensatory training and Nova Vision. *Curr Treat Options Neurol* 9: 41

Pellicano E, Jeffery L, Burr D, Rhodes G (2007) Abnormal adaptive face-coding mechanisms in children with autism spectrum disorder. *Curr Biol* 17: 1508–12.

Pennefather PM, Tin W (2000) Ocular abnormalities associated with cerebral palsy after preterm birth. *Eye* 14: 78–81.

Pennington L, McConachie H (2001) Predicting patterns of interaction between children with cerebral palsy and their mothers. *Dev Med Child Neurol* 43: 83–90.

Perenin MT, Vighetto A (1988) Optic ataxia: A specific disruption in visuomotor mechanisms. I. Different aspects of the deficit in reaching for objects. *Brain* 111: 643–74.

Persson EK, Hagberg G, Uvebrant P (2005) Hydrocephalus prevalence and outcome in a population-based cohort of children born in 1989–1998. *Acta Paediatr* 94: 726–32.

Persson EK, Andersson S, Wiklund LM, Uvebrant P (2007) Hydrocephalus in children born in 1999–2002. Epidemiology, outcome and Ophthalmological findings. *Childs Nerv Syst* 23: 1111–18.

Piaget J (1955) *The Child's Construction of Reality*. London: Routledge and Kegan Paul.

Pike M, Holmström G, de Vries L et al (1994) Patterns of visual impairment associated with lesions of the preterm infant brain. *Dev Med Child Neurol* 36: 849–62.

Poggel DA, Kasten E, Muller-Oehring EM, Buzenthal U, Sabel BA (2006) Improving residual vision by attentional cueing in patients with brain lesions. *Brain Res* 1097: 142.

Poo C, Isaacson JS (2007) An early critical period for long-term plasticity and structural modification of sensory synapses in olfactory cortex. *J Neurosci* 27: 7553–8.

Porro G (2005) Visual field investigation in children. In: Boerehaave Commissie, editor. *Pediatric Ophthalmology II*. Leiden: Leids University, pp. 29–38.

Porro G, Dekker EM, van Nieuwenhuizen O et al (1998a) Visual behaviours of neurologically impaired children with cerebral visual impairment: an ethological study. *Br J Ophthalmol* 82: 1231–5.

Porro G, Hofmann J, Wittebol-Post D et al (1998b) A new behavioural visual field test for clinical use in pediatric neuro-ophthalmology. *Neuro Ophthalmol* 19: 205.

Porro G, Wittebol-Post D, Van Nieuwenhuizen O, Schenk-Rootlieb AJF, Treffers WF (1999) Visual functions in congenital hemiplegia. *Neuro Ophthalmol* 21: 59.

Porter J, Miller O, Pease L (1997) *Curriculum Access for Deafblind Children*. University of London Institute of Education Research Report RR1.

Pott JWR (1992) *Visual Functions in 5 Year Old Children in Relation to a Very Low Birthweight and/or A Very Preterm Birth* [Thesis]. Rotterdam: Erasmus University.

Povlishock JT, Jenkins LW (1995) Are the pathobiological changes evoked by traumatic brain injury immediate and irreversible? *Brain Pathol* 5: 415–26.

Powell HWR, Parker GJM, Alexander DC et al (2005) MR tractography predicts visual field defects following temporal lobe resection. *Neurology* 65: 596.

Prayson RA, Hannahoe BM (2004) Clinicopathological findings in patients with Infantile hemiparesis and epilepsy. *Hum Pathol* 35: 734.

Prechtl HF, Cioni G, Einspieler C, Bos AF, Ferrari F (2001) Role of vision on early motor development: lessons from the blind. *Dev Med Child Neurol* 43: 198–201.

Quah SA, Kaye SB (2004) Binocular visual field changes after surgery in esotropic amblyopia. *Invest Ophthalmol Vis Sci* 45: 1817.

Quinn GE, Fea AM, Minguini N (1991) Visual fields in 4- to 10-year old children using goldmann and double-arc perimeters. *J Pediatr Ophthalmol Strabismus* 28: 314.

Quinn LM, Gardiner SK, Wheeler DT, Newkirk M, Johnson CA (2006) Frequency doubling technology perimetry in normal children. *Am J Ophthalmol* 142: 983.

Rabinowicz IM (1974) Visual function in children with hydrocephalus. *Trans Ophthalmol Soc UK* 94: 353–66.

Rahi J, Cable N (2003) Severe visual impairment and blindness in children in the UK. *Lancet* 362: 1359–65.

Ramadan AA, Hassan AM, Choudhury AR (1997) Hemianopic visual field in children with intracranial shunts: report of two cases. *Neurosurgery* 41: 1449.

Reinhard J (2005) Does Visual restitution training change absolute homonymous visual field defects? *Br J Ophthalmol* 89: 30.

Reynell J (1978) Developmental patterns of visually handicapped children. *Child Care Health Dev* 4: 291–303.

Reynell J, Zinkin PM (1975) New procedures for developmental assessment of young children with severe visual handicaps. *Child Care Health Dev* 1: 61–9.

Ricci D, Anker S, Cowan F et al (2006) Thalamic atrophy in infants with PVL and cerebral visual impairment. *Early Hum Dev* 82: 591–5.

Ricci D, Luciano R, Baranello G et al (2007) Visual development in infants with prenatal post-haemorrhagic ventricular dilatation. *Arch Dis Child Fetal Neonatal Ed* 92: F255–8.

Ricci D, Cesarini L, Groppo M et al (2008a) Early assessment of visual function in full term newborns. *Early Hum Dev* 84: 107–13.

Ricci D, Romeo DM, Serrao F et al (2008b) Application of a neonatal assessment of visual function in a population of low risk full-term newborn. *Early Hum Dev* 84: 277–80.

Ricci D, Cesarini L, Romeo DM et al (2008c) Visual function at 35 and 40 weeks' postmenstrual age in low-risk preterm infants. *Pediatrics* 122: e1193–8.

Ridder WH, Borsting E, Banton T (2001) All developmental dyslexic subtypes display an elevated motion coherence threshold. *Optom Vis Sci* 78: 510–17.

Riddoch G (1917) Dissociation of visual perception due to occipital injuries with especial reference to the appreciation of movement. *Brain* 40: 15.

Robertson R, Jan JE, Wong PK (1986) Electroencephalograms of children with permanent cortical visual impairment. *Can J Neurol Sci* 13: 256–61.

Rogers M (1996) Vision impairment in Liverpool: prevalence and morbidity. *Arch Dis Child* 74: 299–303.

Roland EH, Jan JE, Hill A, Wong PK (1986) Cortical visual impairment following birth asphyxia. *Pediatr Neurol* 2: 133–7.

Roman-Lantzy C (2007) *Cortical Visual Impairment: An Approach to Assessment and Intervention*. New York: AFB Press.

Rosen L, Phillips S, Enzmann D (1990) Magnetic resonance imaging in MELAS syndrome. *Neurology* 32: 168–71.

Rosenberg T, Flage T, Hansen E et al (1996) Incidence of registered visual impairment in the Nordic child population. *Br J Ophthalmol* 80: 49–53.

Ross RM, Heron G, Mackie R, McWilliam R, Dutton G (2000) Reduced accommodative function in dyskinetic cerebral palsy: a novel management strategy. *Dev Med Child Neurol* 42: 701–3.

Roth G (1994) *Das Gehirn und seine Wirklichkeit.* Frankfurt: Suhrkamp.

Rudanko SL, Fellman V, Laatikainen L (2003) Visual impairment in children born prematurely from 1972 through 1989. *Ophthalmology* 110: 1639–45.

Rueda MR, Fan J, McCandliss BD et al (2004) Development of attentional networks in childhood. *Neuropsychologia* 42: 1029–40.

Russell-Eggitt IM, Mackey DA, Taylor DS, Timms C, Walker JW (2000) Vigabatrin-associated visual field defects in children. *Eye* 14: 334.

Sabel BA, Kenkel S, Kasten E (2004) Vision restoration therapy (VTR) efficacy as assessed by comparative perimetric analysis and subjective questionnaires. *Restor Neurol Neurosci* 22: 399.

Safran AB, Laffi GL, Bullinger A et al (1996) Feasibility of automated visual field examination in children between 5 and 8 years of age. *Br J Ophthalmol* 80: 515.

Safran AB, Landis T (1996) Plasticity in the adult visual cortex: implications for the diagnosis of visual field defects and visual rehabilitation. *Curr Opin Ophthalmol* 7: 53.

Saidkasimova S, Bennett DM, Butler S, Dutton GN (2007) Cognitive visual impairment with good visual acuity in children with posterior periventricular white matter injury: A series of 7 cases. *J AAPOS* 11: 426–30.

Saint-Amour D, Saron CD, Schroeder CE, Foxe JJ (2005) Can whole brain nerve conduction velocity be derived from surface-recorded visual evoked potentials? A re-examination of Reed, Vernon, and Johnson (2004). *Neuropsychologolika* 43: 1838–44.

Sakata H, Taira M (1994) Parietal control of hand action. *Curr Opin Neurobiol* 4: 847–56.

Salati R, Borgatti R, Giammari G, Jacobson L (2002) Oculomotor dysfunction in cerebral visual impairment following perinatal hypoxia. *Dev Med Child Neurol* 44: 542–50.

Salomao SR, Ventura DF (1995) Large sample population age norms for visual acuities obtained with Vistech-Teller Acuity Cards. *Invest Ophthalmol Vis Sci* 36: 657–70.

Salt A, Dale N, Osborne J, Sonksen P (2006) *Developmental Journal for Babies and Children with Visual Impairment.* London: DfES/DoH Early Support, Crown Copyright.

Saunders KJ, McClelland JF, Richardson PM, Stevenson M (2008) Clinical judgement of near pupil response provides a useful indicator of focusing ability in children with cerebral palsy. *Dev Med Child Neurol* 50: 33–7.

Saunders KJ, Westall CA (1992) Comparison between near retinoscopy and cycloplegic retinoscopy in the refraction of infants and children. *Optom Vis Sci* 69: 615–22.

Schäfer EA (1888) On electrical excitation of the occipital lobe and adjacent parts of the monkeys brain. *Proc R Soc Lond* 43: 408–10.

Schanke AK (1992) Møte med psykiatriens historie. Lobotomering belyst med kasuistikk. Tidskrift for norsk psykologforening, vol 29. In: Nicholas J (2000) *Congenital Rubella Syndrome: Neuropsychological Functioning and Implications Illustrated by a Case Study.* Norway: Vestlandet Resource Centre, pp.16–13 (available at: http://www.nud.dk/14A2BCED-A8F7-4289-9C76-3ACC218843F9).

Schaumburg HH, Powers JM, Raine CS, Suzuki K, Richardson EP, Jr. (1975) Adrenoleukodystrophy. A clinical and pathological study of 17 cases. *Arch Neurol* 32: 577–91.

Schenk-Rootlieb AJF, van Nieuwenhuizen O, van der Graaf Y, Wittebol-Post D, Willemse J (1992) The prevalence of cerebral visual disturbance in children with cerebral palsy. *Dev Med Child Neurol* 34: 473–80.

Schenk-Rootlieb AJ, Van Nieuwenhuizen O, Schimanck N, Van der Graaf Y, Willemse J (1993) Impact of cerebral visual impairment on the everyday life of cerebral palsied children. *Child Care Health Dev* 19: 411–23.

Schenk-Rootlieb AJ, van Nieuwenhuizen O, van Waes PF (1994) Cerebral visual impairment in cerebral palsy: relation to structural abnormalities of the cerebrum. *Neuropediatrics* 25: 68–72.

Scher MS, Dobson V, Carpenter NA, Guthrie RD (1989) Visual and neurological outcome of infants with periventricular leukomalacia. *Dev Med Child Neurol* 31: 353–65.

Schiefer U, Kolb M, Wilhelm H, Petersen D, Zrenner E, Harms H (1993) Detection of homonymous visual field defects with flickering random dot pattern. In: Mills R, editor. *Perimetry Update 1992–93.* Proceeding of the Xth International Perimetry Society Meeting. Amsterdam: Kugler Publications, pp. 243–251.

Schlosser RW (2003) *The Efficacy of Augmentative and Alternative Communication: Toward Evidence-based Practice.* San Diego: Academic Press.

Schwartz TL, Dobson V, Sandstrom DJ, van Hof-van Duin J (1987) Kinetic perimetry assessment of binocular visual field shape and size in young infants. *Vision Res* 27: 2163–75.

Scottish Education Department (1987) *Curriculum and Assessment in Scotland. A Policy for the 90s.* Edinburgh: Scottish Education Department.

Seghier ML, Lazeyras F, Huppi PS (2006) Functional MRI of the newborn. *Semin Fetal Neonatal Med* 11: 479–88.

Sereno MI, Tootell RB (2005) From monkeys to humans: what do we now know about brain homologies? *Curr Opin Neurobiol* 15: 135–44.

Shapiro SM (2003) Bilirubin toxicity in the developing nervous system. *Pediatr Neurol* 29: 410–20.

Sharma P, Bairagi D, Sachdeva MM et al (2003) Comparative evaluation of Teller and Cardiff acuity tests in normals and unilateral amblyopes in under-two-year-olds. *Indian J Ophthalmol* 51: 341–5.

Sheridan MD (1976) *Manual for the STYCAR Vision Tests.* Windsor: NFER-Nelson.

Sherman KR, Keller EL (1986) Vestibulo-ocular reflexes of adventitiously and congenitally blind adults. *Invest Ophthalmol Vis Sci* 27: 1154–9.

Sherman SM, Koch C (1986) The control of retinogeniculate transmission in the mammalian lateral geniculate nucleus. *Exp Brain Res* 63: 1–20.

Shevell MI, Majnemer A, Morin I (2003) Etiologic yield of cerebral palsy: a contemporary case series. *Pediatr Neurol* 28: 352–9.

Signorini SG, Bova SM, La Piana R, Bianchi PE, Fazzi E (2005) *Neurobehavioural Adaptations in Cerebral Visual Impairment.* Elsevier International Congress Series 1282, pp. 724–8.

Simpson JI (1984) The accessory optic system. *Ann Rev Neurosci* 7: 13–41.

Sireteanu R (1996) Development of visual field results from human and animal studies. In: Vital Durand F, Atkinson J, editors. *Infant Vision.* Oxford: Science Press, pp. 17–22.

Sjöström A, Kraemer M, Lundberg S, Abrahamsson M, Gustafsson E (2001) Polyfocal VEP, a new method for perimetry in young children. *Eur J Paediatr Neurol* 5: A76.

Skoczenski AM, Norcia AM (1999) Development of VEP Vernier acuity and grating acuity in human infants. *Invest Ophthalmol Vis Sci* 40: 2411–17.

Skoczenski AM, Good WV (2004) Vernier acuity is selectively affected in infants and children with cortical visual impairment. *Dev Med Child Neurol* 46: 526–32.

Snowdon SK, Stewart-Brown SL (1997) Preschool vision screening. *Health Technol Assess* 1: report 8.

Snyder LH, Batista AP, Andersen RA (1997) Coding of intention in the posterior parietal cortex. *Nature* 386: 167–70.

Sobrado P, Suarez J, Garcia-Sanchez FA, Uson E (1999) Refractive errors in children with cerebral palsy, psychomotor retardation, and other non-cerebral palsy neuromotor disabilities. *Dev Med Child Neurol* 41: 396–403.

Solomon SG, Lennie P (2007) The machinery of colour vision. *Nature Rev Neurosci* 8: 276–86.

Sommer MA, Wurtz RH (2006) Influence of the thalamus on spatial visual processing in frontal cortex. *Nature* 444: 374–7.

Sonksen P, Petrie A, Drew KJ (1991) Promotion of visual development of severely visually impaired babies: evaluation of a developmentally based programme. *Dev Med Child Neurol* 33: 320.

Sonksen PM (1983) The assessment of 'Vision for Development' in severely visually handicapped babies. *Acta Opthalmol* 157 (Suppl): 82–91.

Sonksen PM (1993a) The assessment of vision in the preschool child. *Arch Dis Child* 68: 513–16.

Sonksen PM (1993b) Effect of severe visual impairment on development. Management of visual impairment in childhood. In: Fielder A, Bax M, Best A, editors. *Clinics in Developmental Medicine.* London: Mac Keith Press, 78–90.

Sonksen PM, Dale N (2002) Visual impairment in infancy: impact on neurodevelopmental and neurobiological processes. *Dev Med Child Neurol* 44: 782–91.

Sonksen PM, Macrae AJ (1987) Vision for coloured pictures at different acuities: The Sonksen Picture Guide to Visual Function. *Dev Med Child Neurol* 29: 337–47.

Sonksen PM, Silver J (1988) *The Sonksen–Silver Acuity System. Test system and 15 Page Instruction Manual.* Windsor: Keeler Ltd.

Sonksen PM, Stiff B (1999) *Show Me What My Friends Can See: a Developmental Guide for Parents of Babies with Severely Impaired Sight and their Professional Advisers.* London: The Wolfson Centre.

Sonksen PM, Levitt SL, Kitzinger M (1984) Identification of constraints acting on motor development in young visually disabled children and principles of remediation. *Child Care Health Dev* 10: 273–86.

Sonksen PM, Petrie A, Drew KJ (1991) Promotion of visual development of severely visually impaired babies: evaluation of a developmentally based programme. *Dev Med Child Neurol* 33: 320–35.

Sonksen PS, Salt AT, Wade A, Profitt R, Heavens S (2005) *The Sonksen logMAR Test of Visual Acuity*. Maidstone: Novomed.

Sparks DL (2002) The brainstem control of saccadic eye movements. *Nature Rev Neurosci* 3: 952–64.

Spencer J, O'Brien J, Riggs K, Braddick O, Atkinson J, Wattam-Bell J (2000) Motion processing in autism: evidence for a dorsal stream deficiency. *NeuroReport* 11: 2765–7.

Squire LR, Wixted JT, Clark RE (2007) Recognition memory and the medial temporal lobe: a new perspective. *Nature Rev Neurosci* 8: 872–83.

Stasheff SF, Barton JJ (2001) Deficits in cortical visual function. *Ophthalmol Clin North Am* 14: 217–42.

Stedman TL (1984) *Medical Dictionary*. Baltimore: Williams & Wilkins, p. 530.

Stein J, Talcott J, Walsh V (2000) Controversy about the evidence for a visual magnocellular deficit in developmental dyslexics. *Trends Cogn Sci* 4: 209–11.

Stewart RE, Woodhouse JM, Trojanowska LD (2005) In focus: the use of bifocals for children with Down syndrome. *Ophthalmic Physiol Op* 25: 514–22.

Stewart RE, Woodhouse JM, Cregg M, Pakeman VH (2007) The association between accommodative accuracy, hypermetropia and strabismus in children with Down syndrome. *Optom Vis Sci* 84: 149–55.

Stiebel-Kalish H, Lusky M, Yassur Y et al (2004) Swedish interactive thresholding algorithm fast for following visual fields in prepubertal idiopathic intracranial hypertension. *Ophthalmology* 111: 1673.

Stiers P, Vandenbussche E (2004) The dissociation of perception and cognition in children with early brain damage. *Brain Dev* 26: 81–92.

Stiers P, De Cock P, Vandenbussche E (1998) Impaired visual perceptual performance on an object recognition task in children with cerebral visual impairment. *Neuropediatrics* 29: 80–8.

Stiers P, De Cock P, Vandenbussche E (1999) Separating visual perception and non-verbal intelligence in children with early brain injury. *Brain Dev* 21: 397–406.

Stiers P, van den Hout BM, Haers M et al (2001) The variety of visual perceptual impairments in pre-school children with perinatal brain damage. *Brain Dev* 23: 333–48.

Stiers P, Vanderkelen R, Vanneste G, Coene S, De Rammelaere M, Vandenbussche E (2002) Visual–perceptual impairment in a random sample of children with cerebral palsy. *Devel Med Child Neurol* 44: 370–82.

Stiers P, Vanderkelen R, Vandenbussche E (2004) Optotype and grating visual acuity in patients with ocular and cerebral visual impairment. *Invest Ophthalmol Vis Sci* 45: 4333–9.

Stiers P, Swillen A, De Smedt B et al (2005) Atypical neuropsychological profile in a boy with 22q11.2 deletion syndrome. *Child Neuropsychol* 11: 87–108.

Stiers P, Fonteyne A, Wouters H, D'Agostino E, Sunaert S, Lagae L (2010) Hippocampal malrotation in pediatric patients with epilepsy associated with complex prefrontal dysfunction. *Epilepsia* 51: 546–55.

Stoerig P, Kleinschmidt A, Frahm J (1998) No visual responses in denervated V1: high-resolution functional magnetic resonance imaging of a blindsight patient. *Neuroreport* 9: 21–5.

Stores G, Ramchandani P (1999) Sleep disorders in visually impaired children. *Dev Med Child Neurol* 41: 348–52.

Suzumura H, Kobayashi A, Saito S et al (1995) Usefulness of automated isoptometry and central three zone testing for visual field screening in children, Transactions of the VIIIth International Orthoptic Congress, Kyoto, pp. 284–8.

Tallal P, Miller S, Fitch RH (1993) Neurobiological basis of speech: A case for the pre-eminence of temporal processing. *Ann N Y Acad Sci* 682: 27–47.

Talvik I, Metsvaht T, Leita K et al (2006) Inflicted traumatic brain injury (ITBI) or shaken baby syndrome (SBS) in Estonia. *Acta Paediatr* 95: 799–804.

Tanaka K (2003) Columns for complex visual object features in the inferotemporal cortex: clustering of cells with similar but slightly different stimulus selectivities. *Cereb Cortex* 13: 90–9.

Taylor MJ, McCulloch DL (1991) Prognostic value of VEPs in young children with acute onset of cortical blindness. *Pediatr Neurol* 7: 111–15.

Taylor MJ, Keenan NK, Gallant T, Skarf B, Freedman MH, Logan WJ (1987) Subclinical VEP abnormalities in patients on chronic deferoxamine therapy: longitudinal studies. *Electroencephalogr Clin Neurophysiol* 68: 81–7.

Teller DY (1979) The forced choice preferential looking procedure: a psychophysical technique for use with human infants. *Vis Res* 14: 1433–9.

Teller DY (1997) First glances: the vision of infants. The Friedenwald award lecture. *Invest Ophthalmol Vis Sci* 38: 2183–203.

Teller DY, Palmer J (1996) Infant color vision: motion nulls for red/green vs luminance-modulated stimuli in infants and adults. *Vision Res* 36: 955–74.

Teller DY, Mcdonald MA, Preston K, Sebris SL, Dobson V (1986) Assessment of visual acuity in infants and children: the acuity card procedure. *Dev Med Child Neurol* 26: 779–89.

Teller DY, Brooks TE, Palmer J (1997) Infant color vision: moving tritan stimuli do not elicit directionally appropriate eye movements in 2- and 4-month-olds. *Vision Res* 37: 899–911.

Tepperberg J, Nussbaum D, Feldman F (1977) Cortical blindness following meningitis due to hemophilus influenzae type B. *J Pediatr* 91: 434–6.

Tomaszewska MA, Gray M, Enqvist J (1996) Problems in building up an integration system. In: de Jong C, Neugebauer H, editors. *Timely Intervention: Special Help for Special Needs.* Wurzburg: edition bentheim, pp. 107–13.

Tootell RB, Dale AM, Sereno MI, Malach R (1996) New images from human visual cortex. *Trends Neurosci* 19: 481–9.

Tootell RB, Hadjikhani N, Hall EK, Marrett S, Vanduffel W, Vaughan JT, Dale AM (1998) The retinotopy of visual spatial attention. *Neuron* 21: 1409.

Treffert DA (2009) The savant syndrome: an extraordinary condition. A synopsis: past, present, future. *Phil Trans Roy Soc Lond – Series B. Biol Sci* 364: 1351–7.

Treisman A (1986) Features and objects in visual processing. *Sci Am* 114B–125B.

Treisman A (1987) Properties, parts and objects. In: Boff KR, Kaufman L, Thomas FP, editors. *Handbook of Perception and Human Performance.* New York: Wiley.

Tremblay K, Kraus N (2002) Auditory training induces asymmetrical changes in cortical neural activity. *J Speech Lang Hear Res* 45: 564–72.

Tresidder J, Fielder AR, Nicholson J (1990) Delayed visual maturation: ophthalmic and neurodevelopmental aspects. *Dev Med Child Neurol* 32: 872–81.

Trevarthen C, Aitken KJ (2001) Infant intersubjectivity: research, theory, and clinical applications. *J Child Psychol Psychiatry* 42: 3–8.

Triulzi F, Parazzini C, Righini A (2006) Patterns of damage in the mature neonatal brain. *Pediatr Radiol* 36: 608–20.

Trobe JR, Bauer RM (1986) Seeing but not recognizing. *Surv Ophthalmol* 30: 328–36.

Troster H, Brambring M (1992) Early social emotional development in blind infants. *Child Care Health Dev* 18: 207–27.

Troster H, Brambring M, Beelmann A (1991) Prevalence and situational causes of stereotyped behaviours in blind infants and preschoolers. *J Abnorm Child Psych* 19: 569–90.

Tshopp C, Safran AB, Laffi JL, Mermoud C, Bullinger A, Viviani P (1995) Automated static perimetry in the child: methodologic and practical problems. *Klin Monatsbl Augenheilk* 206: 416.

Tsiaras WG, Pueschel S, Keller C, Curran R, Giesswein S (1999) Amblyopia and visual acuity in children with Down syndrome. *Br J Ophthalmol* 83: 1112–14.

Tsuneishi S, Casaer P (1997) Stepwise decrease in VEP latencies and the process of myelination in the human visual pathway. *Brain Dev* 19: 547–51.

Tustin F (1972) *Autism and Child Psychosis.* New York: Science House.

Uggetti C, Egitto MG, Fazzi E et al (1996) Cerebral visual impairment in periventricular leukomalacia: MR correlation. *Am J Neuroradiol* 17: 979–85.

Uggetti C, Egitto MG, Fazzi E et al (1997) Transsynaptic degeneration of lateral geniculate bodies in blind children: in vivo MR demonstration. *AJNR Am J Neuroradiol* 18: 233–8.

Uggetti C, Bova S, Egitto MG et al (2001) Il disturbo visuopercettivo nei bambini affetti da leucomalacia periventricolare: studio neuropsicologico e neuroradiologico. *Rivista di Neuroradiologia* 14(Suppl 3): 153–6.

US Public Health Service (1980) *International Classification of Diseases, 9th Revision – Clinical Modification* (ICD-9-CM).

van den Hout BM, Stiers P, Haers M et al (2000) Relation between visual perceptual impairment and neonatal ultrasound diagnosis of haemorrhagic-ischaemic brain lesions in 5-year-old children. *Dev Med Child Neurol* 42: 376–86.

Van Essen DC, Lewis JW, Drury HA et al (2001) Mapping visual cortex in monkeys and humans using surface-based atlases. *Vision Res* 41: 1359–78.

van Hof-van Duin J, Mohn G (1987) Early detection of visual impairment. In: Galjaard H, Pechtl H, Velickovic M, editors. *Cerebral Palsy – Early Detection and Management*. Dordrecht: Martinus Nijhoff, p. 79.

van Hof-van Duin J, Heersema DJ, Groenendaal F, Baerts W, Fetter WP (1992) Visual field and grating acuity development in low-risk preterm infants during the first 2 1/2 years after term. *Behav Brain Res* 49: 115–22.

van Hof-van Duin J, Cioni G, Bertuccelli B, Fazzi B, Romano C, Boldrini A (1998) Visual outcome at 5 years of newborn infants at risk of cerebral visual impairment. *Dev Med Child Neurol* 40: 302–9.

van Splunder J, Stilma JS, Bernsen RM, Evenhuis HM (2004) Prevalence of ocular diagnoses found on screening 1539 adults with intellectual disabilities. *Ophthalmology* 111: 1457–63.

van Splunder J, Stilma JS, Bernsen RMD, Evenhuis HM (2006) Prevalence of visual impairment in adults with intellectual disabilities in the Netherlands: cross-sectional study. *Eye* 20: 1004–10.

Varela F (1985) *Ethisches Können*. Frankfurt: Schatz.

Vicari S, Bellucci S, Carlesimo GA (2006) Evidence from two genetic syndromes for the independence of spatial and visual working memory. *Dev Med Child Neurol* 48: 126–31.

Vision Impairment Scotland (2003) *Vision Impairment Scotland: A New System of Notification of Childhood Visual Impairment and the Information it has Provided on Services for Scottish Children*. Edinburgh: VIS (available at: http://www.viscotland.org.uk).

Vitali P, Minati L, D'Incerti L et al (2008) Functional MRI in malformations of cortical development: activation of dysplastic tissue and functional reorganization. *J Neuroimaging* 18: 296–305. [please provide at least 3 author names]

Volpe JJ (1998) Neurologic outcome of prematurity. *Arch Neurol* 55: 297–300.

Volpe JJ (2003) Cerebral white matter injury of the premature infant – More common than you think. *Pediatrics* 112: 176–80.

Walsh TJ (1990) *Visual Fields Examination and Interpretation*. San Francisco: American Academy of Ophthalmology.

Walthes R (2005) Zerebrale Sehschädigung– eine Herausforderung an die Disziplinarität der Sonderpädagogik. *Vierteljahresschrift für Heilpädagogik und ihre Nachbargebiete* (VHN) 74: 207–17.

Warburg M (2001) Visual impairment in adult people with moderate, severe, and profound intellectual disability. *Acta Ophthalmol Scand* 79: 450–4.

Wässle H (2004) Parallel processing the mammalian retina. *Nature Rev Neurosci* 5: 747–57.

Watson T, Orel-Bixler D, Haegerstrom-Portnoy G (2007) Longitudinal quantitative assessment of vision function in children with cortical visual impairment. *Optom Vis Sci* 84: 471–80.

Wattam-Bell J (1991) The development of motio-specific cortical responses in infants. *Vision Res* 31: 287–97.

Wattam-Bell J (1992) The development of maximum displacement limits for discrimination of motion direction in infancy. *Vision Res* 32: 621–30.

Wattam-Bell J (1994) Coherence thresholds for discrimination of motion direction in infants. *Vision Res* 34: 877–83.

Watts R, Liston C, Niogi S, Ulug AM (2003) Fiber tracking using magnetic resonance diffusion tensor imaging and its applications to human brain development. *Ment Retard Dev Disabil Res Rev* 9: 168.

Waugh M-C, Chong WK, Sonksen PM (1998) Neuroimaging in children with congenital disorders of the peripheral visual system. *Dev Med Child Neurol* 40: 812–19.

Weisglas-Kuperus N, Heersema DJ, Baerts W et al (1993) Visual functions in relation with neonatal cerebral ultrasound, neurology and cognitive development in very low birthweight children. *Neuropediatrics* 24: 149.

Weiskrantz L (1998) *Blindsight: A Case Study and Implications*. Oxford: Oxford University Press.

Weiss AH, Kelly JP, Phillips JO (2001) The infant who is visually unresponsive on a cortical basis. *Ophthalmology* 108: 2076–87.

Weissten N, Wong E (1986) Figure-round organisation and the spatial and temporal responses of the visual system. In: Schwab EC, Nusbaum HC, editors. *Pattern Recognition by Humans and Machines* Vol. 2. New York: Academic Press.

Werth R, Schadler G (2006) Visual field loss in young children and mentally handicapped adolescent receiving vigabatrine. *Invest Ophthalmol Vis Sci* 47: 3028.

Westheimer G (1975) Editorial: Visual acuity and hyperacuity. *Invest Ophthalmol* 14: 570–2.

Westheimer G (1979) Scaling of visual acuity measurements. *Arch Ophthalmol* 97: 327–30.

Whiting S, Jan JE, Wong PK, Flodmark O, Farrell K, McCormick AQ (1985) Permanent cortical visual impairment in children. *Dev Med Child Neurol* 27: 730–9.

Wiesel TN (1982) Postnatal development of the visual cortex and the influence of environment. *Nature* 299: 583–91.

Wigglesworth JS, Pape KE (1978) An integrated model for haemorrhagic and ischaemic lesions in the newborn brain. *Early Hum Dev* 2: 179–99.

Wild JM, Ahn HS, Baulac M et al (2007) Vigabatrin and epilepsy: lesson learned. *Epilepsia* 48: 1318.

Willis DM (1979) The ordinary devoted mother and her blind baby. *Psychoanal Study Child* 34: 31–49.

Wilson JGM, Jungner G (1968) *Principles and Practice of Screening for Disease.* Geneva: World Health Organization.

Wilson M, Quinn G, Dobson W, Breton M (1991) Normative values for visual fields in 4- to 12-year old children using kinetic perimetry. *J Pediatri Ophthalmol Strab*Zhang X, Kedar S, Lynn MJ, Newman NJ, Biousse V (2006) Homonymous hemianopia: clinical–anatomic correlations in 904 cases. *Neurology* 66: 906.

Wong VC (1991) Cortical blindness in children: a study of etiology and prognosis. *Pediatr Neurol* 7: 178–85.

Woodhouse JM, Adoh TO, Oduwaiye KA et al (1992) New acuity test for toddlers. *Ophthalmic Physiol Opt* 12: 249–51.

Woodhouse JM, Pakeman VH, Cregg M et al (1997) Refractive errors in young children with Down syndrome. *Optom Vis Sci* 74: 844–51.

World Health Organization (1978) *International Classification of Diseases and Causes of Death – 9th revision* (ICD-9). Geneva: World Health Organization.

World Health Organization (1980) *International Classification of Impairments, Disabilities and Handicaps* (ICIDH). Geneva: World Health Organization.

World Health Organization (1992) *Consultation on Management of Low Vision in Children.* Bangkok: WHO/PBL/93.27.

World Health Organization (1993) *Management of Low Vision in Children.* Report of a WHO consultation, Bangkok 23–24 July 1992. Geneva: World Health Organization.

World Health Organization (1999) *Global Initiative for the Elimination of Avoidable Blindness.* Geneva: World Health Organization, WHO/PBL/97.61 Rev. 2.

World Health Organization (2001) *International Classification of Functioning, Disability and Health* (ICF). Geneva: World Health Organization.

World Health Organization (2003) *Consultation on Development of Standards for Characterization of Vision Loss and Visual Functioning.* Document WHO/PBL/03.91. Geneva: World Health Organization.

World Health Organization (2007) *International Classification of Functioning, Disabilities and Health– Children and Youth Version.* Geneva: World Health Organization.

Wouters H, Fonteyne A, Lagae L, Stiers P (2006) Specific cognitive profile in a boy with fragile-X syndrome and temporal lobe epilepsy. *Dev Med Child Neurol* 48: 378–82.

Zeki S (1993) *A Vision of the Brain.* Oxford: Blackwell Scientific Publications.

Zemach I, Chang S, Teller DY (2007) Infant color vision: prediction of infants' spontaneous color preferences. *Vision Res* 47: 1368–81.

Zentall SS, Zentall RR (1983) Optimal simulation. A model of disordered activity and performances in normal and deviant children. *Psychol Bull* 94: 446–71.

GLOSSARY

Many of the terms in this glossary were originally defined for adults and may need some modification when applied to children. Nevertheless, they are offered here because these are the terms with which most agencies are most familiar.

ability Ability indicates the capacity to perform certain defined tasks (Fig. 20.1, column 3). In ICIDH (WHO 1980) the term **disability** (ambiguous, see separate glossary entry) was used to describe a lack or loss of ability. The ability to perform defined tasks is different from **participation** in life situations (ICF), which involves interactive engagement with other individuals; for example speaking is an ability but conducting a conversation is participation.

achromatopsia inherited lack of colour vision owing to impaired function of the cones in the retina.

accommodation the facility of the eye to focus upon near targets.

activity In ICF (WHO 2001) the term activity is used for the ability aspect in ICIDH. Both terms are needed. ability relates to the available resources (vision, hearing) in the medical model of disability. Activity relates to the goal (participation) in the social model of disability.

acuity/visual acuity a measure of the ability of the visual system to see, or resolve, the component parts of an image as being separate from one another when tested at maximum contrast (black/white). The measures used are given in the appendix.

adrenoleucodystrophy a rare disorder affecting peroxisomes, with recessive inheritance, causing progressive damage to the white matter of the brain and the adrenal glands.

agnosia lack of a specific higher visual function.

Aicardi syndrome syndrome characterized by absence of the corpus callosum, punched-out areas in the retina, and optic nerve abnormalities, which accompany profound motor and intellectual disability. (Inheritance is X-linked dominant.)

323

akinetopsia inability to see movement. The term has been extended to describe disability seeing movement, for which the term 'dyskinetopsia' has also been employed.

altitudinal hemianopia lack of vision in the upper or lower visual field.

amygdala almond-shaped structures in the medial temporal lobes of the brain, which serve memory and emotional reactions.

anosagnosia not to be aware of an agnosia probably due to damage to the part of the brain responsible for giving insight.

antenatal before birth.

apraxia inability to carry out a specific purposeful action despite the motor capacity and wish to do so.

aqueduct of Sylvius small-diameter canal in the brain which allows cerebrospinal fluid to flow between the lateral ventricles and the third ventricle (water space in the brain).

Arnold-Chiari II malformation downward displacement of the cerebellar tonsils through the foramen magnum of the skull. Type II includes additional myelomeningocele and, in many cases, hydrocephalus.

assessment Assessments of **visual functions** determine a threshold condition for one stimulus parameter at a time. Assessments of **functional vision** determine sustainable task performance. *See also* **scales**.

astroglia small supporting cells in the brain with a shape resembling a star (*astra* = star [Lat]).

athetosis writhing body movement.

attention (a) The ability to appraise a visual scene, identify an element, and attend to it. (b) The ability to limit one's cerebral processing capacity to a specific part of the sensory input. This results in increased sensitivity for the attended stimuli, as well as reduced sensitivity (suppression) for unattended stimuli.

autistic spectrum disorder a spectrum of psychological conditions in which impaired social interaction, limited interests, and repetitive behaviours are prominent.

automated perimetry the use of computerized equipment to investigate the extent of the visual field.

Balint syndrome inability to see more than one or two entities at once (simultanagnosia), in association with impaired visual guidance of movement (optic ataxia) and an inability to shift gaze to a new visual target, despite the ability to move the eyes on command (dyspraxia of gaze), owing to extensive pathology affecting the posterior parietal territory of the brain.

basal ganglia discrete structures in the lower part of the brain.

blindness Blindness, according to the dictionary, means total lack or loss of vision. Unfortunately, its association with entitlement for services has led to the erroneous perception of a black and white dichotomy between those who are 'sighted' and those who are 'blind', while ignoring the large grey area of those with **low vision**. The WHO defines blindness numerically as visual acuity of <3/60 (20/400, 0.05). The International Council of Ophthalmology (ICO 2002) has suggested a functional definition: those who have no vision, or so little that they must rely mainly on vision substitution techniques (e.g. cane, Braille, hearing). In the realm of visual **dysfunction**, use of the term blindness can be misleading because the level of functioning depends more on the task requirements than on the degree of visual impairment. Dysfunctions of visual processing are compatible with normal visual acuity.

bruxism grinding of the teeth.

calcarine cortex the part of the brain in the occipital lobes which serves primary processing of vision. It has an upper and a lower part separated by a cleft, the calcarine fissure.

centrum semiovale an alternative term for cerebral white matter.

cephalocele a congenital defect in the skull through which the brain protrudes into the nose (ethmoid encephalocele) or at the back of the skull (occipital encephalocele).

cerebral visual impairment A cerebral visual **impairment** is a visual impairment caused by a cerebral **disorder**. Cerebral visual impairments are distinct from **ocular visual impairments**. (In the USA the term cortical visual impairment is used and includes impaired visual acuity. The term cerebral is used in this text, primarily because subcortical damage is also seen.)

chorioretinitis (or retinochoroiditis) inflammation, which usually resolves to cause scarring at the back of the eye, affecting the retina and underlying choroid.

clastic lesion discrete lesion which is locally destructive.

cognition cognition involves the processing of information for conscious awareness and decision-making and to prepare for action. Visual cognition builds on visual **perception**. Deficits in cognitive processing result in **dysfunction** of **functional vision**.

cognitive visual impairment impairment of the categorization and storage (memory) of visual information, and the analysis and utilization of this information. (Recognizing that visual perception, cognition, and attention constitute an integrated system.)

coloboma (pl: colobomata) a notch, break, or fissure in any ophthalmic structure.

conjugate eye movements eye movements in which the two eyes move in the same direction.

contrast sensitivity a measure of the minimum difference in subtle shades of grey that can be detected by the human visual system.

convergence/divergence turning the eyes in/out to view a near target, then a more distant target; these constitute disjugate eye movements, which are normally accompanied by **accommodation**.

convergence insufficiency reduced ability to turn the eyes in to look at a near target.

corpus callosum the structure which joins and connects the two halves of the brain.

corticospinal tracts the pathways which run from the cortex of the brain down through the spinal cord to bring about and control movement of the body.

coup and contre-coup coup, in this context, means a blow to the head causing damage to the underlying brain. Contre-coup injury is damage to the brain on the side opposite to the impact on account of rapid movement of the brain inside the skull at the time of injury.

deficit A general term used to indicate either the lack (congenital) or the loss (acquired) of an **ability** or function.

delayed visual maturation visual impairment in the newborn child which abates spontaneously (thus the diagnosis can only be retrospective).

diffusion tensor imaging (DTI) a form of magnetic resonance imaging which identifies limited movement of water in tissues. This facilitates identification of the functional anatomy of nerve pathways in the brain.

dioptre the power of a lens which brings a parallel beam of light to a focus at 1m.

diplegia impairment of movement of the lower limbs caused by dysfunction of the brain, spinal cord, or peripheral nerves. In the context of this book, the principal cause is periventricular white matter damage, resulting in diplegic cerebral palsy.

disability The term 'disability' must be used with caution, since it means different things to different people. In the 'Americans with Disabilities Act', disability is synonymous with **impairment** (Fig. 20.1, column 2); in 'being on disability' it denotes a socioeconomic consequence (Fig. 20.1, column 4). In ICIDH (WHO 1980), the term referred to an ability deficit (Fig. 20.1, column 3). The term 'ability deficit' avoids this ambiguity.

disorder Disorder is a general term to describe any deviation from the normal state of an organ (Fig. 20.1, column 1). It may be a disease (a process), a condition of damage (injury, scar), the absence of a part (e.g. amputation), or a condition of congenital anomaly.

dorsal stream a pathway in the brain between the occipital lobes (at the back of the brain), which serve vision, and the posterior parietal area (at the top of the brain near the back), which subconsciously provides orientation within the visual scene and thereby brings about moment-to-moment visual guidance of movement. Visual search is also facilitated. Damage gives rise to problems finding things in crowded scenes (foreground clutter or background pattern), impaired visual guidance of movement of the upper or lower limbs (or both), and limited attentional capacity.

ductus arteriosus a blood vessel near the heart between the lung and body blood supplies, which short-circuits the lungs before birth, and which closes shortly after birth.

dysfunction This term is used for abnormal functioning caused by deficits of **perception** or **cognition**. A visual dysfunction can exist even if there is no lower level visual **impairment**, or it may coexist with a lower level visual impairment.

dyskinesia diminished capacity to make voluntary limb and body movements, accompanied by additional involuntary movements.

dyskinetic eye movements inaccurate movements of the eyes.

dyslexia specific reading disability despite the requisite intelligence, social advantage, and good instruction.

dysraphism a term covering the variety of types of spina bifida which result from failure of closure of the neural tube during development in the womb.

EEG electroencephalography – the recording of the electrical signals of the brain.

emmetropia normal-sightedness.

encephalomalacia lack of brain tissue owing to prior lack of blood supply.

encephalopathy disorder of brain owing to disease.

ependymitis inflammation of the lining of the cavities in the brain.

esotropia convergent squint in which the eyes are turned in.

exotropia divergent squint in which the eyes are turned out.

extrageniculate visual pathways pathways in the visual brain which do not serve a higher visual function as they do not pass through the 'relay stations' (the lateral geniculate bodies) to the back of the brain (the occipital lobes). These pathways serve reflex vision and other functions related to vision.

extrastriate cortex When sliced, the visual brain which processes image detail has a part with a line (or stria) in it. This is the striate cortex. The visual brain adjacent to this which processes other information such as colour and movement is referred to as the extrastriate cortex.

factor V Leiden a factor needed for clotting. Lack of this factor can cause bleeding.

foramina of Monro the holes between the lateral ventricular water cavities in the brain and the third ventricle (water cavity).

fragile X syndrome a specific disorder (mutation) of the X chromosome which causes a mild to severe intellectual, emotional, behavioural, and developmental dysfunction.

functional brain imaging or **functional magnetic resonance imaging (fMRI)** a method of imaging the brain which detects which parts of the brain are active on account of their using oxygen.

functional MRI tractography (fMRI) brain scanning method which demonstrates functional brain pathways.

functional vision Describes how the person functions in vision-related tasks. It is distinct from **visual functions**, which describe various parameters of how the eye and visual system function.

functioning The leading principle in ICF, the International Classification of Functioning, Disability, and Health (WHO 2001). It stresses that the glass is half-full, rather than half-empty. It replaces the negative terms (**impairment**, **disability**, **handicap**) used in ICIDH. *See also* **scales**.

fusiform gyrus part of the temporal lobe of the brain, which on the right side (in right-handed people) plays a role in recognizing faces.

fusional vergence movement of the eyes in opposite directions, which serves to join up the pictures seen by the two eyes, and thereby bring about the alignment of the eyes to see the object of interest as a single entity.

galactocerebrosidase deficiency a metabolic disorder of the brain.

germinal matrix part of the developing brain where the cells are dividing.

GM1 gangliosidosis lack of an enzyme called beta-galactosidase, which leads to acidic lipid material in cells and progressive damage to the brain.

Goldmann perimetry a method of plotting the visual fields in which a spot of light is moved, and the boundaries between perception and no perception are drawn as contours or isoptres.

habilitation strategies to enhance development when disorders have been present from birth. (The term rehabilitation applies when a function has been lost.)

handicap Term used in ICIDH (WHO 1980) to denote a limitation in **functioning** in a societal context. Use of the term is discouraged, because it has a negative connotation which stresses that the glass is half-empty, rather than half-full. *See also* **scales**.

hemiplegia inability or disability to move one side of the body due to damage to the brain.

hemispherectomy removal of one side (or hemisphere) of the brain.

heterotopia a congenital disorder of the brain.

hippocampus paired deep brain structures responsible for forming short-term memories.

histogenesis a term describing the early development of a fetus in which the inner middle and outer structures of endoderm, mesoderm, and ectoderm develop.

holoprosencephaly failure of development of the forebrain into the two cerebral hemispheres.

homonymous hemianopia lack of vision on one side which is in the same distribution for each eye.

homonymous quadrantanopia lack of quarter of visual field in the same distribution in both eyes affecting an upper or lower, left or right quadrant.

horizontal pursuit horizontal eye movements brought about by following a visual target (*see also* **smooth pursuit**).

hydrocephalus a condition in which obstruction of the normal flow of water (cerebrospinal fluid) is blocked, which results in expansion of the water spaces in the brain, damage and displacement of brain structures, and accelerated growth of the skull.

hypermetropia long-sightedness.

hypometric saccades fast reflex eye movements which fall short of their visual target.

hypothalamus a small but crucial part of the brain which contributes to the control of hormones, temperature, sleep, hunger, and thirst.

impairment Although sometimes used to describe a **disorder** (e.g. cataract, retinal scar), the term is better restricted to the functional limitation (e.g. visual acuity loss) caused by that disorder. Impairments are assessed by varying stimulus parameters, one at a time, to achieve threshold performance.

infarction death of tissue in the body owing to loss of blood supply.

inferior colliculi paired structures at the back of the mid-brain (below the **superior colliculi**) comprising two small protrusions which process hearing

keratoconus slowly progressive conical distortion of the front of the eye, the cornea.

kinaesthetic information knowledge of the position in three-dimensional space of parts of the body with respect to each other and the external environment, independent of the balance system.

Krabbe disease progressive degenerative disorder of myelin in the nervous system with recessive inheritance.

latent nystagmus to and fro movement of the eyes which only occurs when one eye is covered (*see also* **manifest nystagmus).**

lateral geniculate bodies/nuclei paired relay stations in the brain, between the eyes and the back of the brain (the occipital lobes), responsible for vision.

lateral ventricles symmetrical spaces in the brain where cerebrospinal fluid is made.

lingual gyrus part of the visual brain.

lissencephaly (smooth brain) a developmental disorder of brain in which the grey matter is inside and the smooth white matter is on the outside owing to impaired migration of brain cells during development.

loss of vision acquired impairment of vision (visual impairment is the term applied where impaired vision has been present from birth but has not been lost).

low vision This term describes a range of conditions between normal vision and **blindness**. The word 'low' indicates that vision is less than normal; the word 'vision' distinguishes it from blindness. The WHO defines low vision numerically as visual acuity of <20/60 (0.3). The International Council of Ophthalmology (ICO 2002) has suggested a functional definition: a level of vision that benefits from vision enhancement (magnification, illumination, contrast), although vision substitution techniques may be used as an adjunct (e.g. talking books).

lysosomal disorders lysosomes break down waste products in cells. They have many enzymes. If an enzyme is not working, a waste product (such as mucopolysaccharide) accumulates and this causes damage in the brain and elsewhere, causing progressive dysfunction.

macrocephaly a large head.

magnetoencephalography (MEG) a brain imaging method which uses magnetic fields.

magnocellular pathways the pathways between the eyes and the visual brain which have larger cells. These are resilient rapid conducting pathways and serve perception of movement (*see also* **parvocellulear pathways**).

manifest nystagmus to and fro movements of the eyes which are constantly visible (*see also* **latent nystagmus**).

mesencephalon the midbrain.

mesopic dim lighting conditions (photopic, bright lighting conditions; scotopic, conditions with minimum lighting).

microcephaly a small brain and head.

microgyria abnormal dysfunctional area on the brain with small wrinkles.

microphthalmia pathologically small eyes.

mitochondrial disorders mitochondria provide energy for cells. When they do not work, there is functional failure in the affected area. The brain and vision can be affected.

multicystic encephalomalacia multifocal damage to the brain, for example due to an episode of lack of blood supply in which tissue dies back to leave cysts in the brain.

myopia short-sightedness.

neonatal the period just after birth.

nystagmus involuntary to and fro movement of the eyes.

ocular visual impairment An **impairment** are impairments caused by an ocular or optic nerve disorder and from **cerebral visual impairment**.

optic ataxia impaired visual guidance of limb and body movement.

optic atrophy pallor of the nerves at the back of the eyes (the optic nerves) due to damage.

optic nerve hypoplasia small optic nerves due to incomplete development.

optic radiations the visual pathways running from the lateral geniculate bodies to the occipital lobes.

optokinetic nystagmus involuntary to and fro movement of the eyes generated by moving black and white stripes (or similar targets).

optotypes black and white images used to test visual acuity.

orthophoria straight eyes even when one eye is covered.

pacchionian granulations tiny membrane structures which protrude from the water spaces around the brain into the venous blood sinuses, which serve the transfer of cerebrospinal fluid back into venous blood.

pachygyria abnormal wide gyri on the surface of the brain due to abnormal migration of cells during brain development.

parahippocampal gyrus the grey matter surrounding the hippocampi, responsible for encoding and retrieving memories.

paroxysmal ocular deviations rapid-onset, usually short-lived, involuntary movement of the eyes in one direction.

participation Used in ICF to describe how a person interacts with other individuals and the social environment. *See also* **activities**.

parvocellular pathways the pathways between the eyes and the visual brain which have smaller cells. These cells primarily serve analysis of image detail.

perception Perception indicates conscious awareness of the environment through the senses. Visual perception indicates awareness through vision. It is mostly processed in the ventral stream. **Functional vision** builds on visual perception, but also involves **cognitive** functions, such as memory, recognition, integration with other senses, and often conscious thinking, decision-making, and visually guided motor action.

perceptual visual impairment disorder of the processes required to decode incoming visual information (recognizing that visual perception, cognition, and attention constitute an integrated system).

perimetry a method of mapping out the visual fields.

perinatal the period between 22 weeks' gestation and 7 days after birth.

periventricular leucomalacia damage to white matter adjacent to the **lateral ventricles** in the brain, which is a type of white matter damage of immaturity.

peroxisomal disorders rare genetic conditions causing cells of the brain to progressively degenerate. These include **adrenoleucodystrophy** and Zellweger syndrome.

polymicrogyria multiple small convolutions on the brain surface owing to abnormal cell migration during development, which is associated with a range of brain dysfunctions depending upon which area of the brain is affected.

porencephaly cysts or cavities in the brain resulting from resorption of tissue as a sequel to destructive disease such as **infarction**.

probabilistic diffusion tractography the statistical method required for functional MRI tractography.

progressive leucodystrophy progressive degeneration of the white matter of the brain as occurs, for example, in **adrenoleucodystrophy**.

prosencephalon the front part of the developing brain in utero, which becomes the cerebral hemispheres and their contents.

prosopagnosia inability/disability recognizing faces due to damage or impaired function of the part of the brain which does this, namely the **fusiform gyrus** of the temporal lobe, usually on the right side.

psychometric evaluation psychological measurement of brain function.

pulvinar discrete part of the thalamus deep in the brain which plays a part in reflex unconscious visual function.

putamen discrete area deep in the brain, which is one of the **basal ganglia**, and which assists control of movement and influences learning.

quadriplegia/tetraplegia disability moving all four limbs as a sequel to damage to the brain.

refractive error impaired optics of the eye which can be corrected with spectacles or contact lenses.

reticular (activating) system part of the brain stem which plays a part in maintaining arousal and motivation.

retinochoroiditis inflammation causing damage to the retina of the eye and underlying choroids. Causes include infection by *Toxoplasma* or cytomegalovirus.

retrogeniculate visual pathways the white matter pathways between the **lateral geniculate bodies** and the visual cortex in the occipital lobes.

retrograde transsynaptic degeneration visual pathway damage in the womb. It can result in the connecting pathways in the eye disappearing. This results in less tissue in the optic nerve, which can be seen as a cupped appearance in the optic nerve head.

saccadic eye movements fast movements of the eyes.

scales Scales are needed to identify various degrees of functioning. Scales can be distinguished by their direction and type. Scales of dysfunction, handicap, or impairment tend to rate 'normal functioning' as '0' (no loss) and total impairment as '100'. Scales of functioning count in the opposite direction; they rate 'no function' as '0' and 'normal functioning' as '100'. A scale of functioning can accommodate better than average performance and acknowledges that normal functioning implies a reserve for sustainable performance.

schizencephaly an abnormal cleft in the structure of the brain, lined with grey matter.

scotoma an area of lack of vision in the visual field.

simultanagnosia limited ability to see more than one or two things at once owing to damage to the posterior parietal area of the brain on both sides.

smooth pursuit ability of the eyes to smoothly follow a moving target.

spastic diplegia a form of cerebral palsy with weakness and spasticity of the lower limbs. **Periventricular leuomalacia** is the most common cause.

spastic movements limitation of muscle movement due to increased tone (hypertonicity).

stereopsis the perception of three dimensions brought about by the summation of the slightly different images seen by the two eyes.

strabismus misalignment of the eyes, also known as a squint.

striate cortex part of the occipital cortex, which receives the pathways from the **lateral geniculate bodies**, responsible for image processing.

subependymal heterotopias the abnormal presence of brain grey matter beneath the ependyma, which is the layer lining the cavities (ventricles) in the brain.

superior colliculi paired structures at the back of the superior mid-brain (above the **inferior colliculi**) comprising two small protrusions, which process subconscious reflex peripheral visual function.

sylvian fissure/lateral sulcus a cleft in the normal brain which separates the frontal and parietal lobes above from the temporal lobe beneath.

tectal pathways the subconscious visual pathways connecting to the **superior colliculi**.

tentorium cerebelli a rigid structure made up of dura mater separating the occipital lobes above from the cerebellum (which serves coordination of movement) below.

tetraplegia/quadriplegia disability moving all four limbs as a sequel to damage to the brain.

thalamus a large deep brain structure which serves pain perception, as well playing a part in subconscious visual function.

transtentorial herniation downward protrusion of swollen temporal and occipital brain tissue through the orifice bounded by the tentorium.

trigone (of the lateral ventricle) the triangular area bounding the posterior portion of each lateral ventricle, where visual pathways are located.

tuberous sclerosis an inherited condition affecting multiple organs of the body. Brain involvement includes abnormal gyri, calcification developmental disorders, and seizures. Retinal lesions are seen in some cases.

ventral stream the pathways in the brain between the occipital lobes and the part of the temporal lobes, which serve recognition and route finding.

vision enhancement Vision enhancement techniques are used to enhance the quality of the visual information that reaches higher centres. Vision enhancement techniques include magnification, illumination, and improved contrast. They are the predominant techniques used in vision rehabilitation for ocular conditions.

vision substitution Vision substitution techniques use other senses to supplement or replace the information normally provided by the visual system. They include Braille, talking books, long cane, listening, memory, etc.

visual ability deficit A visual ability deficit (visual disability) describes a lack or loss of the **ability** to perform certain tasks that require visual input at a sustainable, supra-threshold level. The term is used primarily to describe a **disability** resulting from visual impairment.

visual agnosia lack of ability to recognize familiar objects or faces, despite sufficient clarity of vision.

visual crowding a lower level of visual acuity measured when observing crowded text or imagery than when observing single letters or images. Commonly seen for eyes with amblyopia.

visual dysfunction Visual dysfunction describes a failure of **functional vision**, owing to an abnormal mode of functioning of the higher cerebral centres that process visual information. Visual dysfunctions may exist even if the visual input is normal. It is distinct from a **visual ability deficit**, which results from normal processing of deficient information.

visual functions Visual functions describe how the eye and the basic visual system function in terms of threshold performance for various stimulus parameters that are tested one at a time, for example visual acuity, visual field, contrast sensitivity. A deficits of visual function is described as a **visual impairment**. Visual functions are distinct from **functional vision**, which describes how a person functions on tasks that involve multiple parameters and sustainable supra-threshold performance.

visual impairment Visual impairment describes a lack or loss of one or more **visual functions**. This can be at the ocular level (ocular visual impairment) or at the lower brain levels (cerebral visual impairment). Ocular and occipital visual impairments can cause **visual disability**. Perceptual and cognitive deficits can cause **visual dysfunction**.

Williams syndrome a genetic disorder affecting chromosome 7, causing **dorsal stream** dysfunction as well as the classic features of an elfin facial appearance, impaired mental function, and engaging demeanour, transient high calcium levels and disorder.

INDEX

Index notes:

Page numbers in italics indicates material in figures or tables. vs. indicates a differential diagnosis or comparison. The following abbreviations have been used:

ABCDEFV, Atkinson Battery of Child Development for Examining Functional Vision
CVISTA, Children's Visual Impairment Services Tayside Agencies
IVH, intraventricular haemorrhage
PVL, periventricular leucomalacia
WDMI, white matter damage of immaturity

ABCDEFV *see* Atkinson Battery of Child Development for Examining Functional Vision (ABCDEFV)
abnormal eye movements, spastic diplegia 198–199
abscesses, neonatal meningitis 63
accessory optic system (AOS) 6
accessory optic tract 6
access to information 218, 245–246
    contrast sensitivity impairment 219–220, *220*
    dorsal stream dysfunction 223–224
    ventral stream dysfunction 223–224
    visual acuity impairment 219–220, *219*
accommodation 98–105, 102–104, 183
    aetiology 104
    cerebral palsy 102, 103–104, *103*
    hypermetropia correction *99*, 102
    management 104
    motor deficits 104
    retinoscopy reflex 103
    visual acuity 104
    WMDI 31–32
acquired neurological injury 21–22
activities of daily living (ADL) 289
    education strategies 228
    school perception issues 243–244
    visual processing disorders 279
adaptation
    multiple disability assessment 187–188
    visual information quality 269
adult models, visual–perceptual dysfunction 108
age of child
    cerebral visual impairment classification 290
    dorsal stream dysfunction 109
American Speech and Hearing Association (ASHA) 250–251
animal single-cell recordings, cortical visual pathways 12–13

animal studies
    functional magnetic resonance imaging (fMRI) 137
    neurophysiology 137
anxiety
    emotional development 168
    psychiatric considerations 179
APD *see* auditory processing disorders (APD)
arterial stroke 22
arteritis, neonatal meningitis 63
assessments
    behaviour *see* behavioural measures
    case histories 190, 191–192
    cerebral palsy *see* cerebral palsy
    challenges to 183–184
    cognition *see* cognitive assessments
    first year of life 70–72
        behavioural techniques 70–71
        electrophysiology 71–72
        see also specific methods
    functional *see* functional assessments
    methods of *68*
    multiple disabilities *see* multiple disabilities
    peripheral vision *see* peripheral vision assessment
    predictive values 74–75
    problems of 22
    visual acuity *see* visual acuity assessment
    visual function *see* visual function
    visual information quality 270
astigmatism 98
athetoid movements, orientation and mobility 233
Atkinson Battery of Child Development for Examining Functional Vision (ABCDEFV) 130, 138, *139–140*
    clinical populations 141–142
    preterm infants 142
    severe cerebral visual impairment 142, *143–145*
    vision screening test follow-up 141